GARY NULL'S

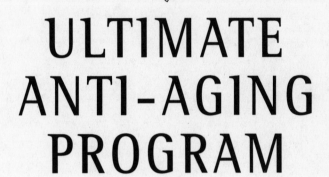

ULTIMATE ANTI-AGING PROGRAM

GARY NULL'S

ULTIMATE ANTI-AGING PROGRAM

GARY NULL, Ph.D.

BROADWAY BOOKS NEW YORK

DISCLAIMER

Readers are advised to consult with health-care providers knowledgeable in alternative/complementary/preventive medicine to determine which vitamins, minerals and food supplements would be beneficial for their particular health needs and the dosages that would be best for them. It is also imperative to understand that certain medications (e.g., Coumadin) limit the type and amount of vegetables you can consume. If you are taking medication, or if you are pregnant or nursing, you must consult your physician to see if anything suggested in this material is contraindicated.

BROADWAY

A hardcover edition of this book was originally published in 1999 by Kensington Books. It is here reprinted by arrangement with Kensington Books.

GARY NULL'S ULTIMATE ANTI-AGING PROGRAM. Copyright © 1999 by Gary Null. All rights reserved. Printed in the United States of America. No part of this book may be reproduced or transmitted in any form or by any means, electronic or mechanical, including photocopying, recording, or by any information storage and retrieval system, without written permission from the publisher. For information, address: Kensington Books, 850 Third Avenue, New York, NY 10022.

Broadway Books titles may be purchased for business or promotional use or for special sales. For information, please write to: Special Markets Department, Random House, Inc., 1540 Broadway, New York, NY 10036.

BROADWAY BOOKS and its logo, a letter B bisected on the diagonal, are trademarks of Broadway Books, a division of Random House, Inc.

First Broadway Books trade paperback edition published 1999.

Designed by Stanley S. Drate/Folio Graphics Co. Inc.

Library of Congress Cataloging-in-Publication Data

Null, Gary.
    [Ultimate anti-aging program]
    Gary Null's ultimate anti-aging program / Gary Null. — 1st Broadway Books trade paperback ed.
       p. cm.
    Originally published in 1999 by Kensington Books.
    Includes bibliographical references and index.
    ISBN 0-7679-0436-2
    1. Longevity. 2. Aging Prevention. 3. Detoxification (Health) 4. Aging—Nutritional aspects. 5. Aging—Psychological aspects.
    I. Title.
    [RA776.75.N84 1999b]
    612.6'8—dc21
                                                99-34050
                                              CIP

00 01 02 03 10 9 8 7 6

ACKNOWLEDGMENTS

Special thanks to: Sally Burton, general text editor; Patrick Jennings, chief science researcher; Lois Zinn, transcriber; Sallie Batson, writer; and Vicki Riba Koestler, creative editor.

CONTENTS

PART VIII ✧

AND IN CONCLUSION

PART 1

CONFRONTING AGING

1

THE GOOD NEWS: AGING IS CHANGING

As Baby Boomers turn fifty, fear of aging has prompted an explosion of interest in slowing, if not reversing, this process. Boomers, and subsequent Generation Xers, are united in their passionate desire to remain young. They work out; they eat foods that are perceived to be healthy; they take supplements; they wear trendy clothes—all to maintain a grasp on youth.

Why is it, then, that some people remain youthful well into what is considered middle or even old age, while others begin to show marked signs of aging in their twenties? In my own family, virtually all the men on my father's side were either prematurely gray or bald. My hair was already thinning and graying at age eighteen and, by twenty-five, I was letting my hair grow a bit longer to make the hair loss less obvious. All the vitamins, supplements, organic foods, and exercise in the world cannot restore hair lost because of a genetic tendency for balding. Like many others, I, too, believed that such genetic programming could not be reversed.

Or so I was taught.

AGE IS ONLY A NUMBER

Like it or not, we begin to age the moment we are born. However, given that our bodies are designed to live productive, vital lives well past age one hundred, this should not be an issue. As a population, we are living longer. This, however, does not mean that we are aging *better*. Hypertension, congestive heart disease, arterial sclerosis, stroke, dementia, arthritis, diabetes, Parkinson's, Alzheimer's, cancer; osteoporosis; menopause; graying and hair loss; wrinkled skin; fatigue; weakness; loss of muscle mass and tone; diminishing vision, smell, and hearing; a tendency to overweight; digestive problems, and loss of appetite—I refuse to accept these conditions as normal.

I assert that, while a youthful attitude is helpful, no one needs to simply accept a decline in vitality—be it wrinkles and balding, gray hair, or osteoporosis and loss of muscle mass and tone—as their fate because they have reached a certain age. Once we accept that age is only a number, there is much we can do to retain, and even regain, our youth.

The good news is that we have done just that. Not once, which could be a fluke, but with four successive research groups—more than a thousand people who participated in four separate nine-month programs and two separate eighteen-month programs.

THE SEARCH FOR A WAY TO LIVE FOREVER

In 1993, I began a quest to better understand what really causes us to age prematurely and develop these diseases assumed to be part of the aging process. Frequently, symptoms of these ailments could be alleviated by dietary changes. Diabetics could better regulate their blood sugar through diet and exercise; osteoporosis patients could restore bone mass through dietary changes and weight training; even patients with cardiovascular disease could reduce serum cholesterol levels through diet, but nothing could effectively change the aging process.

During the past five years, I have conducted studies with approximately five thousand people—one thousand volunteers *specifically* for this project—in my search to create a protocol to slow aging. My goal was to not only alleviate these conditions—lower dangerously high cholesterol levels; help insulin-dependent diabetics get off insulin, etc.—but to find a new way to process disease.

My premise: *A healthy body does not get sick with anything.* And, in this context, a healthy body does not age prematurely.

From this point of view I began my search for effective ways to slow, and even reverse, aging. This book is a distillation of a power-fully effective protocol that, followed fully, stalls aging, regardless of your current age.

THE QUEST BEGINS

Historically, we have considered everything from gray hair and creaky joints to heart diseases and memory loss to be normal mani-festations of the aging process. However, in my travels around the world, I had already seen enough contradictions—even within the same culture—to know that there are things that people do that vary the speed of the aging process, as well as the number of ill-nesses experienced in this process.

My research took me to Italy several times specifically to inter-view hundreds of people about their diets, exercise levels, genetics, as well as environmental and stress factors. In town after town, village after village, I found that people who lived in rural areas lived longer, chronologically, and, more important, exuded a sense of calm, joy, and serenity that I did not observe in those who lived in the metropolitan areas of Milan, Rome, and Naples. This was also true of my visits into the countrysides of England, Scotland, Ireland, and France.

It then became a task of trying to isolate which factors changed when a person moved from the more bucolic countryside to the sub-urbs or the cities, and vice versa. This took years of effort. In the course of my research I reviewed all of the world's available epide-miological research on longevity and interviewed thousands upon thousands of individuals in several countries about their diets and exercise habits, health, environmental conditions, and attitudes about aging. I documented my findings and felt ready to put what I had learned into practice.

THE PROTOCOL EVOLVES

Over the next five years I worked with more randomly selected vol-unteers from Los Angeles, Washington, D.C., Miami, and New York

City. I would experiment with different criteria, but I always used the same basic protocol, which consisted of a pure vegetarian diet.

Excluded were *all* dairy products—including milk, yogurt, and cheeses—and processed foods, refined carbohydrates, simple sugars, artificial preservatives, color and flavor enhancers; foods treated with pesticides and herbicides; carbonated beverages; artificial sweeteners; meat, chicken, and shellfish; caffeine, including coffee, tea, cola drinks, and chocolate, and most salt.

To the uninitiated, this may sound painfully restrictive; however, I assure you, this diet was very versatile. It included a wide selection of whole grains, nuts, seeds, fruits, legumes, fresh herbs, and cold-pressed oils, such as olive oil, flaxseed oil, and macadamia oil. Water was to be pure, free from fluoride, chlorine, and chemicals. And participants were to consume at least one to two *liquid* meals a day, preferably from quality proteins made from rice or soy, plus a wide variety of phytochemicals from fruits and vegetables. I also suggested a number of cookbooks to show people how creative this regimen could be. Part VI—Eating to Live tells you how to completely restructure your eating habits.

My associates and I then measured parameters and created groups accordingly. At one time, we had five hundred overweight people in one group. Other groups created were for those with arthritis, herpes, Lyme disease, chronic fatigue syndrome, high blood pressure, high cholesterol, food allergies, depression, and anxiety disorders. We soon found that people had difficulty sticking with the program as I outlined it for them. I found it ironic that a person who thought nothing of eating fifty french fries or three scoops of ice cream would balk at taking three or four vitamin capsules.

THE LAWS OF COMPENSATION

The basic nutritional and exercise programs formulated in the course of developing this protocol **are not adequate to reverse the damage incurred in the course of a lifetime of neglect.** The laws of compensation stress that, to the degree that we have damaged our bodies—through caffeine, sugar, meat, processed foods, environmental pollutants, etc.—we must supply the body with a like amount of nourishment, from whole, pure organic foods and concentrated supplements, to compensate and rebuild our bodies.

Eating moderately, or taking a daily multivitamin, alone, will *not* undo the damage. That process is so advanced and the damage so incipient that it will require enormous compensation. A little vitamin C, for example, will not repair a body damaged by years of abuse; massive amounts, administered over a couple of years, may.

Society places few limits on what we can do to damage our bodies—alcohol, cigarettes, meats, fried and processed foods, etc. Yet, when it comes to doing something good for our bodies, such as eating healthy, nourishing foods, exercising, even taking vitamins and supplements, we limit ourselves. Remember this warning when you read what I recommend for this anti-aging protocol, when you hear yourself say, "What do you mean I have to take . . ."

We are ultraliberal in *creating* disease and radically conservative in the areas of preventing and treating it. To live longer and healthier, these conditions must be switched.

Nevertheless, if you *only* follow the diet from your teens, you would double your life span. Once you reach your mid-twenties, you need the diet and nutritional supplements, exercise, and stress management to stave off aging. Just imagine what is possible if you integrate the *entire* program into your life while you're in your twenties, thirties, or even forties!

Yes, I can teach you how to retard and even reverse aging even if you're in what is statistically old age. I've even developed a repair and rejuvenation protocol that has proved affective in reversing ailments in people over sixty. Some of the participants have joined in my study as their last chance for relief before resigning themselves to living out their lives in nursing homes.

SUCCESS AND FAILURE

The highest failure rate (95 percent) occurred in the study group comprised of people who had been diagnosed with chronic depression. Those participants couldn't make it through the first month. A group of overweight individuals fared only slightly better, with a 90-percent failure rate after three months. One group had nothing wrong with them. Here, there was a success rate of about 40 percent.

Less than half of those participants finished either six months or a year with the program.

I then reworked the protocol, this time adding an exercise program. This included forty-five minutes a day, six days a week, of power walking, and three sessions of weight training per week to build muscle mass. The addition of this physical component improved our success rate by approximately 7 percent across the board.

The next alteration in the protocol was the addition of stress management techniques. This included a variety of techniques, including biofeedback, hypnosis, guided visualizations, and positive affirmations. I had thought that behavior modification technology would support, and even increase, participants' ability to adhere to the program; however this did not result in more people sticking with the program.

So, we looked toward their home environments.

ENVIRONMENTAL OUTREACH

We began to teach people how to clean up their personal environments—one more place to lessen their exposure to toxins. They learned how to go through each room of the house getting rid of hidden toxins by removing carpets, particleboard, and other unsafe materials. People learned how to properly insulate their homes; how to get rid of dust and mold; how to shop for and use healthy cleansers, such as apple cider vinegar for washing windows. They learned to replace chemical-laden toothpastes, mouthwashes, and cosmetics with biofriendly products.

We held in-depth workshops on the advantages of full-spectrum lighting, and taught people how to garden using diamide-rich earth and praying mantises and ladybugs in lieu of toxic pesticides for their houseplants and gardens. We covered shopping for all-organic cotton sheets, blankets, and bedding in place of products made from chemically treated fibers. This became a very popular part of our protocol. Any time we would announce a meeting on this topic, there would be a 95-percent attendance level.

We discussed the vital importance of good nutrition. I spent a tremendous amount of time reviewing the world's literature and doing my own research to see which nutrients could best benefit us by stopping disease processes like cancer. I found more than a hundred different fruits and vegetables that could do that and listed them in *The Clinician's Handbook of Natural Healing*.

I researched foods high in phytochemicals to balance the body's natural hormone levels. These were given in juice form, which provided higher bioavailability, so that the person doesn't lose nutrients due to poor digestion. Then I considered foods that help to cleanse and detoxify the body, and talked about garlic, onions, shallots, and other sulfur-rich foods that can eliminate harmful bacteria, parasites, and viruses from our intestines, blood, and liver. Earlier in life, many people damaged their bodies by taking drugs or drinking alcohol; this was an effort to reverse that damage by repairing the cells. Part of the protocol then included flooding the body with organic fruit and vegetable juices spiked with various nutrients from aloe vera to vitamin C to stop mutagenic activity, end DNA damage, cleanse the system, and ultimately repair the body.

The final step in this process was rejuvenation. We found that antioxidants, as a family of nutrients, were very important. Some came from the foods themselves, but much more was recommended in the way of supplements. I gave much higher than usual doses of what people would normally take. Vitamin C, for example, could go from 5,000 to 20,000 mg or higher per day. In some cases, individuals went beyond protocols of what could be taken orally and began to take nutrients intravenously, including high levels of vitamin C, glutathione, and aqueous vitamin A (a water-soluble form of vitamin A), plus selenium and B complex. This was determined to be particularly beneficial for people who had hepatitis, herpes, cytomegalovirus, Epstein-Barr virus, cancer, and AIDS.

Hundreds of people, under the supervision of their physicians, used these protocols with remarkable benefits. In fact, one of these individuals would later become a co-instructor in my program as a nurse practitioner. After earning a doctorate in nursing and spending twenty years in the field, she developed hepatitis B, herpes, Epstein-Barr, mycoplasma, and cytomegalovirus. Today she has none of these diseases. She is completely well. This would not have happened through diet and vitamin supplements alone, as she had been diligent in those areas. She did not see any concrete improvement until she began the intravenous vitamin protocol.

This nurse is not alone. There are hundreds of people just like her who eliminated viruses, bacteria, and diseases completely from their systems, solely by following the program I have developed for you.

This taught me that, in many cases, proper diet alone was not enough, nor was exercise or stress management. These treatment modalities did prevent a person from additional injury and assault to the system, but they could not undo the damage already done from years of abuse or neglect. When I saw that these people were making enormous strides with the more rigorous procedures, I realized that my protocols would have to become more intense.

But there was still something missing. Despite the benefits, many people continued to drop out. I did a hair study on 707 individuals in a nine-month period. Those who actually stuck with the protocol had a success rate of more than 90 percent in reversing balding, graying, and thinning. Some individuals who had been bald for more than thirty years had a new head of hair.

Other things changed as well. Diseases were reversed—arthritis disappeared, energy increased, sleep improved, and allergies were gone. I knew that the protocol definitely worked. What I didn't know was how to get people to stick with it. I did another study on reversing the aging process.

This was a huge study done for the first time in the United States with before-and-after photographs, blood and medical workups, and journals to record daily results. We followed participants' progress, and, every three months, added an additional regimen to their program. Those who followed the program rigorously and stuck with it for the duration of the study experienced remarkable benefits. Women who were fifteen years postmenopause became menopausal again. Wrinkles began to disappear. Bags under the eyes and jowly chins were gone. Gray hair became black, thick, and lustrous. Libidos returned and muscle tone came back.

At our final meeting, one woman said to me, "I have my youth back, something I never thought possible."

Many didn't achieve these results because, once again, few stayed with the complete protocol. Still wondering why, I decided to do other studies. I did a second one-and-one-half year reversing-the-aging process group and a second hair study group, again with phenomenal results for those who adhered to the program. I knew

I had at least answered one basic question—can we slow down and reverse the aging process?—with an unequivocal yes.

But I had not yet found an answer to my second question: Why aren't people sticking to something that can so benefit them?

Then it occurred to me: What I had omitted was what I would now find to be the single most important part of the entire program—modification not only of the behavior but of the existing beliefs as well. Our belief system is what creates our impression of reality which, in turn, determines whether or not we are able to stick with a program. That's why we have overweight people who are unable to stick to their diets, people who engage in mindless daily acts that can lead to self-destruction.

What I did next was to create a program for self-empowerment. In this program, I would take a topic; for instance, the subject of starting over. We talked about what has been lost in life— relationships, loved ones, jobs—and discussed ways of letting go and getting back into life. I realized that people frequently don't receive unconditional emotional support at home or at work. More likely, they're surrounded with toxic thoughts and negative, cynical, and bitter attitudes. You can't be happy until you think happy. And you can't be angry unless you think angry. Many people do not think before they act.

I created a program to help people think, reducing their chances of flying off the handle. I also took a look at the strengths and weaknesses of the twelve-step recovery movement, and created some eighty different two-hour lectures. I went from holding these sessions monthly to having groups meet on a biweekly basis. These study groups would deal with behaviors, beliefs, and values, as well as the physical components of the program—diet and exercise.

I quickly saw that this was the missing ingredient; there was now a 90-percent success rate among people who stayed with the program. I found that if a person just followed the diet or exercised regularly, they would not stick with the program. However, if they dealt with the more important issues, they would stick with the diet and exercise.

I took small groups of twenty-five to fifty people off to my ranch in Texas and, more recently, to my home in Naples, Florida, for intensive cleansing and rebuilding programs that lasted for one to two weeks. Here, people had no responsibilities other than to relax in a supportive environment surrounded by people who were there to encourage them, telling them how capable they were of making proper choices with their life and health. No negativity was present, only unconditional sharing. In addition, they had a chance to experience what it was like to eat gourmet vegetarian meals every day and juice up to twelve or fourteen glasses of fresh organic fruit and vegetables a day. People lost weight; they got their energy back; they began to understand how they had created their own problems. For many, this was a revelation.

Participants in these intense detoxification programs had a 97-percent success rate. They stuck to the program, and they had the greatest overall reversal of aging.

WHAT'S AHEAD IN THIS BOOK

I cannot list every thought related to every question raised in these study groups. There is not enough room to permit me to include details of eighty-six *different* self-empowerment series, some with as many as fifty questions. What I have done, however, is select some of the most popular questions—more than enough to get you started on your own anti-aging program.

I have given you a complete, in-depth look at how I would view each question in the larger context to show you the various ways in which you can answer them. Take your time with this book. Don't rush through it. Come back at different times to the same question to see how many ways you can look at the problem. Over time, as you open yourself up, you'll find more and more positive solutions to negative problems.

In the end, I have developed a program that helps people with every imaginable issue. It is not merely designed as an attack against disease but rather as a means to rebuild a person's health through diet, detoxification, exercise, stress management, and self-actualization.

This last component—self-actualization—was not part of the protocols employed by the early study groups. Whereas the majority of participants in those groups did not stick to the program, more than 90 percent of the people who come to our program now stay with it.

Louann Pennse, who has assisted in teaching the study groups, has worked with more than a thousand people in the last three years. She teaches five days a week, and I with her, three classes a night, and she gives me her feedback as well as that from her participants. As a result, I have been able to determine what people are using and not using in the program.

After working with more than five thousand people these last ten years, I have been able to filter everything down to an understanding of what we have to do to change the way we age. This I will share with you.

BONFIRE OF THE CALENDARS

Much as bra burning was emblematic of the feminist movement in the 1960s, I see calendar burning as the sign of these times, as more and more people—of all ages and types—disregard their chronological ages and, rather than seeing the years that they spend on this planet as a countdown to death, adopt this life-transforming program that teaches all they need to know to stay biologically young and in peak performance for all the decades to come.

2

WHAT'S *YOUR* PLAN TO STOP AGING?

Could you imagine starting your own company without detailed operational and financial plans for the first one, two, five, and ten years of business?

Or starting off on a vacation without first mapping out every detail of your trip—where you're going, how you'll get there, where you'll stay, how much you'll spend?

Or waiting until your child is a senior in high school to sock away money for a college education?

Preposterous, you say.

So why is it that so many people neglect to plan for aging? I'm not talking about a retirement plan; I'm talking about physically aging.

As you've probably realized, you're never too young to prevent this process. In fact, the earlier you commit to the anti-aging programs, the easier your job will be. However, most people aren't even aware that they are aging until they are in need of repair.

While the younger you are when you start caring for your body the better it is, there is no age limit to begin this program. Participants in the study groups that provided this pioneering data ranged from 40 to 91. The most important thing is to start *now*.

WHERE ARE YOU RIGHT NOW?

We all have heard motivational speakers and infomercial gurus advise corporate executives and entrepreneurs, "Plan your work, then work your plan." This wisdom also applies to matters of health and aging.

So, how do you make a plan for reversing aging? Start out by taking stock of where you are at this moment. Take inventory of your physical, mental, emotional, even spiritual assets and liabilities, so that you'll be able to structure an anti-aging program that targets your own needs.

There are three immediate tools you can use to form the foundation of your anti-aging program. First, if you're not doing so already, start a journal. Second, take stock of your life, and third, take an objective look at your body. The latter two are not one-time exercises. You'll do this at least once a month as a matter of habit, so that you really *will* know where you are . . . right now.

MY JOURNAL, MY FRIEND

I'm not talking about a "Dear Diary, Today I had lunch with so-and-so." I mean a serious journal not only of your activities—what you ate, how you exercised and for how long, etc.—but your feelings and thoughts, your hopes and dreams as well. Yes, dreams. *Young* people dream . . . regardless of their chronological ages.

The purpose of keeping a journal is to maintain a regular inventory of your life, especially with regard to reversing the aging process. Areas you may want to address in your journal include:

- A food journal, documenting everything you eat and drink; when you ate or drank it; what you were doing at the time, and how you felt before, during, and after you ate.
- A record of your exercise regimen, i.e., how far you walked or ran; what exercise program you did at the gym—how long on the treadmill, etc.; your pulse rate; respiratory rate; and any physical sensations.
- Vital statistics—height, weight, and overall measurements. If you're working with an exercise coach, personal trainer, or medical practitioner to monitor your health as you begin this program, ask to be assessed to determine your lean-fat ratio and bone density. Have these measurements taken every few months and record them in your journal.

You might also write about conditions in your family and work environments, *anything* that will enable you to redesign your life. I know a man who became an optometrist, joining his father in a thriving practice in New York City. While he was very good at his profession and kept the office open—and growing—even after the death of his father, he expressed the fact that he had very little passion for the field. As we talked, I asked him what motivated him to follow in his father's footsteps. Surely, at one time, there had been some desire to become an optometrist. He grew quiet, reflecting on his career choice. Then he spoke: "When I finished high school, I wanted to be an actor. I went to college planning to major in theater, but once I looked at the realities of becoming a successful actor— and knowing that I would like to have a family and a nice home—I started thinking about something I could do that would give me the money to have that life. I knew that my dad had done very well in his practice, and I knew he'd be pleased if I came into the practice. I guess what I'm saying is that I became an optometrist by default."

I asked him what he would do if he could do anything that pleased him. I also suggested that he write this down, in elaborate detail, creating a vivid, memorable picture of his ideal profession. And he should make note of his conditions of satisfaction—the things he could *not* do without; conditions that, if not met, would make the job unacceptable. About three months later, I saw this man happily scurrying down the street with a shopping bag filled with books. "You were right," he said with a grin. "I was so miserable in my job, and had been for so long, that I didn't even notice it. When I started writing the description of my perfect profession, I just made lists. Then I looked to see if there were any patterns. I showed my lists to my wife, who admitted that she was a little anxious over my thinking of changing careers in my mid-50s—our kids were about to head off to college—but she agreed to play along with me. I really don't think she thought I was serious. Now I'm studying for the LSAT. I'm going to law school."

The more he wrote in his journal, the more he delved into the question of what he would do if he could have any job in the world, he determined that law might be his niche. "I've always thought that lawyers are actors who make better money," he joked. Turning serious, he added, "I've been interested in how the judicial system works since the Sixties and the Civil Rights movement. I don't see myself becoming the next F. Lee Bailey, but I do believe I could be very happy in a general practice; say, with Legal Aid, or one of those organizations that help people go up against their landlords."

Now he was using his journal to plan his course of action, investigating what it would take for a man who'd been out of school since 1965 to get into law school, and getting an appraisal of his optometry practice as the first step toward its sale. Indeed, the profits from the sale of the practice allowed him to follow his own dream without disrupting his family's plans. Five years later, he is now practicing law with a small firm that specializes in tenant advocacy and is younger and healthier and, above all, happier that he has been in thirty years. All this from a few pages in his journal.

TAKING A LOOK AT YOUR LIFE

This is when you determine where you are now with regard to your relationship with the people in your life, where you fit in your universe. The following chart provides you with a blueprint designed to develop a clear picture of the state of your life. In your journal, write your responses to the points and questions in this inventory. From this point, you will be able to make the changes in life and lifestyle that will enable you to reverse aging.

Don't approach this as if you're taking a test. Instead, work on a few points—two or three, or five or six, if you're up to it—every day until you've completed the process. And remember: There are no right or wrong answers. This is an inventory, not an inquisition!

STOP HIDING, START LIVING

1. Beyond working for a standard of living—what other more essential goals could you be working toward:

    (a) Study; mastery
    (b) Enjoy nature
    (c) Hobbies
    (d) More time for family

2. To what do you completely commit yourself?

3. How do you handle failure and crisis?

4. Do you positively affirm that others and yourself must meet certain standards?

5. What standards do you have?

6. Do you try to validate yourself by proving yourself all the time? In what ways?

7. What happens when we live in denial of our other self?

8. When we only feel good by being accepted by others, what are we feeling?

9. If you have experienced love and still need love, what then are you seeking?

10. Success gives you . . . Failure gives you . . . Where will each take you?

11. What rules don't we want to obey anymore?

12. Who in your life is toxic and who is healthy? How do they affect you?

13. Describe ten negative messages you give.

14. How do you show your negativity?

15. Can being too confident trigger negative reactions in others?

16. How will changing directly affect you?

17. Do you focus on the strengths or weaknesses of yourself and others?

18. When and where do you waste time?

19. How much personal variety do you allow?

20. How do you access your spirit?

21. Do we think higher thoughts but act out the lower self?

22. What do we do with those parts of ourselves that we don't like and don't want to acknowledge?

23. Do we blame others for what we have repressed in ourselves? How do we do this?

24. Are we fooling others about what and who we really are? How? Why?

25. Which is more important—

    (a) What we think of ourselves?
    (b) What others think of us?
    (c) Why?

26. How do you cope with loss?

27. Are you more than your parents? How do you show it?

28. What family failings do you still blame yourself for?

29. Your original spiritual energy was manifested by your parents. Was it a valued, cherished feeling? If not, how do you feel about it?

30. Which is more real to you? Why?

    (a) The thought of something
    (b) The feeling of something
    (c) The emotion of something
    (d) All of the above

31. How much free expression have we allowed ourselves?

32. Which is correct to you and why?

    (a) We do stupid things because it's all that we know.
    (b) We've used it successfully in the past.
    (c) We are emotionally compulsive and obsessive about someone or something outside of ourselves.
    (d) We get attention and if we get nothing else, it has its benefits.
    (e) We focus our energy on others, then blame them for not having energy left over for ourselves.
    (f) We are a system of mirrors reflecting back to other more essential persons.

33. Our ego distorts and denies what?

34. What can you do without a lot of money?

35. How many right choices did you make today?

36. How do we affirm ourselves?

    (a) Quietly
    (b) Meekly
    (c) Apologetically
    (d) Affirmatively
    (e) Demandingly

37. How well do you do everything? What determines the quality of your effort?

38. What purpose have you created for your life and legacy?

39. How do you feel about uncertainty?

40. What determines how and what you think about?

41. Which is more relevant—the circumstances or your view of them?

42. How much do you need to achieve harmony?

43. We hide or run from what? Why?

44. What is more important—the event or our response to it?

45. What happens when you don't want anything from anybody?

46. Do we give exclusively in order to receive exclusively?

47. What constitutes success?

48. How much new or old experience are we prepared to accept?

49. Do we honor our individual capacity for experience?

50. Which fantasy do you enjoy? Why? Can you actualize it?

51. What negative influences do you still allow or encourage in your life?

You'll find more of these thought-provoking exercises later in this book. Use them with rigor to create a lifetime of age-reversing habits for yourself.

TAKING A LOOK AT YOUR BODY

Before we can truly make major changes in our lives, we must be willing to modify our outlook and gain deeper understanding of ourselves. We must first learn to have a sense of Self, as well as a love of ourselves. Also, we must know what we look like.

Most people haven't a clue what their bodies look like. Oh yes, they look in the mirror to shave or put on makeup, to see if their clothes are on straight. They look at themselves as though looking at a headshot—from the shoulders up.

As you begin your anti-aging program, you must take a close look at your body. All of it. If you can't trust yourself to be objective rather than critical of your body, I recommend that you ask a trusted friend or family member—an anti-aging buddy—to do this exercise with you. Record and date what you see in your journal for future reference.

- Stand in front of a well-lit, full-length mirror, nude or wearing a bathing suit or underwear.
- Study the shape and condition of your body, from head to toe; front, back, and both sides. You'll need a large hand mirror—or another pair of eyes—to accomplish this.

- Look at your skin. What is its texture? Is it dry, oily, wrinkled, smooth? Note any blemishes or scars, edema, discoloration, or moles.
- How is your muscle tone? Do you appear to be lean, muscular, or flabby?
- How do your shoulders, chest, and abdomen look? Toned or soft? What about your shoulder blades and lower back? What does your derriere look like?
- What is the condition of your hair? Is it dry, damaged, oily, shiny? Straight? Curly? Thick? Thin? Are you balding and, if so, where? Is it gray?
- Pull a strand of hair from the back or crown of your head. Does it feel smooth or rough? Stretch it out as far as possible. Is it strong and pliable or weak and brittle?
- Look at your fingernails. Are they smooth or ridged? Are they strong or weak? Is the nail bed a warm pink (indicating ample blood flow through your fingers) or is it speckled with white or dark spots? Are the cuticles pliable and soft?
- Is your posture erect and strong, or are you stooped over?
- Are your shoulders straight, relatively parallel with the floor, or are they shrugged up around your ears? Do they slope downwards?
- Do your knees meet evenly? Are you knock-kneed or bow-legged? Are your legs flexible and aligned so that you stand relaxed and centered?
- Do you stand with your feet facing forward, positioned directly under your hips?
- Study your feet, assessing your toenails by the same criteria as your fingernails.
- Are your feet and toes callused or is the skin smooth and supple? Are there bunions, hammertoes, flat feet, bone spurs, or any other condition? Is there thickened skin on your heels? Are your arches and insteps strong?

CHANGE IS THE CHALLENGE

Age reversal requires a certain amount of dedication and commitment to change, something not everyone is willing to do. Alice applied to my age reversing program on a dare: her best friend had insisted that she come into the program because she was a heavy smoker and serious coffee drinker. Reflecting on her experiences in the study group, she wrote: "It was a challenge to give them up so I could get in. It was like a dirty bet with myself that I could do it."

Writing about the benefits she received from the program, Alice expressed her appreciation not just for the protocol itself but also for the support groups that gave her the backup and coaching she needed to stick with it. She wrote:

The following are my benefits:

1. I gave up smoking cigarettes and started exercising.
2. My skin texture changed from coarse to smooth.
3. I lost almost all of my facial and neck wrinkles.
4. I got color back into the skin on my face.
5. I went back to school to become a mathematician.
6. I no longer feel faint if I must wait a while before eating breakfast.
7. The quality of my sleeping is profoundly restful, as it was in my thirties, even if I wake up on occasion to use the bathroom.
8. I no longer fear old age, Alzheimer's disease (which my father now has), or life in a nursing home. They just don't seem like "fairly immediate" doom to me. I feel that I am in charge of these "options."
9. I have violent reactions to certain face creams, which shows me that my system is too pure to process certain contaminants.

The very fact that you're reading a book that offers the ultimate anti-aging program indicates that you have at least a passing interest in staying young and healthy. Whether you'll be able to accomplish the results I offer is another matter. Are you up to the challenge? Are you committed to making the changes in your life, taking the steps necessary for age reversal to happen?

Ask most people if they want to become healthy, and they'll say, "Sure I do. I don't want heart disease, arthritis, depression, cancer, hemorrhoids, wrinkles, diabetes. I don't need that." Fair enough. But putting a time frame on when they'll begin to make the changes they need to make is another thing. About 98 percent of the people who listen to my radio show, attend my lectures, or read my books don't actualize what I talk about.

As part of the research to develop this anti-aging protocol, I conducted a year-and-a-half-long hair study to help people grow new hair and reverse graying and thinning. Seven people who completed the protocol now have new, thick hair. In addition, their wrinkles are gone, and they have overcome all kinds of illnesses. Although 140 people initially enrolled in the study, only seven finished. That's an infinitesimal percentage. What happened to the other 133? They were unwilling to follow through because they were not willing to make true changes.

What you say you want to accomplish is immaterial if it doesn't match what you do. What you *do*, rather than what you say, tells me who you are. If what you do and what you say are the same, then you're in balance. But most people say they want to be healthy, then do unhealthy things. Well, if you do something that's immoral, you're not moral. If you do something that's unhealthy, you're not healthy. We've got to stop the games. We've got to stop deceiving ourselves.

EARLY EVIDENCE OF AGING

More than one-third of the American population is chronically ill. And that's an understatement, because it assumes that you're ill only at the point of diagnosis of a classically defined disease. That figure doesn't take into account the idea that you can be 80 percent unwell before the first symptoms of disease manifest.

It may take twenty years for enough tumor cells to show up on an X-ray or mammogram. At the time of the diagnosis, you're at the end stage of a healing crisis, not the beginning. Your arteries could be 90 percent occluded before you find symptoms of angina or some other condition. It might take forty years for an occlusion to get that bad. You're told it was caught early, when, in actuality, you got it at the end. So, we've got another 100 million people walking around who are processing disease that is not yet diagnosed. Then we have another 50 million people, bringing us up to 90 percent of the American population, who have the early stages of disease. These are our youth. Take a hundred ten-year-olds at random, and you will find that 50 percent of them already have the development of old age disease. They already have the beginnings of coronary heart disease, arthritis, loss of smell, sound, or taste, due to overstimulated lives.

Those of you who are baby boomers—forty years old and over—didn't grow up exclusively on a junk-food diet. You played outdoors and got plenty of exercise, and you probably had junk foods a couple of times a week, but not at every meal. Most of today's children eat junk food—or at least highly processed food—at every meal. Rather than daily physical activity, most spend the bulk of their time in sedentary pursuits, watching television or surfing the Internet. And they live in an overly excited, toxic environment. That's why their health is so much worse than those of us who grew up in earlier times—even as recently as the 1950s and 1960s—before fast foods and microwaveable meals.

To put it in perspective, 90 percent of the American population contributes to a 1.3-trillion-dollar disease budget. We are increasing our health care costs at a rate of almost 13 percent per year. In other words, the greatest single increase in our gross national product is in medicine. Trouble is, we have little to show for it as far as cures. Any improvements in heart disease have been because of lifestyle improvements, not medical ones. Same for cancer. People are making changes in their lifestyle that are helping them to prevent the disease. So prevention is the only vehicle that accounts for a change. And still we're increasing the disease rate every year.

In the 1970s and 1980s, people became upset when skyrocketing defense budgets reached $250 billion. Imagine $1.3 trillion. That's six times the defense budget. That's more than all of our food, education, and military spending combined. Next year, it will be $1.5 trillion. And within ten years it will be $2 trillion on disease. None of that goes toward prevention.

Only a tiny percentage of the American population is healthy. And it is no accident that they are healthy. They work at it. You have to work on being healthy, just as you have to work on disease. Both processes are based upon the choices we make.

So, when will you change? You'll change when you lose it all, when you realize one day that you've made the wrong choices. Think of how many times you changed because you lost everything. Yet, when you had warning signs along the way that what you were doing wasn't right, you didn't pay attention. You had to hit bottom before you were forced to change. Then you did so grudgingly. "Okay, I guess I'll change."

Well, there's no power in that. That's not a good motivation.

Think of people in relationships. A woman who has been coming to my health support group on Fridays is in an abusive relationship. Her boyfriend has been nothing but a living hell in her life. At one point, he threatened to kill her, slamming her up against the wall just because she was late coming home. We told her to return to class only if she was willing to change, but she was not ready for that.

Another person in the class, Joel, has changed. He finally started to unclutter his life. This after twenty years of being around me with little progress and growth. Finally, I told him directly, "Today you've got to change, Joel. I don't want you here for another twenty years doing nothing." So, he went out and shaved his beard and cut his hair, which is something he had not changed since high school, despite suggestions from many of us at the center. He also cleaned and organized his apartment and uncluttered his life.

Breaking old patterns of behavior takes courage. You have to stop thinking about everything else that's a distraction. Otherwise, you have a thousand exits along your path. You keep reaching for the exits instead of going forward. Now Joel is going forward.

If Joel could do this, why couldn't the woman go home and tell her boyfriend that he was not to be in her life any longer? She couldn't do that because she didn't want to. It was not that she couldn't. *Can't* shows no choices. Her choice was to *need* him in her life. That's the choice she makes, knowing the consequence.

When she rejoined us later that evening, did she not say she was shaken? She said, "I just went home, and he slammed me up against the door. He raised his fist to me. I ran out past him. And he said, 'I'm going to kill you.' " I told her to go to the police and have this man arrested and to get a restraining order on him. But she wouldn't do it. She said, "He'll be helpless. He won't know how to survive."

Think of how many times you've made an excuse for someone else's toxic, negative behavior or lifestyle. You felt you were redeeming yourself through suffering by acting as a chronic caregiver, knowing the other person would then create a codependent relationship with you. A toxic codependency never becomes positive. You're only going to get hurt. And the other person's not going to change if you're going to be responsible for him. If you're going to cook his food and give him a free home and free clothing, why should he change?

So, here we have a situation where Joel was finally willing to take a step out of his malaise and depression and start to do something with his life. One evening of doing that was worth more than twenty years of coming to my talks.

You've got to do something, not think about it. We're a society that overthinks. We're all waiting for someone to provide us with an answer so that we can act upon what we know we should do, instead of looking for the answers ourselves and then acting.

Better to act on something that doesn't work out than wait for that one correct answer. Everything is a learning process; there is no perfect answer in life.

Perfection does not exist anywhere in the universe. Everything is imperfect.

We intentionally blur the difference between what we need to see and what is there. Therefore, we can always dream about what we feel is perfect when it is not.

Joel is now in the process of changing. He has taken the first step, and that gives him confidence to take the second. He was stepping in his mind, but he never actualized it. Now he is.

But the woman in the group hasn't actualized change. She has brought only toxic men into her life for the past ten years. That prevents her from getting on with her career. Why does she do that? Because as long as she continues to believe that she needs to help these people who don't deserve her help, she can say, "My life is worth something; I suffer for other people." Wrong choice. But as much determination went into saying, "No, I won't get this person out of my life," as there would be to get that person out of her life.

These are not mindful decisions. They are reactionary decisions.

I now challenge you to make the mindful decisions to make the changes in your life to grow younger, not older, with each passing day.

GOAL-SETTING 101

Before you get down to the business of reversing how your body ages, you must set some parameters—specific, *measurable* goals—to mark your progress. You've already taken physical inventory of your body in the exercise described in the section, Taking a Look at Your Body, (page 20) and you've begun the inquiry into the emotional and spiritual components of your life in Taking a Look at Your Life (page 17). Use your responses to these exercises as a foundation for the following Introspective Reflections.

Make your descriptions as vivid, as dynamic as possible. The clearer the mental image you create, the more likely you will be to achieve this goal. In short, decide how high you want to fly. What do you want with your life? What would it take you to get out of bed every morning with a positive attitude? Do you want to feel better, be healthier, live longer, and have freedom from health problems? Don't settle for poor health or a weak immune system!

Then write about how you want to feel physically, emotionally, spiritually. In vivid, graphic detail.

WHO CAN HELP WITH HEALTH?

Ultimately, you are responsible for your own well-being, but having access to proper health-care practitioners is an essential component in all health maintenance, including a program designed to halt and reverse aging. A good holistic medical practitioner who provides educated guidance as well as treatment can be invaluable, both in times of crisis and, for prevention, during times of wellness.

Alternative health practitioneers can help define any weak links in your body's structure and function and then direct you toward optimal care. There are numerous approaches, but some general guidelines bear mentioning. A good holistic medical practitioner will perform at least three basic types of analysis before recommending any treatment modality:

1. Take a complete medical history, including health conditions of your parents and grandparents, as well as other family members.
2. Perform a physical examination that goes beyond conventional methodologies.
3. Carefully analyze the results of appropriate laboratory tests taken at the time of the history-taking and physical examination.

In addition, you—as the consumer of these health-care services—have the right to expect the practitioner to include some or all of these techniques in his or her repertory:

- an approach that treats the person as an organic whole, not merely a collection of ailing parts;
- an orientation toward optimal health and sensitivity to dysfunctions that signal an imbalance in the individual;
- the demonstrated ability to listen carefully and skillfully classify any relevant symptoms in order to arrive at the best possible diagnosis and treatment plan;
- as many noninvasive diagnostic techniques as possible;
- an awareness of the potential diagnostic value of even very minor signs and symptoms in the prevention of major dysfunction;
- a preference for noninvasive over invasive treatment programs (for example, administering substances orally rather than intravenously or by injection, except when a condition mandates a more direct route);
- recognition of the importance of strengthening the body's resistive capacities and an interest, wherever possible, in attempting to repair any malfunctioning organ or gland rather than to replace its function with supplementary secretions;
- familiarity with a combination of treatment modalities, including nutritional supplementation, exercise, stress management, and lifestyle changes, to help the person regain balance;
- a willingness to refer the individual, when the condition warrants, to other medical practitioners whose specialized knowledge in a given area may provide the most valuable restorative program; and
- an acute awareness of the importance of the individual's own attitude toward health, aging, and disease, and a willingness to communicate clearly and openly with that individual.

The alternative health practitioner should expect you to be an active, committed participant in your health care, not a passive patient who accepts everything the doctor recommends without question. Therefore, it is your responsibility to ask all the right questions in order to get the vital information you need to help you contribute to your healing, and anti-aging process.

- What, specifically, is being treated?
- How do you know this is the problem?
- What are some realistic goals in my situation?
- What is the projected time frame for treatment?
- Does every patient who has this condition get exactly the same tests and treatments?
- What are my weak links?
- Are these tests and treatments relevant to my body and condition?

TYPES OF PRACTITIONERS

It is not my policy to recommend a specific practitioner or treatment modality to a person. I do, however, believe that it is vital that you have the information needed to make informed choices. The quality of a doctor's care depends on both the physician and the patient, and mutual compatibility. Therefore, I am supplying you with guidelines to some of the modalities that are viable alternatives to orthodox medical practices. I do not discuss chiropractic and osteopathy, nor do I profile nutritionists, although an experienced holistic nutritionist may be enormously helpful in enabling you to maximize the nutritional potential in your diet. Instead I concentrate on modalities that readers may not have easy access to.

Acupuncture, chelation therapy, clinical ecology, homeopathy, naturopathy, and orthomolecular medicine may be extremely useful treatment protocols as you reverse aging.

Acupuncture This school of medicine comes from China, where ancient scholars learned to open up blocked energy pathways, or meridians, so that healing energy, called *chi*, flows directly to the particular point in the body where it is needed to stimulate the body's innate healing powers. While in many states an acupuncturist must also be a medical doctor or osteopath, licensing requirements vary from state to state. Acupuncture is especially good for pain management, musculoskeletal problems, nerve and circulatory problems, and addictive behavior patterns. Cost of treatment may range from $50 to $100 per visit.

Chelation therapy This is a relatively new medical science, started only about twenty-five years ago. At this time, more than one thousand physicians, including many board-certified cardiologists, are using this modality, which involves an intravenous drip of a chelating agent known as EDTA. This stimulates destruction of free radicals, which are apparently the primary causative agent of the aging process itself. By slowing down the destructive potential of the free radicals, the cells are able to heal themselves. As cells heal, they are more able to fight off infection and disease. Objective data supports claims that chelation therapy can even open up the arteries. Improved vascular circulation in people with blocked arteries, especially those to the brain and the extremities, has been demonstrated following treatment with this modality.

Chelation therapy costs about $100 per visit and the course of treatment generally includes twenty to forty treatments, depending upon the severity of the condition. People are beginning to receive this therapy as prophylactic treatment to slow the aging process. The therapy, however, is not without its problems as patients, especially those with kidney disease, must be monitored for renal function. Physicians must be certified chelation therapists to perform this procedure.

Clinical ecology   Clinical ecologists closely examine the relationship between the elements of a person's diet and any symptoms they have been experiencing. For example, a person's irritable bowel may be the result of milk consumption. The practitioner will be able to identify this causative factor by examining all the foods, inhalants, and liquids the patient consumes, testing them alone and in various combinations, to determine which may be causing a physical or mental reaction. This therapy has proved to be helpful in relieving symptoms of arthritis. Clinical ecologists generally use a four-day rotating and elimination diet, preceded by an initial five-day fast in a controlled environment. This tends to be broader than treatment by traditional allergists. Cost is comparable to that of a clinical physician, ranging from $100 to $150 per visit, depending on the state. The initial visit may cost between $125 and $500, depending on which tests are performed and the time required.

Homeopathy   Based on the principle that the causes of illness may follow a law of similars, homeopathy calls for a healthy person to be given a dilute amount of a specific causative agent to help the body rebalance itself. If a person has a head cold, the practitioner would administer a substance that would cause a head cold in a healthy person; in a sick person, this substance helps to cure them. Homeopathy is particularly useful in treating fevers, bacterial infections, toxicity, and the cumulative effects of alcohol, drugs, tobacco, caffeine, or sugar. It is not recommended in treatment of cancer, AIDS, heart disease, and other chronic illnesses. At one time the prevailing form of medicine in this country, homeopathy is now limited in scope, as a result of an intense drive against it spearheaded by the American Medical Association and allopathic medicine. Renewed interest in this treatment modality has brought this practice to the fore. Licensing requirements vary; in some states, the homeopath must be a medical doctor in addition to his homeopathic specialization. Cost of homeopathic treatment runs between $45 and $125 per treatment.

Naturopathy Naturopaths can treat most conditions. They are not, however, permitted to perform major surgery, although they may perform some minor procedures. This modality is centered in the botanical sciences, using herbs and tinctures, with a wide variety of natural immune-stimulating properties. Naturopaths also utilize muscular and skeletal bodily adjustment. They use a much broader basis for diagnosis than do conventional allopathic physicians. Licensing requirements vary from state to state. Cost of treatment is relatively inexpensive, in the neighborhood of $100 to $150 per visit.

Orthomolecular medicine The goal of this medical specialization is homeostasis, or balance, of the chemicals that occur naturally within the body without using synthetic drugs that might interfere with natural processes. Orthomolecular medicine practioners are conventionally trained medical doctors—physicians and psychiatrists—who utilize this technology as part of their practices. Frequently they use a high-dosage vitamin regimen, far greater than the average physician would presume to prescribe. Orthomolecular psychiatrists have had striking success in treating schizophrenics with megadoses of niacin (B_3), vitamin B_6, and vitamin C. Cost of treatment is comparable to that for conventional physicians.

PART 11

USING WHAT WORKS

3

WHAT PARTICIPANTS IN OUR STUDIES ARE SAYING

As I've told you, during the past five years, there have been some five thousand participants—one thousand *specifically* for this anti-aging project—in the controlled scientific studies that provided the data for the protocol detailed in this book.

The average age of these dedicated participants is forty-three—with one group including children, and another targeting older adults, ages sixty to ninety-two. Of these, approximately 55 percent were female. Most were middle class—schoolteachers, civil service workers, mid-level managers, computer technicians, etc. Approximately 20 percent had advanced degrees, with professions such as psychology, social work, law, dentistry, chiropractic, nursing, accounting, and education. Another 20 percent were in the lower income and education brackets; these people worked in offices, retail stores, and at trades.

Here's what some of these amazing people have to say about their experiences in the program.

In December 1994 I found out I was HIV-positive. Like so many people, I went through a deep depression, hopelessness, guilt, fear, and anxiety. At the same time, I had to make believe everything was fine, since no one in my family knew.

The first time I heard your name was from a gentleman selling vitamins at Queens Mall. He was giving me the advice to not take AZT because you said it was toxic, and he asked me to listen to you, but I had no idea when, where.

At work, my office is separate from another, and one day, I walked in and heard you on the radio, got the station, and listened in my own office. Then I realized it was the same person the vitamin man had told me about. I've been a faithful listener ever since, so naturally, when you announced this program study, I signed up.

It's very hard to change, but you have encouraged me to do so.

Since starting in the group almost a year ago, I've been taking the supplements and your Veggie Green Stuff capsules. I've become more conscious of what I eat, so much so that my kids are "upset" at you because I don't buy meat anymore—maybe once a month. But then, on the other hand, if I'm going to eat something I shouldn't, they will say to me, "What would Gary Null say?" and I'll stop.

I have a lot of respect and admiration for you—your honesty, integrity, the truth you share to help heal the world.

To summarize the changes in me from this program: I go to the bathroom regularly, whereas before I was always constipated. I feel better, more positive. The other day, I went to my mother-in-law's and ate her meal. It must have had MSG or something in it, because I got such a headache—which never happened before. I listen to my body now—its reaction to the things I eat. I'm encouraging my husband and kids to eat healthy and change their lifestyles also.

I know this is just the beginning, but I thank you for your dedication, your time, and your guidance for those of us who are searching for a better life.

My T-cells haven't changed much, but I trust God and your testimony that people have been brought to HIV-negative. This is my goal—to be healthy, physically, mentally, spiritually, and be around a long time to enjoy my children, husband, and life itself.

—Nancy N.

I have improved in terms of energy, most significantly. I have also found I have much more patience and my relationships have improved. At work, I have become more efficient and I have more energy to do activities on the weekend. All in all, I find that when I keep close to the protocol, I feel and function much better.

—Joel K.

So much has changed since I entered your study, and I thank you for the wisdom and enlightenment you have shared with me and the others in our group.

My story is long, but I will try to be brief. In February 1996 I went to a holistic medical doctor. My symptoms were: I was tired and "drained" all the time, especially after eating. After days and days of intradermal skin tests, it was clear that I was allergic to almost every food and inhalant on the planet. The situation looked bleak.

Then I read your book, Who Are You Really?, *in April 1997. It opened my eyes to recognize my true life energy. In your book you give such good examples, and I recognized myself as a dynamic, supportive energy in absolutely the wrong profession. I have been a lawyer for fourteen years.*

When I joined your study group in July 1997, I was asked to write an answer to the question, "How do I live and experience life?" Looking back on my answer then shows how much I have changed in my thinking. In the summer of 1997, my answer was: "I don't. I'm a workaholic. Life sucks. I'm trapped—on a treadmill, worn out, mentally and spiritually dead."

Wow! I cannot believe that was how I answered that question. I was criticizing myself and angry with myself and others. Then, in September 1997, I accepted a full-time teaching position at a graduate school. Then I struggled and questioned, why isn't everything "all better now"? I was carrying two full-time jobs—teaching and lawyering.

Today, less than a year later, as I write to you, I am more peaceful and aware. I am in transition and I accept and honor that. Now I see that at first I was trying to make a quick change—to jump from full-time lawyering to full-time teaching. It was impossible to do. I had obligations to finish. I couldn't leave everybody stranded. You taught me to begin to plan for the change.

Now my plan is to let go of the old way and make peace with where I was and what I was. I accept and approve of myself. I recognize that I cannot make a radical jump. I was trying to change too fast.

Now I'm finding a solution—giving myself time. I'm giving myself time for self-learning, yoga, and meditation. I am saying no to any new law obligations and I'm finishing up with the old obligations.

I'm finding a balance here, because now I know that even greater change requires mastery. I'm going someplace on a path better than where I was. I am focusing more on being present in the moment. I trust myself and my intuition. Instead of old voices and preconditioning controlling my life, I choose nurturing thoughts.

Now, when I meditate each morning, I say to myself, I forgive and I am forgiven. All is well. What is it that I need to know about my career? I am peaceful and kind and gentle to myself and I accept that I am in transition, and I don't criticize myself.

Thank you, Gary, for this protocol, the nutritional products, self-empowerment videos, and for being so wise that you chose Louanne Pennse to lead our support group. She is an inspiration to all of us.

—Geri L.

My energy level has improved during this year-and-a-half–long Reversing the Aging Process study. I require less sleep. The ability to maintain a more intense mental alertness, over an extended period of time, has increased,

Vision at 71½ years of age has remained stable, without the need of eyeglasses. Gum health has improved, and my nails are strong and growing more rapidly. My hair root color has become a speckled brown, black, and gray, where it was previously white. It also grows more rapidly.

Skin wrinkles are lessened and skin texture is smoother and softer.

Sexually, my aging process has been reversed. Use of Eternal brought about premenopausal conditions. I experienced sweats, fuller breasts, and vaginal lubrication. Intake of Passion affects my sexual responses. The intensity of those responses are greater. I also experience sexual stimulation from visual sources. These responses are at a level that had been fifteen years ago.

I started taking Greens and Grains recently. Since that time, I lose only a few hairs when I shampoo. My nails are stronger and are growing more rapidly than previously.

I'm always searching to determine how I can function more purely in order to manifest my true being. Who Are Your Really? made me aware of why I function as a Dynamic Asserter and how to do that more proficiently. You stimulate self-recognition. Especially important is the toxic people I've removed from my environment. Those who are family I have to endure—at times—and have set new rules for dealing with them.

May 12, 1998, marked twenty-four years since I became a Nichiren Shoshu Buddhist. The only purpose of chanting, "Nan myoho renge kyo," is for personal enlightenment. One can only be to others what they are to themselves. For me, the chanting opens and cleanses energy patterns. Only then can rebuilding of positive energy occur.

Thank you, Gary, for being such a devoted host of this fun and joyous voyage.

—Marsha W. C.

For the first four months of the program, I resisted taking the supplements. All my life, I never took any vitamins and supplements other than what was in the natural foods. I had been eating only natural foods and nothing else. I bought all the required items on the protocol the first night after class. But they stayed on my table untouched for the first four to five months. Finally, I decided that I am in the program already, I might as well go with the flow. I also created more faith and trust in the program. The whole thing was a challenge to my belief system to take factory-made products as foods and as nutritious aids. I was open to change, and new ideas gradually sunk in me over the course of the program. I let it happen.

Physically, I am more than ever in touch with my energies within and the energy of other people. Prior to the program the energy field was unknown to me. I took a couple of courses in Pranic healing and in Chi Gong.

Awareness of this issue even helps me in my business. I evaluate the employees who work in my business. During the day, if I observe that they are not present or their energies are low, I send them home to take care of themselves. I didn't do this before. I used to try to get a lot produced during the course of the day. Spiritually, I got in touch with my emotions, which I had piled up under a bunch of factual stuff. I had been ignoring how things affect my feelings.

I put myself in this program again because I wanted to be in a support group to detoxify and because I have benefitted from the program. I am not finished. I believe that some changes happen as a result of a process and some other changes can occur very fast. The change in eating habits, lifestyle, or spirituality can only happen as a result of a process. They require time and exposure. And the support group provides this for me.

I do not have any "obstacles" in my life. I do not look at my life this way. I am looking at where I want to develop to from here and where I want to move on to. I have done everything I've ever wanted to do in my life and I do not have any wish lists to work on, or to be attached to. At this stage of my life, I am inquiring into what I can leave behind and what is my legacy. I want to contribute. I must decide in what way. My passion is in the environment and probably in alternative medicine. I have decided to get out of the business I am in and move on to something that I can directly impact and contribute. That is my challenge. I am in the group because I have benefitted from it. Repeating it will not be the same experience. Probably, more than anything else the group has helped me not to ignore myself emotionally and spiritually.

I am also benefitting detoxifying my body. I have learned a lot of small detailed but important information about foods and health.

—Mavash

When starting the program, I was pretty well mentally readjusted. Three years ago, my own beliefs were validated as far as not conforming to what the society demands from you, just being a freer thinker with no restrictions. Physically, I work a lot of hours, so I didn't find the time to take care of myself as I should have. On weekends I enjoy outdoor activities. After starting the program, I am more aware of the need for daily exercise for the physical, mental, and spiritual aspect in growing and becoming whole.

I've had a hard time in the spiritual area. After having been pushed out of the Catholic Church at an early age, I have had bitter feelings toward the Church and no desire to return. After having children, my wife wanted to bring the children up Catholic, still respecting my feelings. I feel my own spirituality, even though it is not channeled through some bureaucratic system. I am at peace with myself and follow the values I believe are correct. I still feel something lacking in this area, like I need to do more.

I am on a new plane of thinking. A higher level, clearer, sharper, more relaxed, able to control anger better. When I wake in the morning, I'm on, not having to wait for a cup of coffee to start to function. It was easy eliminating coffee. Also I feel less limited than before just from my own limitations I put on myself. That's gone—the sky is the limit. I am able to solve problems better just being more focused and less frantic, just clearer thinking. Everything just seems less difficult, enabling me to enjoy life much more. After using protein supplements and weights I am back on track feeling lighter and stronger with more energy and endurance. From time to time I've been having problems with my energy levels.

Also, my hair is thicker and faster growing, skin is clearer and healthier looking, nails are thicker. Although not channeling my beliefs through a fixed system, I do feel more at peace with myself. I feel on a higher plane after making these changes in my life. I don't feel I need the rules and regulations from a given religion or the guilt or suffering that's expected of you. Though I feel I would like to find another religion different from what I learned in my past just to expand my mind.

The changes I have made were not as difficult for me because I truly want to better myself and make up for the past abuses of my body and the pollution that has accumulated for so long. After making these changes and feeling so much better, it is clear that this is the way I want to live the rest of my life, no doubt. The change was a little different for my wife, who had seen me transform into a new person. She had a hard time adjusting to this, but the change was all positive in my eyes anyway, and now she sees that I am a better, more honest person. I tell it like it is, I don't hold back and accumulate negative emotions.

As far as diet goes, I really did not have a hard time eliminating the bad stuff after learning how it affects the body. Though switching to the new diet has been a constant learning process, I still have a way to go. Sometimes I feel weak and tired, most likely from my diet, but it's becoming easier. People look at me drinking my juices and look at me kind of funny, but I don't care because I know I am better off than them just by drinking the juices.

My hours at work make it difficult to get the physical part done, but I just make time the best that I can, always being aware of the need to incorporate the physical aspect of the program. It's hard not to make these changes after learning what we have in the program. I find now it's impossible to go back to my old ways.

After feeling the positive changes and growing every day and looking forward to a longer, healthier life, it's like I have been reborn. I would also like to run the marathon in 1999, because I don't think I could be ready in 1998. Still I'm going to train now. I love life now. Where everything was pretty much a drag, now I'm on a higher plane looking to go higher and meet harder challenges and learn and better myself as I go and grow through life with my new life's program.

Thank you.

—Edmund H.

One of the issues I felt difficulty in overcoming was the guilt surrounding my mother's death. I worked with her in her treatment to seek an alternative approach and although she complied initially, in the long run she didn't want to maintain the dietary and lifestyle changes. I felt there were perhaps other ways or approaches I could have pursued in her care in retrospect, but that's all in the past. I felt I could have even contributed to her demise, but I learned I have no control over other people's actions.

After four years of living with this guilt I finally let go. Today my father has mild coronary disease, which I feel is partly due to the loss of my mother. I am helping him but understand now that I can explain the options, make suggestions, but ultimately the decision is his own what course he chooses to take.

Physical challenges were prematurely aging skin and hair loss, also fifteen or so years of acne. Today my skin is softer, smoother, and more youthful-looking. My acne is gone. It is rare to see any hairs on my pillow, because the excessive hair loss has ceased. Finding my purpose in life is an issue I am working on still. But I'm following my instincts and intuition and this is providing insights along the way. Like doing the things I enjoy doing, rather than what I may have been conditioned to do. The forgiveness letters and the emotional work were very helpful in the letting go of the guilt of my mother's death and the past as well. Again, the appearance of my skin, hair, and no longer having any acne is a big improvement. Regular exercise along with dietary changes have made for a better-toned body. Although at one time I trained with weights approximately two to two-and-a-half hours a day, three to four times per week for almost ten years, eventually I slacked off, and today I don't exercise as long so I don't get burned out or bored. I do different things in addition to weight training, biking, mambo dancing, meditating, and have a more balanced approach so I could continue for the long term. The program provided me with options I wouldn't normally consider. Because I've been able to let go of the past I look forward to a brighter future. As a result of the physical and emotional work and changes, I've made more time to focus on the spiritual.

Although I'm still not sure what my purpose in life is overall, one aspect has been to serve. As a political activist in my spare time I do work around political prisoners. The people I've come to know, the knowledge I've gained, the personal growth I've experienced have exceeded my contributions, as well as the work I've done for the community advocacy organization.

After visiting the stock exchange on Wall Street as a youth, eventually I took a job on Wall Street. I saw myself or created an image for myself that I should be in the business world. Working on Wall Street was an atmosphere that was oppressive and depressing. We worked long hours and then were demoted for our troubles. When I discovered how Wall Street carried its money I realized this was not my ticket out of my perceived poverty. I wanted a life better than my parents, who struggled in factories and odd jobs. I suppose I was overcompensating. I left Wall Street and studied the things I enjoyed—anthropology instead of business. Learned a new language. I am pursuing my interest and intuition, and although I felt a bit apprehensive at first and received many criticisms initially the changes I've made feel great.

I have adopted an organic vegetarian diet, I exercise approximately five days per week. During my fourth month of the program I was feeling somewhat fatigued and began to exercise less, but the extra antioxidants helped. I used to feel stagnant and that I wasn't growing.

Today, I am taking on challenges I probably wouldn't have dreamed of in the past—particularly around my activism with regard to political prisoners and other issues. I do temp work for a community advocacy organization and prefer jobs that potentially serve the community.

Today I see myself as having a future in which I am open to all sorts of possibilities and not confining myself to preconditioned notions. I find myself willing to explore different things and not just playing it safe as I did in the past. Initially taking risks felt scary and things usually didn't turn out as planned; however I've learned to reflect, learn from the situation, and look for new ways to make improvements.

I have learned from the chances I've taken, I feel less apprehensive and look forward more to the challenge. I'm not sure where my pursuits will take me, but at least I'm more open to the unknown and am willing to challenge boundaries, where in the past I probably would have barely even considered, let alone pursue. As a result of the changes I've made I feel more connected or engaged to people and things around me. Sort of like being part of a process in the larger scheme of things I'm still learning to comprehend.

—Benjamin V.

I will be sixty-four years young soon and I was thinking about retirement before I started the program in February. I also lost my job because of downsizing (company moved). Now I feel energized and know that retirement is not what I am looking forward to.

In July I will start a twelve-week training program and will join the work world again and life. Physically, I have lost fifteen pounds, converted to a vegetarian diet, and I powerwalk! I feel better now than I have felt for a long time. I did dilation four years ago because of severe angina. I have been free of the angina; I am taking all the recommended supplements and vitamins. I have high blood pressure and cholesterol, am overweight. Spiritually I am more attuned to my surroundings, try to learn more about other people, their customs. Also, I get in touch with my own beliefs and thoughts. Try to help others—if they want my help.

When I started the program, I was mostly interested to learn to avoid old age diseases and to avoid possibly having to go later into an old age home. Now I know that I do not have to acquire the diseases that most older people succumb to. I want to live an active and healthy life—and now I know that it is possible if I continue the program that we started tonight, and I will continue! It taught me, live a clean and healthy lifestyle: Avoid all the bad foods, negative emotions, negative people. I have no problems avoiding the meats, dairy, and my favorite—chocolate. There are some negative people around me, but their negativity has no influence on me, because I do not let it happen. I am now in control of diet, emotions, and my life! I have become more tolerant, see my life in a different light, do not make fast judgments.

I am sure that I will overcome my high cholesterol, get off my blood pressure and thyroid medication, reduce to my normal weight. I will be healthy and enjoy my life with my children and friends—old and new—for a long, long time. I want to help other people who are willing to learn from my experience. I want to join others who have the same healthy goals in life. I want to enjoy an active lifestyle, nature walks, powerwalks. The only way I would not be able to achieve this is by defeating myself with self-doubt and getting off the program and teachings. No doubt there will be setbacks—but I will not let it deter me from achieving my goal!

—Wilma W.

Growing up I was taught one way of being healthy: by eating the correct foods. However, on joining the program, I've learned so much about how the body works and is nourished by other nutrients and the process the body goes through. My belief was not quite correct. It was a challenge to change my lifestyle, but mentally I know it was the right change. As the weeks went by, I realized the changes, which were the results of sticking to my diet and knowing it worked for me, the way it was supposed to. I was always ready to help anyone who wanted to make this change in their life, and reaching out to others made me feel good, with some satisfaction. I am focused in my thinking and usually set a goal in my mind and really go after it to allow it to happen. The effect of what was told to me in the program made a complete change in my life, and I am able to rationalize problems in the way of health, not any major one, and conquer the problem.

Today I am a better person in shape as I feel much healthier than before. Many of the nutrients I took, the juices, and the habit of eating organic vegeta-

bles, grains, and fruits gave me phenomenal results. My hair is not as gray as before. Patches have come out with the original black renewed hair; my skin is subtle, firm, and younger-looking. My nails are soft and pink. The arthritis in my fingers diminished, and I don't have those dizzy spells as before.

It's my belief that my cholesterol is much lower. I have lost seventeen pounds. I still have to do more in the line of exercises, but this is due to an ailment in the leg. My outlook of appearance is much more appealing to others, as they tell me I look younger. I feel great internally and externally. This physical change is of great importance to me as my health is my happiness. I can do much more at home, as I have more energy. I sleep two hours less and I do not feel fatigued as before. At times, I would feel sloppy on the job, but after attending the classes, I am more alert, think clearly, and am always energetic.

I conquer negative emotions by having a passion for what I want, and carrying out my energy to the positive thought. Being here I am more connected with the Higher Being. My prayer life is meaningful to me and others. I share my time with others in their grief and pain, and I can always refer to an encyclopedia, my magnets, and communication with Him. He is always there for me when I need Him. I feel that innermost relationship spiritually.

Behavioral patterns have changed, as I do not have any hatred in my heart for people anymore. It does not get me anywhere when I can change the negativity to something positive by assisting and giving myself in a situation. Really, I do find comfort, peace, and satisfaction when I can reflect myself in a manner that would be pleasing of others. They would see and imagine me the way I am. It is my belief that whenever you can do a good deed or say a good word to someone or of them, it is the correct way in mind and body. I am a more focused person in my thinking, and I am able to solve problems I may face on my own. Also, I help others who are in need of it. My body feels more youthful, healthier, and always moving onto a happier life. I am free of sickness and I feel great. I am more spiritually connected and my life is more meaningful of a happier, prayerful life.

I have been worried about my high cholesterol due to many years ago and time, again this problem existed. After my body gave me the symptom last year, as I could not breathe properly, I would take Q10 and smell peppermint oil, but it would persist. This is when I made a decision to solve the problem. After taking the green juices, red stuff, and nutrients, I do not have the breathing problem, so I believe my cholesterol has dropped somewhat.

My sister got over her asthma after forty years of her life. She was always in the hospital emergency, and at one time the family thought we would lose her, but she feels great now. I feel much more healthy and I feel I'm living a *much more meaningful life. This change was with results and I intend to keep on it all my life. I see there is a way of life taking good foods and with supplements and exercise, one has to be on the way to good health.*

—Hyacinth F.

I was timid and giving into other peoples' opinions and not speaking up for myself. I was happy letting my husband make decisions—at least the small ones. Now I speak for myself and am involved in every aspect. I went to a massage course and will set up my own place in October when I come back from vacation. I am no longer depressed!

I lost fifteen pounds and feel great. The energy is up. No more migraines. The age spots are fading. The edema is much less and I can tolerate the heat better. My arthritis has improved. So has the irregular heartbeat. My skin looks much younger; also my hair looks better. The compliments of other people are proof nobody believes that I am sixty-five. I am exercising aerobics and re-bounded and starting weight training.

I am reading books about Chinese philosophy and way of life. Nutrition and yoga. I feel connected to the people I care for (older people who need help). This program made me aware that I am great and make good decisions. We consolidated our debt to a low interest rate. I took care of an older sick person against my husband's will and she rewarded me with her life insurance. I feel I can do what I want to achieve.

When I began the program I had to stand up to my husband, who does not believe in this program. He fought me tooth and nail and gave me every argument in the world. I convinced him that it was the right thing for me because of my body and my health and that I was going to do it no matter what. He still wants his meat and potatoes, but slowly he tries vegetarian meals. He drinks a juice in the morning and tries tofu. I still have a hard time to get the juicing and exercise in every day. I still have to get more variety in my cooking. I have still a way to go.

—Marie Q.

The major issues that challenged at the start of this program were procrastination, lack of focus in my life goals and objectives, getting and maintaining a better clarity of my thoughts, and to stop letting family problems and pebbles

in my path deter my objectives. I also had to overcome the lifelong allure of the foods I normally ate.

Physically, I needed to lose weight, lower my cholesterol level, gain more energy, get my body in the best physical condition possible, and correct my slight anemic problem. Spiritually, I lacked self-love. I didn't spend enough time in meditation or prayer and lacked a proper focus on my Higher Self or a Higher Being (e.g., God).

My mind has gained tremendous clarity. I am now able to better focus on the objectives in my life that are important to me. Procrastination, although not eliminated, has been lessened to a degree—I now do most things right away. I have eliminated attending association meetings unless my presence there will contribute tremendously to the meeting. I have made my family take on more responsibility. I am now not so selfish or self-centered, but the me today is now entered in every equation as a primary focus of decisions I make. I have eliminated some of the people and places I used to attend regularly. I have not eaten any meat—except fish—since the first week of the program (that was tough). I do not crave what other people eat anymore, although at time I am tempted to taste (but do not do so). I am now able to tell people I am not eating any meats and do not care how they see it.

My energy has improved. I have not yet checked my cholesterol, but I have no doubt that there has been a tremendous improvement. I have not lost much weight, but my muscle tone in my arms and legs has improved. I am a lot less tired on less sleep, and I now wake up at 5:30 A.M. instead of 6:30 A.M. My breath is no longer atrocious. My skin is not as dry or peeling as much as when I started.

For a time, at the beginning, my whole body ached and my joints cracked constantly—wherever I might have suffered an old injury, now the pain is gone and the joints are cracking less. I am eating a lot less food now than before.

Spiritually, I am now able to meditate a lot longer and do not fall asleep as quickly as before. I am also now able to pray and get deeper into the prayer. I still need to focus more on my Higher Self and speak more directly to the Higher Being (God the Father).

I have still not overcome all the obstacles, but it's an ongoing process. At times, I feel I have not lived up to my abilities and achieved the things I was born to do. But I realized that I have to find myself and improve my health to do all I was put on this Earth to do. I am in the process of overcoming a tremendous financial problem. I also have to overcome more than fifty years of doctrine on culture of eating all types of meat, fish, chicken, lobster, etc. Overcoming constant family problems or the wants of friends, the demands of *my job and civic associations. The above problems are still present but to a lesser degree.*

—Neville B.

When I first joined the support group, I was aware and was struggling to change the way I was conditioned to think. Not just health, but the way I view the world. A lot of the things that were raised in class about guilt and making excuses was taught to me several years ago. Being in this group, in a way, made me see that I have gone a long way. I remember when I had excuses after excuses and never wanted to make any changes. The pain it caused me was great. I wasn't progressing. So when people in the group raise things to me about something I might be doing wrong, I am not so fast to attack them but, always and I mean always, remember that they are coming from the position that they want to make me better. I know that and I know how hard it was for me to get to that stage. It's an everlasting struggle. It is my opinion that the first step is helping yourself and one that I'm willing to take.

Over a year ago, I was working out and one day I just stopped. Looking back at it now, I realize I was not motivated. Since joining this group, I realized that my reasons for working out were wrong. I used to work out to look good, and I found myself working out hard. But when I didn't see the results that I wanted, I quit.

Working out should not be for looks, but used as a way to stay healthy. It was only when I started to think in those ways that I began to love working out. See, because there was no pressure for time. Every day I went to the gym and benefitted. It made me relaxed, vibrant, and, yes, it made me look good.

This group made me see that my mental and physical state is one and the same ways. I struggle to change my lifelong views and must change my view on staying healthy.

P.S. Since joining this group, I feel great, better than I felt in many years.

—Milton J.

I started with feelings of guilt. I was apprehensive, spending time in the past. I was influenced by my environment, having trouble actualizing. I felt disorganized, struggling with relationships, commitment, finances, and self-image.

Physically, I was gaining weight and feeling achy. My skin was blotchy, hair graying. I was losing my good exercise habits. I was a recovering smoker.

I did not think spirit was essential. My spirituality was awakening; I knew it existed, and believed in it. However, it was not an integral part of my life.

I have become more aware of my mental process. This has enabled me to see why I was behaving in some negative ways. I lost fifteen pounds; my skin is clearer. My hair seems darker. My digestion is better. I used to have polyps in my lower intestine and they are gone. My life is more affirmed, being able to help others. I feel more worthy.

I came to the program to change my diet and attitude in order to detox. I had done some work in these areas previously. However, I seemed to be sliding back to my old ways. The detox program seemed like a good way to get started again. I was a little apprehensive about the completeness of the program. After about two weeks, I changed my diet, leaving behind meat, dairy, and sugar. This was relatively easy in that everybody was supportive. I have to give myself credit for making my family and friends supportive. Listening to Gary, I had been exercising regularly for three years. However, I have stopped exercising. I am still struggling with it even though I am active on the job.

I have gained many insights into the meaning of life and actualizing. I see myself integrating more in the future. Right now I feel like I'm letting myself and the group down. I can do a lot better. I see myself joining the running club. Mentally, I think I am getting it. I think I might be able to do more with myself and find more meaning in my life.

—Michael M.

Mentally, I was chronically depressed. I felt hopeless and lost. When I looked in the mirror I kept thinking and knowing that I was just getting older and uglier and sicker. I was only twenty-one!

Each day I would wake up feeling as if I was in an eternal jail, expecting nothing good to happen, only people who I resented and who didn't love me to meet. I had nowhere to go. I felt that if I didn't have anyone to go somewhere with, it would be pointless to do it by myself. So I stayed home a lot and did nothing. I was so bored with myself, I just slept most of the day. I had to think whether something I would do was productive or not. Trying to only do productive things, like reading about business law all day, and having no fun at all made me even more depressed.

I wasn't aware at the time that I ended up doing nothing all day because I was so bored. I had nothing to look forward to, nowhere to go, couldn't conceive of what to do, and was always saying to myself that I couldn't do it. I *couldn't go to the bookstore in Manhattan because I didn't want to spend the $3 for the train ride. I couldn't get a date because I was too ugly and unlovable. I couldn't be healthy because I didn't have enough money. I couldn't be happy because I was so hopelessly sensitive to criticism and always being made fun of for unknown reasons. I felt sorry for myself a lot. I sang all of my favorite depressing songs over and over to myself. Often I cried before I slept. I hardly ever laughed; I isolated myself from meeting people and didn't smile very much.*

Another big issue was that I had very low self-esteem. Being a Creative Assertive, I am always somewhat insecure, but I really thought of myself as unworthy of any success. I couldn't even look a person in the eyes when I talked to him. I let people talk to me in condescending ways. I let them tell me how stupid and no good I was, and I believed it. That came from my family. I had no friends.

Physically, I was underweight, had acne all over my face, dark circles under my eyes, weak feeling. I had bad indigestion. I couldn't eat grains or starchy foods without having an itchy reaction on my face, with more pimple eruptions afterward. I felt bloated after meals. I ate a lot of fat, which made me feel sluggish, and added to my feelings of depression. I had been weight training at home for about two years, but I could not get any muscle mass. It took all of my strength to squat one hundred pounds ten times. I slept about twelve to fourteen hours a day. I had many outbreaks of herpes cold sores, especially when under emotional stress. Felt tired a lot—couldn't wake up early in the morning. Spiritually, I was very selfish. Didn't care about anyone but myself.

Now I feel good for no reason many times. I look forward to each day, wondering whom I will meet. I do my best not to hold grudges. Don't feel sorry for myself, don't tell myself I can't get a date. I say to myself, "Come on, baby, you can do it" instead during difficult times. Don't sing sad songs anymore, only uplifting ones. Can squat 170, deadlift 170 for twenty reps without much trouble. I gained twenty pounds. I am more muscular now, have more endurance. No herpes itch. I think more about helping others. I bought gifts for my sisters for the first time in their entire lives for their birthdays. I don't talk about myself to death to other people, and I have forgiven all the people who hurt me. Not angry and bitter about anything.

—Oscar L.

It has been very easy for me to do and follow each step of the program. I have been listening for over eight years and had followed Gary's advice, books, and protocols ever since. This has been an opportunity to do it more in depth. I had been very physically active; this is just a step forward to move my life where I want to be.

The program has helped me to focus more in my emotions and feelings and have control over my adventure, instead of focus on someone else's opinions. It has brought a center to my life as a whole. I am a happier person, I relate to others more easily, and have more flexibility. Mentally, I have a lot more focus and clarity. Everything is a thought away, and I am able to accomplish almost anything that I want to. Physically, I have a lot more energy and feel like I am worth a million!

When I started the program on January 16, 1998, I had candida and a cystofibroid breast. Today I am free of it. I feel completely healthy and full of energy. My skin has improved in clarity, it's softer; my hair is fuller and thicker. I feel a sense of wellness, well-being, am happier and more centered. My body looks healthier; I lost some unwanted fat. I am leaner and in great shape. I am pleased to have joined this program.

I would recommend it to anyone who would like to improve their health. I am thankful to Gary Null for sharing his time and knowledge with us. Thank you very much and keep up the good work!

—Elizabeth P.

Although I had no labelable (or at least labeled) major issues at the start of the program, I noticed, in general, a better mood. Changes got made—I started being firmer about my boundaries, making sure my work got done before taking my daughter out to the playground. Thus, calmer existence. I had been going away every weekend to avoid my husband (divorce situation). I saw this was draining me and decided to stand my ground. I started giving myself more space from the other "Playground Moms" who let their kids do things they didn't like and then bemoaned it—and stopped wondering if there was something wrong with me.

The fun things—I played a softball game, because I wanted to. I stopped relationships with four people who had lied to me/shown contempt, etc. I seized an opportunity to do something new I wanted to—plastering a house—by offering to help a friend.

I had been too busy worrying and thinking I needed to "solve the prob-

lem" before doing anything. I noticed that I didn't even consider looking at what was working, positive goal orientation—that in me caution was so strong, "what I want" never even saw daylight above a very pessimistic assumption of "what I can have." I realized this (me) was the biggest influence in making my life bleak. Even though there were some people putting pressure on me that I was blaming—that getting rid of their stuff would only leave me more effectively running from my fear, pain—more comfortably addicted but not joyful.

I see people's "stuff" more clearly, helping me let them be more easily, if that seems appropriate, or challenge them if that seems appropriate. Today I told a woman (who I knew post facto had abused her child physically and emotionally) who was going to have the child (who I know) evaluated for attention deficit disorder that she needed to face the fact that the child had emotional patterns produced from her experiences and not to be drugging the child to avoid (under the hypothesis "it's genetic") responsibility. I am not unconsciously running around wasting my emotional energy looking for people's approval/attention. I never was a conformist in my behavior, but there was a stress in wanting to be liked.

—Briseis G.

I had a lot of confusion and was pretty depressed. I had also felt alone and disconnected. My house was suffering and my business also. I had the hardest times making decisions. I felt as though I was a pinball with almost no control over things going on around me.

All the time this is going on I was a great actor. I tell you, not much fun at all. I was overweight, approximately 195 pounds. No desire to do anything— just go to work , try to do my job, spending more time trying to get out of doing things than actually doing them. My back was in constant pain. I felt bloated.

Spiritually, I felt very alone with no place to turn. I was always looking for something, but failed to touch anything. Very mad for no reason.

I am no longer depressed. I don't need to talk about how bad life is because now it is great. I have very little trouble making decisions. I was seeing a person to help me. This I started in October. She said many times that in all her years no one had made the progress I had in such a short period of time. I no longer see her.

Physically, my shape has changed dramatically. I went from 195 when we started, with no energy, to 160 now. My weight has been stable for about six *weeks. I used to wake up every few hours at night. Now I sleep straight through. I guess this is more mental than physical, or maybe a combo of both. I sleep about five hours a night and have more energy than ever. I take the exercise pretty seriously (actually, it's a lot of fun). Before I had all I could do to get off the couch. I would be winded for nothing. Now I ride a bike about forty minutes every day. I have no more back pain and I can button all of my pants.*

I was listening to the AM station before Christmas and heard Gary mention new programs forming. This is something I felt I needed but was afraid to do. So what I did was just call before I had too much time to talk my way out of it. I tell you, from that first meeting on, every day is better then the day before. I have a cabinet shop and my work is no longer painful. I almost look forward to going. I have recently opened a new business also, and it's been a lifelong dream. I no longer see it as impossible. It is a fireworks company and I know now I will have no problem seeing this through.

At first my family was afraid I was joining a cult. Now I am asked questions on a daily basis. I receive a lot of support. I had no idea life could be this good. I like to help people around me and look forward to doing as much as I can.

—Anthony N.

I was struggling in January—not feeling in sync, needing to move in a direction, not sure about the direction. I knew I was moving in a positive direction but thinking that I needed to make some decisions about my life. I felt more confused, disoriented—why am I doing a lot of things and not happy with the results? Physically, I felt fat and ugly, with a double chin. My complexion was darkening, my back was hurting, my tongue was coated. My clothes didn't lie correctly on my body. I had a smile, but my singing had stopped (sort of—I sing for myself).

My digestion was off. I was spiritually connected to higher powers and yet I was still searching. I did not really know how I would spend my next seventy-five years. (I'm forty-eight now.)

This is my year. I am making more strides in my life than I have perhaps in any other year. I am feeling more clear on a daily basis. I am feeling and thinking and remembering more. I am more in touch with myself. These things have occurred because I want them to and because I am constantly working to have them manifest. I am providing space for mental clarity. I am working on it and it is happening. My body is changing. I am working hard to make it happen. The program, I think, is a major factor. I continue to exercise more and more and I feel good about myself. So far I've probably lost twenty pounds, but muscle takes the place of some of the fat. My complexion is returning to its natural state. My back has fewer blemishes and hurts less often. My breathing is deeper. My memory is improving (somewhat). I can perform more strenuous exercises. I look into the mirror and now I think there is hope. I'm getting pretty again :) I'm liking my physical body more.

As the fifth child in a family of nine, I have always been the person who tried to bring sanity to insane family situations. Always the one who tried to negotiate, work things out. Striving for balance maybe. The giver—I remember as a teenager I was feeding hungry children (who didn't belong to me) in our community, working with youth. Concerned about making a difference, this spirit led me into counseling, and now for over twenty years I have been counseling and assisting people to change their lives. While very gratifying, I always wanted more. Now I understand as I change myself more, I will be more effective in what I do. As I change me more and I open myself up to what is most gratifying for me, I become more in tune to my needs, and their resolution. I am able to affect more people in a positive manner. I will be communicating to masses of people—motivating, uplifting, and nudging, pushing toward behavior modification.

—Adele B.

In April I was offered a chance to teach piano to a group of adults in an adult education program at a city high school. I accepted and am now teaching a group of thirteen people on Monday nights. A year ago, I probably would have refused to do it, but now that I am doing it, I can see a future—teaching or performing music; getting back into music, doubts and all. I've begun studying with my old music teacher and spending a lot of time at the piano, and deciding how to teach my class. It is something that just happened, *but I felt good enough to try it (even though the negative tape was playing in my mind). Another thought occurred to me—if I fail or the job is not renewed, so what? I can keep studying and try to teach elsewhere. This is a big step for me.*

Physically I have gone from doing little or no exercise to five days a week. I use a NordicTrack, hand weights, and recently began jogging. This is a major step for me because I have always hated exercise, hated gym classes in school, couldn't do most of what was expected, and I had a father who was bigger, stronger, and much more athletic than me. I've always been repelled by gyms and the whole jock mentality. I now am starting to believe that just doing it is important, not how good or how athletic I should be.

Spiritually, I am trying to find some connection with life—rather than a just "go with the flow" attitude. I don't accept major religious dogma but am very excited by music, art, theater, etc. Music (composing, performing) is, in one sense, a form of meditation. You need that quiet space.

I have had to overcome a negative attitude, fostered by a negative or non-supportive family environment—not abusive, but closed. I am small, my father was big. I was weak, he was strong. He played sports, I played music. My relatives are generally bigger than me, and this really developed into an inferiority complex.

I guess I suffer from what you call the "small man syndrome." All through high school and college I was smallest of my friends. This, combined with a negative attitude, has been very hard to overcome. I am still working on it, a work in progress. I have made some progress and am supported by my wife. I feel this has held me back in life, music relationships, and having a positive outlook. This is definitely a work in progress.

—Fiore D.

At the start of the program, I was almost mentally paralyzed. I thought that my career was over. It was a major challenge to change the outlook of my life. I have many health problems; among the most important were high blood pressure, high cholesterol, enlarged prostate, and hemorrhoids. I was under medical care, and it seemed that treatment was taking me nowhere. I had the belief that for me there was nothing left in life. I was waiting for my Maker to take me away.

I reexamined my life. I felt the rush of energy. I restarted my engine. I discovered that there was a life ahead of me. I discovered new interests and I started living again. One of the first things I did with my new burst of energy was start an exercise program. My healthy habits made me lose weight. As I saw my progress, I became more committed to the program. Needless to say, I recuperated my health in every way.

I am so amazed that at my age, I am accomplishing things that I thought I never would. I thank God for putting me on the right track of good health. I feel that now I am more in touch with myself. I found new purpose in my life and my energy and optimism is spread to others. Friends and relatives see the changes in me and request my advice.

One of the biggest obstacles was inside of me. I have procrastinated *for so long that it took a monumental effort to get organized and committed. The second obstacle was clutter in every way. I have examined my life and little by little I started uncluttering my mind of preconceived ideas, or unhealthy habits, and of physical clutter. I became less angry and fearful, and when anger and fear stoke me, I've examined my feelings and tried to find out why I was feeling that way.*

I have forgiven everybody that has hurt me in the past. I understood that the only thing that was hurt was my ego. I have realized that by taming my ego I can free more energy and use it in positive ways. I see myself now and in the future healthy and active, helping other people to reach their goals. I have embarked in new tasks that I never dreamed of. Now I am into biking, camping, and hiking.

—Magno O.

When I called to join the program back at the end of October, I was at the end of my rope. I had been struggling with thoughts of suicide for the past four months and was hoping that being in the program would give me the lifeline I so desperately wanted and needed. I'd been out of work for a year and was feeling hopeless about my situation. I had no unemployment benefits left—my boyfriend was supporting me—and felt useless and worthless.

I was seriously considering signing myself into a psychiatric hospital. That is something that I'd never considered in my forty-three years of living, since I know all too well how mental illness is treated and am against using drugs as a first line of treatment (if at all).

My first meeting was a bit overwhelming, since I didn't start at the beginning of the group, but I caught up and began the program. It was difficult to afford the supplements, but my boyfriend was supportive and able to help out a bit every week. He was willing to help in any way since it was painful for him to see me in such a state and it made him feel so helpless. The biggest change occurred after a month of being off sugar and dairy. After that point and to this day (eight months later) I have not had the deep depression return.

The questions I was asked to answer, and reading the life energies book helped me make some major life changes. I applied to, was accepted, and graduated from the Cornell Cooperative Extension Master Gardeners Program. Most people who go through this program are retired because it's held on Wednesdays out on Long Island from 9 A.M. to 4 P.M. Basically, you can't hold a regular nine-to-five job (as I've done for most of my working life) and be in this program. I decided I should just do it now and not wait. I got a job taking care of two children for a friend and was able to have a small income (better than none). I also moved in with my boyfriend of nine years.

I also eventually began doing a work/study with the Tri-State Healing Center, working with Diane and Ray, that I enjoyed and appreciated very much. It felt so much better, not having to take more money from my boyfriend.

Also, I started a community supported agriculture organic produce project in my hometown and now have eighty members. I gave lectures, started a CSA newsletter, and helped get an article about CSAs published in Newsday. I now need to find a larger location and hope to get another 120 members. These are things I might have dreamed about doing but would never have thought possible. I always thought my place in the universe was to help people with their dreams and that (1) I didn't have any dreams or (2) if I did, there was no way they would come true.

This brings me to the present and what I can now say is, I wish I could start the program all over again! The reason is because (like Gary said) I did great with the questions, making life changes, and the spiritual parts, but I didn't deal with the diet and exercise parts of the program as I could/should have. I would like to be a buddy for a new person on the program because I'm a good example of what can happen (great and not so great). I now realize that I want and need to get up to speed with the diet and exercise parts of the program so I am able to keep up with the life changes I've made so far. If I don't, I can see illness around the corner. I won't have the strength to keep up with myself! I realize that I have to get out of my mind (so to speak) and into my body.

I had been sexually and physically abused periodically throughout my life, starting as early as age seven (and possibly younger) and stopping approximately twenty years later, and because of that have always had a desire to be bodyless. This program has helped me get my self-esteem to a place where I'm ready to go to the next level of healing. It's all a matter of me getting out of my own way since I am my biggest obstacle.

As far as the future goes, I am not sure what it will bring, but I know it's going to be a lot more positive and fun than the first forty-three years. I thank Gary and Luanne, and everyone else connected to this work, many, many, many times.

—Suzanne Z.

When I was young, I suffered from severe chemical and food sensitivities. The orthodox methods (antibiotics for my strep throat) offered no help. Staying off most foods prevented the occurrence of extreme allergic reactions. I still was not feeling good. This was weakening every aspect of my being (cognition, physical strength, moods, state of mind). I had a pale complexion and dark circles under my eyes.

When I got involved with Gary Null's allergy program, within two weeks of green juices I was feeling remarkably better. Now it's been nine months and I can eat almost any food. The clarity of my thinking is better. My "light years"—I have no more moodiness, depression, lethargy, or poor complexion. Instead, I feel vital, healthy, and alive.

In the future I see myself helping other people through my experience. I will continue to learn about internal energy. Perhaps I will get a Ph.D. in Oriental medicine. I will take my own hardships and the lessons that I learned from them and use them to help others.

—Peter A.

The obstacle that I had to overcome was that I always followed Null's wellness program, but I was a comfort addict and did things in moderation. Now, I am more disciplined and able to handle the challenge of discomfort. I've been following my health detox program continuously and find it enjoyable and pleasant to do.

On the physical level, my dentist told me my gums looked the healthiest he had seen in me when I went for my half-year visit. I told him about your health detox program and the protocols that I took; he wasn't interested. My friends tell me that I look so good, they are inspired to get healthy themselves.

I now have a youthful appearance and rejuvenation of glowing skin and hair. I lost about twenty-five pounds and five inches from my waist. I've been cross training almost every day in my rotation routine. I went from walking three miles to jogging five miles. I do about one hour, ten minutes walking and running stairs in a stadium. I bike about sixteen miles on weekends. I'm also weight training and have been taking judo and jujitsu for twenty-five years.

I have more energy, strength, vitality, and alertness due to this program. My health is excellent, I'm never sick or fatigued, and I no longer have sinus problems. Many people and friends have been complimenting me about my well-being and positive attitude. Many come to me seeking health and nutritional advice, but when I tell them what they have to give up (coffee, sugar, smoking, wheat, dairy, alcohol, negative attitude), most change their minds. Some end up making gradual changes, and I help encourage them to do their best.

On the emotional level, I use meditation, hypnosis, affirmations, and creative visualization to destress. I no longer let toxic people run my life and/or seek their validation. I've been letting go of many things and getting clutter out of my life. I've become more detached from my possessions, am laughing more and slowing down my lifestyle to the speed of nature, which has increased my awareness. I have become more spiritual, kinder, gentler, humbler since the program began. My intuition and psychic abilities are much sharper from eating, drinking, and juicing organic foods.

I'm no longer afraid of challenges and uncertainty in my life. I am better at self-actualizing rather than just talking. I judge people for what they do rather than what they say.

—Steven H.

I started this program at a point where I had become totally obsessed with my weight and body image. This obsession led me to exercise extensively and have such a rigid control over what I ate. There was no joy in any of this for me. My obsession left no room for my family or friends. Everything I did had to fit in around my rigid schedule. This obsession was just replacing a lot of pain I had inside me. If I kept myself busy with exercise and a rigid schedule, I didn't have to deal with any emotions, not sad ones or good ones.

I heard Gary Null on the radio for the first time last October, he was talking about detoxification. I know my body wasn't that toxic, but mentally I was struggling. The thing that interested me about what Gary was saying was that his detoxification program was mental as well as physical and spiritual. I joined the next available support group with my husband, because I felt if we could do it together, it would really be helpful.

Once starting the group, and following the protocols, my self-esteem started to improve; I started seeing my thought patterns in a new light. If I could replace my negative thoughts with positive ones—what a change might occur! Now I find myself continuously reinforcing positive affirmations to myself and to others, and I believe more and more opportunities are being open for me. I'm more flexible and relaxed, I'm enjoying myself more, and I'm constantly making changes and looking for ways to improve my life.

I have increased my body fat to a much healthier level. My sex drive has increased as well. I have also started to cut back on so much strenuous exercise and add more yoga and learn Chi Gong, which I needed to help balance me physically. My cholesterol dropped fifty points and my HDL went up to a very healthy ratio. I believe this was due to the elimination of dairy products, as I was not eating any other animal products before. I am sleeping about one hour less a day. I used to be a chronic gum chewer and candy eater. I would crave sugar through the day. Now these cravings are gone and I can't imagine ever desiring those things anymore.

In the future I see myself becoming more of who I am. I plan to study Feng Shui; I've started studying Chi Gong. I plan to continue looking inside myself and questioning things that prevent me from honoring my true self. I'm looking forward to this journey.

—Didi S.

I first met Gary Null in January 1997. I am amazed at the changes that have occurred since then. I should start by describing the life I led prior to that meeting. I drank ten cups of coffee a day or more. Lunch would be a hero or pizza. Dinner, I could think of nothing better then a burger and french fries washed down with a cold beer—more than one. If not for Chinese takeout, I never would have eaten vegetables. In short, I consumed all the vital chemicals not found in nature. I was a toxic mess, a blob sitting in front of a TV set with one hand on a beer and the other in a bag of chips. I was 380 pounds and killing myself; worse, I was very unhappy. I knew something had to be done, but what?

On January 12, 1997, I arrived at Gary's Paradise Gardens, fully committed to do whatever "this nut" wanted for two weeks. That first day, I had no appreciation of the changes I would undergo. For fourteen days, I was happy. I lost sixty pounds. For the first time in my life I was detoxified. In February, I was back in the real world, enjoying a new lifestyle. All my food came from the health food store. I realized a healthy body and a healthy mind went hand in hand. If I put toxic food in my body, I would have a toxic mind.

I now identify myself as a vegetarian. Quite simply, I do not eat meat or dairy. Those few times I cheated, I felt awful. In the past year I have had meat six or seven times, all at social occasions—Christmas or Thanksgiving or when invited to dinner. While I looked forward to these parties and thought I would enjoy the food, I found that I have changed. I no longer like the taste of meat. The next day, it always made me feel sluggish.

The next step in my health evolution was to buy a juicer. My days now begin with green tea and vegetable juice. They give me a shot of "energy" I never got from coffee and a Danish. I can and use powdered juice and find them to be very good. I find juicing helps to keep me connected. Gandhi did not have to spin his own cloth.

The most important part of my day is exercise. Every day without fail, I work out. I run or walk forty minutes to an hour every morning. In the evening I lift weights or do Chi Gong. This for me is the most essential part of each day—if I have a hard workout, everything falls into place.

I now set goals for myself; doing this I must be careful—frustration and negative thoughts creep in when I do not achieve these goals in the time limit I set. My life is better than it was and getting better each day. I know that I still have a long way to go, but I will be in good shape soon.

—Kevin F.

When I began the protocol, at issue was my general attitude of skepticism regarding whether I would indeed be helped by this program. And whether I was capable of following the protocol laid down was another issue I thought very hard about. How could I manage without eating meat? I was also a worrier, and the general direction of my health was of concern to me. Worrying about my health did not, of course, help the situation. Lack of energy and insomnia, also flatulence caused by a spastic colon. There was also stiffness in the legs, which to me indicated a sign of arthritis. Indigestion, dizziness, and leg cramps were virtually a way of life for me, and despite numerous lab tests and doctor's visits, relief at best lasted only for a short time. All of the above contributed to my desire to seek help for my physical condition.

After almost a year in the program, I have become more confident about my health in general, and I can see marked improvement in mind, spirit, and body. Having followed the program almost religiously, including the meditation techniques, I find that my mind is more focused and my memory has definitely improved. The most obvious result I have noticed is the increase in my energy level. With only six hours of sleep I can complete a full day without feeling tired or lethargic. My skin is also much smoother than it used to be, and the liver spots that once covered my neck and chest are barely visible. My fingernails, toenails, and hair grow very fast and have to be trimmed more often than before. The constipation, indigestion, and bloating have been greatly reduced.

—Winston W.

I was glad when I heard of the opportunity to start in a support group with Gary Null. Over the last ten years, I started gaining weight and became a couch potato. Three years ago, I was diagnosed with hypothyroidism and started using Synthroid pills. I used to get spells of tiredness almost every month that sent me to bed to sleep in order to feel better. I knew that I needed to do something different but did not have enough motivation to do it on my own.

That's why getting into the support group was a big difference for me. I can say that the challenges that I was facing when I started the program were dealing with low self-esteem, low motivation to move forward, eating the wrong foods, and being unable to lose weight. I also felt the passion that I used to have when I was younger had diminished. I needed a different perspective in my life.

After I started the program and continued the protocol, I felt less tiredness. I am exercising now and I feel great. People tell me that I look thirty-five years old—I am now forty-six, with a grandson. My skin is smooth and I feel young. I don't get headaches and I am in a good health. I have some cysts in my breast that I believe will disappear with the change of eating habits. In the past, I used to wear my glasses for reading; now I remove them. My blood test came out much better than the first test.

The program has helped me be more relaxed and assertive. When I am facing a problem, I look at it with a different perspective and know that it will be solved, even if it isn't at that particular moment. I get less angry with people and don't feel that I need to compete. My thoughts are more clearly to the point without getting into too much rationalization. Since I started the program, I felt depressed only once and I faced it and it was nothing. My self-esteem has been raised and I am able to look at myself without self-blaming.

I feel now more motivated to get involved in different things; to be adventurous and allow the child within me to come up. For example, I heard of a workshop for the preparation of the Latin American Feminist Women Conference, to take place in 1999 in Santo Domingo. Since I am Dominican, I decided to go and find out what it is all about. It was a nice trip and I came away with more knowledge of what is going on concerning women, children, and family issues in Santo Domingo.

—Gilsia P.

As an artist, I felt that my focus was not up to my ability (with the years that I've put into training, more than twenty-five years). Prolific thoughts should

have been in prolific works. After listening to Gary Null for three years on the radio, I decided that this could only help me focus and get to the work I needed to do.

Since I've been in the program five months, there have been many changes. I have lost ten pounds. My energy, which was low, has increased. I'm not as tired as I was previously. I talk less and finally I find myself listening more to what people are saying (particularly in my family). I did not realize how angry I was until we had to write ten letters to people who caused us some kind of pain. After that exercise I was truly able to let go of the anger, and able to speak to my exhaustion without feeling anything, pain or otherwise. While I've always been a mediator, trying to understand why people do the things they do, I no longer care to understand them. I don't need them in my life—now I please myself first.

When I began this program I wasn't sure what I wanted to do—become less toxic, enabling me to focus on what I needed to do for me. What's important is that all my life had been the need to create with word or with paint. Two years ago I changed my schedule as a full-time teacher to part time and replaced my painting full time. Since then I painted, but not full time. Hence my entrance in the program. I realized I needed to focus my energy and thoughts to create and decided this might be exactly what I needed. It was more than what I envisioned. The questions we had to ask ourselves and answer honestly helped to create an environment for change. I used to be a sweet junkie and now I can walk by cakes, pies, and cookies without feeling deprived. I find I eat many more raw vegetables—something I had not done before.

I am rarely tired. I walk now more than I have done in the months before beginning the program. My energy level is higher and I feel great.

—Mimi V.

I did not have any physical constraints that I was aware of. The introduction of the detox program made me aware of my mental restrictions more so than physical. To learn how to focus and not be sidetracked by obstacles was my starting point. I did not know or understand how my energy or relationships would or could affect my perspective of life. This stage of unwillingness allowed me to be happy in my ignorance.

I learned how to get toxic people out of my life. I leaned how to strengthen my attitude, be patient and not respond with negativeness. I look at myself in a new light of happiness and motivation. I have learned how to be happy with myself.

Physically, I am stronger from exercising daily. I am a martial artist and I am able to do things other people I work out with are unable to do (handstand pushups, dips, and pushs into having my body parallel with the floor).

—Barry R.

At the beginning of the program, I was challenged with learning how to think clearly, to learn to focus and how to plan. Staying away from toxic people and not letting myself get carried away with their problems. It is a slow process, but I'm under control. The challenges that I have at home, in my marriage, I look at with courage, not indifference. The learning process is an everyday affair.

My letting go of meat has improved my digestive problems, which I've had since childhood. I found out also that I have an allergy to corn that we consumed daily. Learning to eat organic food has not been easy. My conscience reminds me every time I go against the rules. Letting go of sugar has been great. Detoxifying my system is still an ongoing process—my brain fog is slowly going away.

—Marjorie A.

I had been listening to your program for many years; but when my husband and I retired at age sixty-two, Myron began listening to your show. When he heard the call to participate in the study, he talked it over with me and we decided to go with it with deep sincerity. We happily bought juices, changed our water system to a filtration under the sink, joined a gym and connected to organic food sources. It became a total change in our daily routine—a new way of life.

As we proceeded with the protocol, we noticed big changes in our energy. I couldn't lift any weight at first on the machine cycle. Now I can handle forty-five pounds pull down, five pounds bench press, sets of fifteen at a time. We do all kinds of lifting, pressing, pulling, and our muscles are bulging.

My skin glows with health. People stop me and notice a different quality in my look, but they can't put their finger on it. My chiropractor says that my skin and look are significantly different and youthful. The contact and attention to my own body and the speed at which I can respond to what my body needs is marvelous. My nails are stronger and more youthful. I experience increased strength and endurance and continued, good energy. I also have a new attitude of optimism. I have experienced more rapid hair growth. My gums are healthier and firmer and my teeth do not decay. I also experience improved sleep patterns. I do not stuff myself with poisonous herbicides, animal products, etc., and the juice is visibly energizing as I drink it.

So many of our friends are manifesting illnesses and at the moment, the two of us are emanating good energy and good health. That is worth all the effort. We will continue in this maintenance protocol for life. It is a sensible concept to move toward wellness and prevention, rather than indulgence in illness.

I have begun piano lessons and am given a complex new piece to work on because my mind is seeking challenge. Myron and I dance western square dance at a challenge 3A level. We are alert and aware of the political and cultural ramifications of the protocol. We think that these positive results are only the beginning of what is possible for us as productive, creative, service-oriented seniors. We have joy and optimism, humor and openness, and that makes our lives full of possibility.

—Wilma H.

I am an artist. I am very excited. Tomorrow my husband and I are leaving on a two-week Baltic cruise with friends. We were married forty-five years ago. We never did anything fun like this. Our friends do it often. We are both work-aholics, and love what we do. Having fun has been work for us. Also, my diet is limited because of food allergies. I once got amoebic dysentery on a trip. I worried about getting colitis away from home.

Gary, I am the woman who told you that twenty years ago the head of gastroenterolgy of a New York City hospital said, "Barbara, get rid of your colon, and get on with your life." I started listening to you. By 1980, I had changed a lot. After my last colonoscopy, I saw a computer printout of the inside of my large intestine. It was "pink and purty." Now, being in the program, my colon is perfect. I question whether there really is such a thing as colitis, or is it just sensitivities to different things?

Back to our trip. My husband and I never have been together for two solid weeks without work projects. We will have fun!

—Barbara K.

Following your protocols for the reversing the aging process study has significantly improved my health in many ways. My weight is maintained at 110

pounds effortlessly. It used to fluctuate a lot. It was as high as 130 pounds at one point several years ago. This 110 pounds is the weight I maintained when I was nineteen–twenty-two years old. It's wonderful!

I require one hour or more less sleep per night than I did before the study. Now I sleep more soundly and feel more alert and energized during the day. I have gotten no colds or flus since I have been in the program. This is a welcome change! I had been going to a dermatologist before the study for acne and rosacea. The topical medication he prescribed for rosacea did not help it. Also, he prescribed tetracycline to be taken on an ongoing basis for acne. I refused to take this. I believe that the protocol for the study was a much safer and more effective treatment for acne. Acne is no longer a problem for me and the rosacea has significantly improved.

I find that I look and feel younger now than I did before starting the program. People often assume I am ten or more years younger. I'm so grateful for this. My skin is more clear and healthy. My hair is silkier and seems thicker. Also the number of gray hairs growing in is becoming fewer and fewer. This is great! Menstrual pain has lessened very significantly. I used to take Tylenol about every four to six hours for the first forty-eight hours of my menses. I take no medication now whatsoever, and experience at the most only mild discomfort. Also I no longer have the premenstrual puffiness and headaches I used to have.

Emotionally, I'm better able to deal with day-to-day stress and traumatic events. In general, I feel more calm and positive than I did before the study. I am fully committed to using what I have learned to maintain my health and perhaps improve it further. I have been sharing what I have learned with others and I'm grateful for the joy of watching them benefit too.

—Marlene D.

The improvements in my overall health have been amazing. It is difficult to really believe in something until you actually put it into practice and notice the results for yourself. I used to suffer from severe seasonal allergies. During the night, I would not be able to breath easily since my sinuses would swell and make it difficult to breathe. One nostril would get so clogged that it wouldn't work properly. In a few days I would develop headaches and a bad case of halitosis. This caused me to withdraw from speaking with people at the office, since I did not want them to notice my breath. I had tried going to ENT doctors, but they always told me these were ragweed, pollen, or dust allergies that I

had to live with. Then they would give me a prescription for some nasal spray and send me on my way. Needless to say, these were only temporary and artificial remedies. Since being on your strict protocol, I have not had these allergic attacks during spring or fall!

I have also noticed that my mental sharpness is better now then it was when I was twenty-eight years old (I'm presently forty-one years old). I've noticed this because when I was twenty-eight, I tried going for my master's degree in electrical engineering while working full time. I was not able to focus to the level required for maintaining a B average or better. I've been in graduate school now for three semesters and I have a GPA of 3.25. In this past spring semester, I registered for two courses while working on a project in the office with a very tight schedule and lots of pressure. One of the courses required commuting to the campus thirty minutes away. On both courses I received grades of B. My friends admire my effort, but what they don't know is that I have an edge they don't have; I have more energy, have an optimal diet, and I'm putting all these health benefits to good use.

I've also expanded my physical activities to include bicycling and playing tennis. I recently played someone eleven years my junior in a tennis match. I did not get winded and we had to play a tiebreaker. This also I remember not being able to do at age twenty-eight!

My emotional well-being was terribly challenged a few months ago, but I think I was able to get through it because of what I've learned from you. I want to thank you very much for all you've done for me and others.

—Miguel P.

Being involved with my study group has established a new dimension in my life, which is I'm a new person. Over the years I do recall you stating that in the order of priority, one's belief system was first and foremost; second, stress management; third, exercise; and diet last. On September 25, 1996, at our first session, you specified that diet represents 15 percent; exercise, 10 percent; stress management, 25 percent; and behavior, 50 percent. This time it was loud and clear—maybe because it was quantified, especially with behavior and stress representing 75 percent of the package.

The tools and techniques that were shared in our biweekly meeting were invaluable because it allowed those of us who went through the exercises to get to know more about ourselves and examine our conditioned minds. Also to see where we have been the source of our own suffering and limitations in our lives. I've never been at such peace with myself as I am now, having a "can do" attitude with what matters to me and what is important to me. Reexamining my beliefs, values, and perceptions has provided tremendous benefits with regard to my interactions with others; where they might attempt to manipulate, control, or induce feelings of guilt it has not worked, and not being a victim to these mind games is very empowering.

The greatest challenges that I encountered during the entire process was to integrate the suggested dietary intake and consistent exercise with my schedule, so the most number of juices I had gotten to was approximately six. My present occupation requires me to be on the road driving to be in and out on various appointments in various areas, so preparing and taking enough of the juices with me during the day was not as consistent as I would have preferred it to be. In spite of it all, the number of sleep hours that I'm able to get by on has reduced to approximately five hours per night. My energy level has never been better and focus with clarity is greater.

I am certainly looking forward to going into the advanced stage of the Reversing Aging Process if you decide to continue, because I know there are greater strides I'll be making with the continuous growth and process in my life.

—Ivon

Changes on the physical level due to the Reversing Aging Study: much less muscle soreness, especially upon waking and also after physical work. Less lower back pain, which has bothered me for years. An increase and leveling of energy throughout the day. Better digestion and quicker transit time culminating in better-formed stools. My skin looks better, eyes clearer. I didn't consider myself overweight, but my set point went from 192 to 186 pounds, and I am physically stronger. Faster hair growth, a bit more hair on legs. If I do get a rare cold it is of short duration (one to three days). I feel comfortable with less chiropractic adjustments. Very little of the old, lingering lethargy after rising in the morning. A marked diminishment of allergic reactions.

On the emotional and mental level: an improvement in mental alertness. My mind feels stronger, more new ideas. Fewer periods of brain fog. An improved outlook on life because I am proactive. An improved awareness of stress and its impact on my health. This is an area in which I need to do more work. I have become more aware of my lifelong need for control and its harmful effect on my psyche and physical health.

Answering the questions posed to the support group has effected my relationships in several ways. First with myself: the questions increased my awareness of the fact that many people and events have negatively impacted my life and that I don't have to buy into these agendas. My best course is to honor self first, and this is not selfish. Don't be afraid to say no. Change and growth come with some pain and I have been in a comfort zone. Don't beat up on myself, accept errors. I have more belief in my abilities. I must not only know, I must actualize.

On relationships with others: I have distanced myself from members of my family who are hostile and negative. I have begun to set limits, to say no. It has at times been painful. I am working on letting family members know how I feel about their actions. I realize that my future doesn't lie in my present job. I have been more forthcoming in presenting my views regarding management problems within my company. The value of kindness and caring is clear. Humor and lightness goes far.

—Charles M.

Since starting this program in January, I have had positive changes both physical and mental. Starting with the physical changes, the constant rash I had on my face from lupus has completely cleared up. I have had the rash for the last two-and-a-half years, and I was told the only way to clear it up was with antibiotics. I also suffered from extreme fatigue. I have cut out 1.5 hours of sleeping. Also migraine headaches that I got often have almost been 100 percent eliminated. My concentration level at work has greatly improved, along with a general feeling of overall calmness.

As far as the mental part, this has been my most accomplished detoxing. I have been able to totally eliminate an abusive father and brother from my life. This is the most liberating feeling!! I put up with so much from them for years; now that part of my life is gone forever!

Having dealt with that situation has also opened my eyes to the kinds of relationships I have been in. All my relationships with men have been abusive. I have never been treated with kindness or respect. I will never let anyone treat me that way again. I have learned that I am good and that I am deserving of kindness and love. This is the greatest feeling. I have also reevaluated my friendships. I have eliminated the ones who were users and takers.

I have also uncluttered my household. I have gotten rid of bags and bags of clothing. I have given many knickknack types of junk to an animal group for a garage sale. So many happy and positive things have happened over the last few months, that have changed my life for the better. My life is better now than it has ever been. I am very grateful for this program.

—Laura B.

I have been transformed by the experience of the program. Physical and mental changes have taken place that I did not, could not, anticipate. I have found it easy to stay on the diet and supplement regimen. I have no problem staying away from meat, dairy, and wheat. I eat out in restaurants far less than I did. I enjoy shopping for organic products in health food stores and take pleasure in cooking. My wife has come to enjoy the meals I cook and has taken to shopping for organic produce and groceries in the local health food stores.

My closest friends and family members first were upset with my dietary changes. They had their negative comments about the number of supplements I take. However, I know the benefits of the changes.

With the first two weeks of the program I saw and felt significant changes in my body. I no longer had the bloated feeling in my stomach. My energy level increased. People think I'm eight to ten years younger than I am. I have comments about the radiance of my skin. I lost twenty pounds without dieting! I've packed on five to seven pounds of muscle. My workouts are energy-filled. I lift more weight than ever before. I run three to four miles, three to four times a week. I jump rope for fifteen minutes every day and practice martial arts three times a week. I've added to my evening social schedule during the week and I meditate each day—all on six hours rather than the eight hours of sleep that I used to require.

Emotionally and mentally I have made changes that make me feel like a kid again. I have a positive outlook on life. I see life as filled with endless possibilities. I have begun to explore career changes and see myself adding to my professional life. I'd like to become a personal trainer. I began classes in the study of philosophy. I have a sense of calm about me, an inner peace without anxiety or preoccupation with the past or future. My relationships with my wife and others have improved. I have learned to accept others without the need to change them. I have eliminated toxic people and activity from my life. I want to share this with others. However, I will never impose my "way" on them. I have become a better human being and have come to enjoy who I am.

—Nick J.

I am a hepatitis B carrier and I would like to not be infected with this virus anymore, and have more energy. I feel my energy level is more even. I do not have those high and low yo-yo–like energy levels. I also started having mercury fillings removed, which eliminated this frequent hazy feeling I feel in my brain.

I am a person who has problems being consistent and focused. I do get some major goals in my life accomplished, but a lot of others I start, then I stop it. I wanted to learn to be fluent in Spanish and I would start studying, but after a few weeks I would stop, and eight years have passed and I still can't speak Spanish. The reason for this behavior I believe is because I am interested in so many things that when I start something, I would be working at it for awhile when another activity would appear and distract me. I would stop whatever I was doing and be off on a different path. Then when I look back at my life, I realize that I have accomplished very little. Had I concentrated on one thing at a time I would have accomplished more in the same amount of time.

I know my first goal is to heal myself from hepatitis. That means doing what needs to be done listed in the program and obtaining the job that is what I want to do because only then will I feel that I am honoring my life and time. This I feel is an important part of my healing, because the anxiety and guilt that I feel now for not doing what I want affects my healing process.

I see myself a year from now filled with energy and health to live every day able to fulfill my goals. I want to feel that every minute of my life is lived with purpose and direction.

—Junglien C.

At the start of this program, I was feeling very depressed, because I had been struggling with CFIDS for almost ten years. I had been to many physicians (both holistic and conventional) and felt that they were not really dealing with my whole being—just a few body parts such as my thyroid, liver, etc. I would look around me and just feel so lonely and overwhelmed because it seemed like everyone else was enjoying their lives much more than I was. I really felt stuck and rather hopeless.

Physically my body was very depleted. One doctor several years ago told me he didn't know how I made it through the day because I had zero energy in my meridians. I had to force myself to get through each day because I have a husband and two sons. I gave my family all I had and often there was noth-

ing left for me. (I know now that my focus was misdirected.) My hormones were out of balance. My thyroid was not functioning well and my adrenals, lymphatic system, liver, and gastrointestinal systems were all out of balance. I had very bad PMS every month; for almost two weeks out of four I would be achy and bloated. I would go to bed exhausted and wake up just as tired.

Spiritually I didn't feel very connected to the world. I guess I felt that life was passing me by and all I had was this struggle called chronic fatigue. I still volunteered and gave of my time to causes but always wished I could do more.

Mentally I am feeling much more hopeful about my future. I am now convinced that I am a good person and say to myself over and over how proud I am of myself. Even though I feel that I have always been a kind person, I feel that I am even kinder and more giving because I really like, no, love myself. I feel that by saying the affirmations that we were taught I have a much more positive attitude about my abilities. I realize that a big part of my problem has been self-esteem or lack thereof, and now I feel my self-esteem is really blossoming. I feel more confident asking for what I want from other people and am much less shy about talking in public. Another aspect that has improved is that I no longer feel tearful as much as I used to. I know that by feeling stronger mentally I am also helping my immune system to heal.

I have been working hard to detoxify my body and have been faithful about doing the program because I knew it would work. Finally I found someone who understood that I am much greater than the sum of my parts. My gastrointestinal system has improved considerably, e.g., I am no longer bleeding rectally and have much fewer episodes of diarrhea. My PMS is down to a day or two as opposed to two weeks of agony. I can get through more days now without the overwhelming need to take a nap in the middle of the day. I have been exercising for about twenty minutes, five to six days a week, and feel a definite improvement in my stamina. My body feels more toned and my muscles feel much stronger. I recently learned that I have the beginnings of osteoporosis and I am also working with a holistic gynecologist to build up my bones.

I have taken a deeper interest in my religion and have felt very comforted by being a part of a group. I have been seeking out people to help who are suffering and have given them information about natural forms of healing. Recently I gave four friends information about how to prepare for and recover from the various surgeries they were undergoing using nutritional protocols. They all seemed grateful for my help, and it made me feel very satisfied. I find that I really enjoy helping people.

The greatest obstacle that I had to overcome was not believing that I was *worth the time to invest in changing my life and healing my problem. At first it was hard to physically get myself to the bimonthly meetings, but once I got there it was always worth the effort. It seemed like an expensive proposition in buying all the supplements, but I changed my priorities and decided that it would be worth all the expense, and I realize it has been. My family, especially my children, did not like all the changes I was making in the food I was buying, but I did it anyway. Now my boys are beginning to respect what I am trying to do because they see that I'm feeling better. I see myself as becoming a happy person totally. I feel very focused as to my goal in improving every part of my life.*

One of my biggest goals for the future is finding my passion in life, and hopefully finding employment in that field. I feel now that I have the tools necessary to achieve this. Another goal of mine is to totally overcome CFIDS, and actually be healthier than people around me who have no so-called illnesses. I thank the program so much for putting all the necessary components into this study group.

—Iris S.

Where do I begin to convey to you how listening to you and being part of the study group has changed my life? It hasn't been easy, and I haven't done it perfectly, but I'm not going to be hard on myself. I've actually done really well, even if I've had my slipups. I've lost about twelve pounds and gone down about two or three clothing sizes. I've never felt better. When I really stick to it, I feel the best. The juicing has probably been the best thing that I've incorporated into my daily life. What a difference that has made. I feel more energetic and can get by on less sleep, so I have more of my day to be productive. Just that alone is a major coup!

The first thing I noticed, and probably most important to me, was not having any menstrual cramps. My body barely goes through any noticeable changes, and it doesn't distrupt my life the way it used to. I haven't taken any kind of drug—not so much as an aspirin—since beginning the program eight months ago.

My facial skin has never been better. I don't even get the one or so monthly breakouts that were just commonplace. I have a pretty regular exercise routine, which is great. I've been able to get rid of a lot of "stuff," including clothes that I had no need for that were just taking up my living space. That's an ongoing process.

What I love the most is that people are asking me what changes I've made in my life, and I'm able to share with them what I've been doing. People want to hear this information. Even if they are not ready to make the changes for themselves, they are listening to it and noting what is possible. I'm living proof! I've been talking to people I never thought I would and saying smart things like never before because my confidence level is high.

It just makes sense not to eat any animal products, or even use any kind of animal products. It just makes sense to eat a live diet. Processed foods were—and still are—only being produced to make money. There is nothing good about them. Being healthy is so simple, I can't believe the road I had to travel to figure it out. But I'm grateful I've discovered the answers now; it could have been another thirty-seven years.

I look forward to sharing information with as many people as I can. That is what is most important not to hoard this valuable knowledge, but to get it out there among the masses. It can't be said enough. The world will have to change when people start making changes themselves. For this I thank you and look forward to continuing to listen to you and your ideas.

—Amy O.

In the beginning of the program, I felt that I was in a bad state of mind. I felt limited by the hepatitis that I have. Now I don't care about the disease I have in my body. I don't seem to care about my morality as much. I understand that the most important thing is my attitude. If I keep a positive attitude, I know things will be all right. To be aware of myself and the things around me is the only thing that counts. To understand that to have compassion for myself is to have compassion for others and vice versa.

Hepatitis was my physical challenge at the beginning of this program. Now the challenge is me and how I can change to be a better person. I guess this is what my challenge has been all along.

—Joel K.

I have gained awareness that I used to be fearful with other people in interactions with them. In the same context, I had a strong need to be approved of, loved and admired. Now, I no longer fear others and I realize that I do not need love from others. I realize I can, through my own personal positive achieve-

ments, manufacture my love for myself, and I have been doing these things—
and I feel so very, very comfortable in the presence of all others, and I just am.

A number of different people say that I look very well. I feel very well
generally. I believe my stamina has increased, and I am starting to do some
strength exercises for my upper body.

—Murray G.

Since beginning this program, for the first time in my life I am able to see
myself as a loving, beautiful, complete, whole person, and I see all of these
things in myself. I accept myself and I'm making choices because I want to
make them. I'm enjoying myself, and exploring all the things I've always
wanted to do without fear.

I have decided to have closure in all my unfinished business. I've registered
to go back to school, and I'm excited about doing that. It's taken me so long.
All of a sudden, I have a list of things I want to do, and I'm taking one step at
a time. I see myself starting projects—helping children, counseling, and sharing all I know about the changes I have made in my life. I see myself challenging me to run the marathon.

I see myself making a transition from living in New York to another space.

I have uncluttered my life, and I continue to do so. I need less and less
accumulation of stuff.

Physically, I feel lighter; emotionally, I love myself more and more. I see
myself being self-sufficient about the work I want to do—starting an organic
cleaning business, learning massage therapy, and doing holistic counseling are
the goals I'm focused on for the next five years.

I look younger, more energetic. When I started the study, I didn't exercise
enough. I was about ten pounds overweight and had no energy by the middle
of the day. I had acne on my cheeks and forehead and my skin wasn't healthy
at all. By the end of the study, I did the Avon 5k Run and felt wonderful. This
propelled me to join the New York Road Runners Club and run in competitions.
My skin looks wonderful, and friends and family have commented on how
great I look.

I never had a problem changing my diet. My issue was the mental/emo-
tional challenge and realizing at this time in my life I'm actualizing my goals
and living without stress and negativity, and that cocreating my life is something that is so easy to do. I feel blessed that I'm doing it, negotiating with
myself and accomplishing the daily goals I'm setting for myself.

I have turned my life around from one of mediocracy to one of purpose and fun.

—Lindsay P.-T.

Throughout the course of this protocol, many changes have taken place for me. Answering the questions consistently has created a shift in behavior patterns that, while not entirely assimilated, I surrender to what is an ongoing process in the future. Gary, you said that the class would be determined through natural selection, and the reasons I am in it thus far are that my choices come from an idea you stated at the beginning: honoring our happiness. I have learned to be completely true to myself and, slowly but surely, my life is beginning to be organized around this principle.

Interestingly, serving the happiness is the constant, while every circumstance, condition, and choice is always changing and the challenge I find now is in not being so affected by their good or bad outcomes. So, the future is entirely shifting by what I determine now, from eating habits to eliminating past-based destructive ways of being that would otherwise sabotage choices.

The paradigm, as you have created it, is a future that can alter the quality of life on this planet for all our world family, as it embraces life itself versus the old world paradigm that destroys life. I see with new eyes that were strengthened from the inside out, while my heart is filled with gratitude from what has been revealed to me.

Specific measurable results of my participation in this study:

A. PHYSICALLY:

A ten-year complaint of chronic cysts on ovaries during PMS and menstruation. Prior to starting the protocol, a medical doctor recommended surgery to remove them and wanted to prescribe birth control pills to reduce inflammation. This pain inhibited movement and desire to exercise, as well as creating excruciating difficulty with bowel movements. Within three months of protocol, all symptoms disappeared and the problem became entirely nonexistent.

Years of inability to sleep—I could go days without needing rest—I discovered I had a thyroid condition that could cause a premature heart attack, as well as outward symptoms of bulging eyes; nervous disposition; easily angered over the slightest issues; cravings for sugar that were out of control. Since the protocol, I desire sleep at a regular hour and rise without an alarm clock at exactly six to seven hours from sleep time. The bulging is greatly reduced and seems gone, and my disposition is so excited about life and much more peace-ful. (I am able to control the level of excitement also.)

Chronic soreness in the throat area, with swollen glands every few months it seemed, has disappeared since I began the protocol. I only experience that familiar lump-in-the-throat feeling when I don't say what I really wanted to say to someone.

Breathing difficulties from secondhand smoke inhalation, from apartment neighbors. I often had painful breathing and shortness of breath. Since the protocol I breathe with no discomfort or pain or any kind. I have doubled my capacity for breath, which is evident when I sing, because my phrasing is be-yond belief in length and ability, compared to what it used to be. I have made unreasonable requests of management that I was afraid to before starting, and now have gained progress and cooperation to limit smokers to their rooms only. (They had been smoking in hallways, elevators, and stairwells.)

My skin has gone through major shifts and continues to as I experience this protocol. When I began, it was rough and dry, with no blemishes except during menstruation. Now it is like silk and blemishes are slight at the time of menstruation.

Cravings for foods completely ran my life. At times I felt helpless to their destructive ways. Gradually, with the protocol, my willpower became some-thing I never knew existed that now makes choices from what honors my life.

The sugar cravings are not completely shifted, as I still desire sweets at the onset of my menstrual cycle. (As children, we ate nothing but candy in our household from morning to night—the worst kinds—as we did not like the diet of canned foods and instant potatoes with meat our dad offered.) Now I no longer eat what in my past was okay. Sugar is now replaced with fruit or fruit-sweetened products or barley-rice sweeteners. This is forever shifting. Neither do I desire to eat dairy foods, whereas in the past I ate cheese or yogurt every other day.

I look and feel fifteen years younger.

B. MENTALLY:

Before the protocol, I was often lethargic, in attitude and spirit. I was run by negativity and resignation. Nothing seemed to go my way and probably never would. I lacked an ability to focus and think clearly. I was a big reaction machine. Poor you if you crossed my path on a PMS day or you fooled me. My anger ran me. It kept relationships with men nonexistent, and friends at a distance. Everyone was out to get me, or so I thought. I swam and sang, despite this lack of luster in me. It was all just a superficial experience of life and happiness. The rut I kept digging got bigger and bigger.

In the beginning of the program, I became increasingly self-aware, to the point of embarrassment that I was ever that rude or hostile to someone. It is so easy to apologize and admit my wrongs immediately. I take notice when an old habit wants to engulf me, and I discipline myself to take the other direction completely—whether it be to table a disagreement or choose a food that honors me.

I wake up with a jolt of joy and I sleep from exhaustion. I am noticing that I am pretty reliably happy most of the time, and, in the face of challenge, a newfound resilience takes over, and I know I can handle it. I am further from giving up than I could have been a year and a half ago.

Gratefully yours.

—Juliet H.

Being on the protocol has helped me physically and mentally. My yearlong bouts with allergies have ended. I no longer suffer from seasonal attacks of hayfever brought on by pollen, ragweed, and other allergens. The flu and colds I got with every change of season have also diappeared. Numerous aches and pains experienced when bending down, reaching, or lifting are gone. I sleep better, wake on time, and take these functions for granted, where previously they were unpredictable and problematic.

My body has changed considerably, so much so that the list of improvements seems endless to me. But more dramatic has been my change of mind. I no longer suffer from mind fog. My concentration does not lag when listening to someone speak or while reading, and my writing has improved. Since all three are inextricably linked, the change has been hard to believe.

I now feel I'm more tolerant and understanding of those I choose to be with. I am able to stand outside myself, seeming to witness changes in behavior and attitude I was not aware of previously. My social skills are such that I no longer see unexplained behavior as threatening or strange.

This did not happen overnight, nor did it happen solely because of the diet, the juices, or even the exercises. It happened because both phases of diet and exercise complemented the classes taken and meetings held to clear up questions and problems that occurred during different phases of the program.

It was during these meetings that I began to change former concepts of self. Questions were handed out to take home and think about. A lot of thought had to occur before they made sense, and any attempt to answer or even understand them was futile if you—I—did not think hard. These ques-

tions dealt with the existence of who you were, or who you thought you were, challenging not only conscious beliefs but ones held without being aware of them. Initially, thought brought on resistance, but the more I grappled with the questions, the more meaningful my responses. They forced in me an openness of mind that could no longer cling to the shakey precipice of the easy reply.

What has followed has been a profound sense of why and how I dealt with the world around me and where I could obtain some of the answers.

—Norman P.

In February 1997, I had brain surgery due to a tuberculum sellaw meningioma. The tumor wrapped itself around my pituitary gland, destroying my optic nerve. I am blind in the right eye and have limited vision in the left. My thyroid gland is not producing its hormone (hypothyroidism).

I started on the protocol in September—eight months after having a craniotomy—twenty hours of surgery—with complications that had me in intensive care for three days. (I did not have the strength to brush my teeth; I was so weak I could not walk.) I joined the Natural Running and Walking Club and, ten months after surgery, I discontinued all the steroids, seizure pills, synthroid, laxatives, antiacids I'd been taking. I had a pill for and to counter complications.

Due to my participating in this program, I no longer talk about my illness. Instead I speak about my new health. I am more positive in my thoughts, behavior, and speech. My medical doctor cannot understand how I have recovered physically, emotionally, and mentally in such a short time. Gary, I am doing great. I am happy. I am legally blind—so what?

—Frank E.

I have a psychiatric history that spans more than thirty years and includes five hospitalizations. The first lasted for ten months, and subsequent hospitalizations ran from two weeks to one month. I have been on psychiatric medications for most of this time.

I have a goiter and an inflamed thyroid from lithium and mild tardive dyskinesia from Stelazine. I often wanted to stop taking medication but was told by my doctors that the standard approach for anyone who has been hospitalized several times is to remain on medication for the rest of his or her life. I did attempt to go off medication several times, but without true support from others, I was not successful.

Last year, before I heard of your study group, I once again pushed to stop medication, but each time I brought up the subject, I was told, "This is not the right time." During the summer, while changing the dial on the radio, I heard you speaking about a meeting that would take place that night to form support groups, one of which would involve individuals with depression. Although I was not very familiar with your ideas, I decided to attend. At that time I was taking Wellbutrin, Stelazine, and lithium. I was just beginning another attempt to stop lithium.

Today I am off all psychiatric drugs. I have been off lithium since July and off Wellbutrin and Stelazine since November. I did this without my psychiatrist's knowledge, and only informed her in January that I entered the new year 1998 free of all psychiatric drugs.

I feel balanced, happy, excited by life. I am less confused and clearer in my thinking, with improved recall. Since November, several crisis situations have occurred, which I have handled well and without undue stress. Most surprising is the return of a range of subtle feelings, which must have been suppressed by all the drugs. I see myself emerging from a pit. Before me I see a horizon that continues to expand. One step leads to the next. Sometimes I may fall, but I am resiliant.

Early in the study, almost immediately, your views and energy touched me in some way that enabled me to gain trust in my own perceptions. It is as though a part of me that had been captive to the psychiatric view that I was "sick" was set free to reclaim my health and to renew confidence in my own experience. I was then able to get off the medications, to explore the questions of each meeting, to write forgiveness letters, to write affirmations, to let go of negative thoughts more often.

I did stray from the diet and had a gangrenous gallbladder removed in March—which may have been partly due to Premarin that I had been taking for five years and have now stopped. I am now back on the diet, and will soon begin exercising again. I am also in the process of ending therapy.

I believe that, in my twenties, had I stayed clear of the psychiatric profession and its drugs and, instead, worked on mental attitude, focus, and goals, I would not have started down the slippery slope leading to greater and greater dependence on medications. I also believe that the experiences that led me to the hospital were valid, spiritual experiences for which I was simply not prepared.

Thank you for a new beginning.

—Patricia F.

It is a privilege to be part of your research program. Since the first week of applying your protocol, I began to experience a series of changes in my life. My vision has improved; I gained energy, and my memory has improved. Now I have better control of my life.

In general, this protocol has helped me to grow physically, emotionally, and spiritually. I hope for more to come!

—Joseph J. L.

When I came into the study, I was not self-assertive. I would keep my opinions, my emotions, my needs inside to avoid conflict and uncomfortable situations. This was because I always felt "less than" or incapable of doing things. In other words, I had no self-confidence.

I failed in college, and my previous image of a gifted, smart student was replaced for many years by a belief that I was no longer special or smart. I decided I couldn't learn anything difficult, so I made this belief come true by not making a 100 percent effort at college. I was afraid to fail; I believed I would fail, and so I failed. This was carried over into all aspects of my life. I adjusted by lowering my expectations—keeping my challenges easily manageable—so that I would not fail.

Every day I replayed past mistakes, situations when I could have acted better, situations that caused me pain or embarrassment, and I would feel bad all over again.

Physically, I had begun to see my metabolism slowing down. Previously, I had no problem maintaining my weight. Now I was gaining weight and looking out of shape. I was beginning to look older than my years.

About five years ago, I noticed my hair thinning. While it is not important to have hair, I believed it to be a sign of ill health. I wanted to be so healthy that I could grow a full head of hair.

Now that I look back, I had smoked for more than half of my life. I could feel the effects of smoking on my body—reduced endurance; clouded thinking; low self-esteem. I had no ambition or high-energy drive.

Since joining the study, I have come to believe that I am both hero and architect of my life. There is no waiting for some magic to happen. I am the magic.

With regard to physical conditions, I have lost twenty pounds and have the best muscle tone in my entire life. I have stopped my hair loss. Bursitis in my right knee is greatly diminished. I can exercise more and exert my knee more than before, I don't have the swelling or discomfort I had before.

I would have afternoon drowsiness and mental fog between 2 and 4 P.M. I do not have that anymore. I am also able to increase my energy levels through simple breathing techniques—and also because I now believe it is possible for me.

I sleep an hour or two less per night. My recovery from infections, colds or flu is amazing. I was able to rid myself of pharyngitis without any antibiotics in less than a week. Flu would have lasted a week. Now—if do feel sick—I am able to knock it out in two and a half days. All of the symptoms are not as great as before.

I am able to exercise longer and with greater ease. Recovery from exercise and exertion is greatly improved, i.e., when I have a heavy workout day, I am not as sore or fatigued the next day. I am able to do several activities in one day and not be exhausted afterward.

—Andrew K.

Thank you for creating this protocol.

The changes I was able to make during this protocol were more marked than any changes I have been able to make in several years. When I followed the protocol closely—September through February:

- *I lost twelve pounds.*
- *I lost several inches from my hips and waist.*
- *My blood pressure dropped to 102/60.*
- *My self-confidence and energy level rose to a new high.*
- *My sense of security, that I could cope with new situations, increased.*
- *I received many comments on my shiny hair.*
- *People commented on how nice my skin was.*
- *I had a more focused, steady sense of energy.*
- *I was less dehydrated.*
- *I didn't get headaches, whereas before I usually got at least one severe headache a month.*
- *Overall, I felt more competent, confident, positive, and clearheaded.*
- *I was able to focus on other goals in my life.*

It is clear that my stated goals continue to be missed, despite all of the "preparing" I had done.

The act of succeeding in your protocol was the biggest step I have taken in years. I had taken your suggestion to join the weight-loss group, conscious of my desire to lose weight but not really aware of how the extra ten or twelve pounds bothered me. When I succeeded in losing twelve pounds, the psychic burden that was lifted seemed more like a hundred. That, in combination with the pointed exercises that we did in the group, raised my self-esteem, to use that trampled word. I felt better and stronger than ever. I had learned to cope with and compensate for the way I look, except for those few extra pounds, so I would always hide myself. My new mode is, "I feel energetic, attractive, and strong."

This was such a palpable improvement for me that I felt like a different person and the people around me really noticed. They saw the physical change immediately, which I thought was funny because, as much as the weight bothered me, it was within the norm enough that I didn't think anyone else would notice. But people especially noticed how I seemed stronger and happier. When I lost my job, it was perfect timing, and I was unfazed.

As is my tendency, the moment I had more energy, I took on more efforts. In the course of this process, I have come to see myself more clearly. I have always been very energetic and enthusiastic, as well as ultrasensitive. As you can see, that combination can make someone vulnerable. I am a person who lives so much in the moment that I have had trouble with gaining perspective or disciplined long-term thinking, although the level of self-discipline I have shown during long periods of my life for artwork and physical training might seem to belie this. I am a typical creative assertive as described by various traits, but mainly dynamic supportive. The main challenges for me have always seemed to be the practical concerns to taking care of myself, food, clothing, shelter, finances. All of this has led me to a new place in this moment, in reference to the protocol and my life. I am able and strong enough to see "doing my artwork" as the organizing principle, and everything can follow from there.

The protocol requires that I commit to a workout routine, which I can usually do for a limited period of time. The protocol is practical and easy, and I had great satisfaction and success with its routine, i.e., I had a job. Now, I must rise to the challenge of making my own routine and making it long-term—a day at a time.

There are other important challenges that face me now that do require courage, as you spoke of the other night, because, as you quoted Henry Emerson Fosdick, "He who chooses the beginning of the road, chooses the place it leads to."

There is one other point that I want to address and that is that I went through the weekly questions in the context of other questions that I have been working on and found they are extremely focusing and practical. They really cut to the heart of the matter and are critical to the age-reversing process. When I missed doing them, I really felt the drag in terms of slow grasping of the entire process of the protocol. The questions are pointed, relevant, essential and practical.

For me, the biggest challenge will be to acknowledge the limitation that I cannot do everything and have the courage and consciousness to choose.

I really appreciate your giving your time to this process. Thank you.

—Elaine R.

Since I began to follow this protocol, I have lost twenty pounds—178 pounds, down from 198—without eating any less food. In fact, I eat more healthy food and burn it off more quickly.

My sleep is now more restful. I sleep more soundly and wake up more alert than before beginning the program.

My hair is growing in a lot faster than before—almost twice as fast, in fact. I am growing new hair in the front of my head, which was bald before, and I had a bald spot on the back of my head but now it is gone.

I suffered with lower back pain into my left buttocks, sciatica with pain so bad I could not walk for two days. This is gone now.

I think more clearly now, and I think good, positive thoughts.

Sexually, I am more alive than ever. My erections last sometimes two hours and I feel more passionate when I make love. It is like I am seventeen all over again. I share more in a physical way with my mate than ever before. Sex is great again, not a chore.

I have more physical energy than I ever had before. My muscular strength has almost doubled. I can lift more weight and work out longer with more strength than ever. I can play and work longer without tiring.

I was an alcoholic for twenty-two years and every cell in my body was toxic. I have overcome my addiction to sugar and food. I am free of that chain now, and eating fresh, organic fruits and vegetables and green juices daily. This has taken away my craving for sugar and has replenished my body. I look forward to each new day with joy and happiness instead of anger, pain, and fear.

—Joe O.

I have learned that I should really watch the things I eat because why would I want to put something harmful into my body? Everything around us has an effect, and it is up to us whether we choose to accept it. I have also learned to take one day at a time and live it to its fullest, and that everyone gives of an energy—some good, some bad, depending on who we are around. We can change this energy, so you don't want to be around people who put themselves down, and you don't want people who feel sorry around because they can have an affect on us.

—Donny R.

From this program I learned to use my energy more efficiently in a positive way—toward God, my family, and all people—to honor life, spirit, mind, and body. I've also learned that power, money, and greed are things that keep you a prisoner in your life. Nourish your body and mind with foods that provide health, not disease.

—John R.

One Sunday morning about a year ago, I woke up, ate breakfast, got dressed, and started to go out. I looked for my car keys but could not find them. I went downstairs to look for my car, and it was missing too. I realized that I had left the keys in the trunk lock and my car had been stolen.

Later I was listing to Gary Null and he mentioned the Reversing the Aging Process group. I knew this was what I had to do. I called up, and luckily there was room for me. I had been juicing for almost a year—not organic. I also was taking supplements. I was ready to begin the protocol. Once I began the program, I started to feel better. I didn't get sore throats in the morning after taking 5000 mg of vitamin C at night.

I decided that I was going to start living like a human being instead of working all the time like I had been doing. I had taken the month of August off and told my toxic baby-sitter I couldn't pay him so much. Shortly after I stopped working, I fell in love, and started going out with a man, for the first time since my divorce eight years earlier.

I was very happy. I was praying to get my car back, and looking for it. One day, I went for a walk and was pulled to go by Our Lady of Mount Carmel

Church. I walked a different way than I would have walked ordinarily and, miraculously, spotted my car. I was so grateful to get it back, and the experience increased my faith in God.

Of course the exercise walk was part of the program.

Now, I am facing the challenge of building a relationship with my boyfriend and creating harmony between us and my wonderful, exuberant son, Sam. I am working less and spending more time with Sam.

I still need to work on my weight and overeating—especially when writing for my job. I am sleeping better now, especially if I exercise a lot. Anemia, which had been a problem, has not gotten worse.

Also, I still need to work on having more respect for myself and deal even better with toxic people in a calm, confident way and give my knowledge effectively to others. I am a work in progress, and I still have a long way to go.

—Virginia R.

At twenty you have the face that God has given you,
At forty you have the face that Life has given you,
and at sixty, you got the face you deserve. . . .

Last year, this time on BAI Radio,
Gary mentioned an orientation and I felt I had to go.

So I showed up with my sidekick and I knew in a flash
He's talking to me to the Big Apple bimonthly I'd dash.

Just sign on the dotted line so we know you commit,
Show up in your sneakers and shorts and don't try to quit.

If you want to be a fox . . .
You're gonna have to detox.

Oy vays uh meer! No more bagels with a shmeer!
As a species we're full of feces.

No dairy, pesticides, caffeine, or wheat,
Your homework will be checked, so don't try to cheat.

I was introduced to aloe Vera, Phil, Sam, Ian and Jill,
All colors, shapes, and sizes—no one's "over the hill."

Since my teens already a vegetarian so I thought I was cool (huh)
Harboring anger and resentment, parasites, and stubborn as a mule.

Whether in lead be Louanne Pennse, George, or Gary
All agreed dispose of old patterns and you don't have to marry.

Seek in yourself, both the solution and cause
And don't react too quickly, but take time to pause.

When we no longer say and do what we feel and know
We limit our Options and counter the natural flow.

Identify and cut loose toxic people in your life
Be it boss, father, mother, neighbor, sister, brother, husband, or wife.

Banish Imbalance and Disharmony and let your love light shine.
Control engaging in meaningless responsibility and "no pearls to swine."

I wanna dance in my magnetic pants.
Where would I be without pycogenol, quercetin and Suprema C?

Having more fun in the buff
Thanks to Red and Green Stuff,

But gotta stay on guard,
Thanks to potent rock hard.

I surrendered my fears,
Shed some tears and took off five years.

It's about dignity of choice
and honoring my inner voice.

Thank you, it's been an honor and privilege to share with this group.
Now it's time to actualize, spread my wings, and fly this coop.

With joy, entitlement, self-esteem, and pride,
Peace, love and Null Trim,
It's been one helluva ride!

—Lisa H.

It comes to me as a complete surprise that I am writing this letter to you. It never occurred to me that I would meet you, or even be a client at your healing center, but life is full of surprises.

I am grateful for this program because I feel it has put me on the right path and I feel fantastic! I have more energy, think clearer, and, best of all *thanks to hypnosis I have stopped smoking—my husband, too. I have also stopped eating meat and feel very good about this accomplishment.*

Within this year, I have done a lot of work on myself, of which this program is a very positive part. I continue to work and make many positive changes.

Thank you for your insight, courage, and unselfish sharing of your knowledge. God bless you!

—Muriel C.

Where to begin? This program has been a life-changing experience, even though I had begun some of the components of the protocol—detoxing and using nutrition—to control my lifelong asthma symptoms for about a year and a half before joining this group. For most of my life, I had relied on pharmaceutical drugs that appeased my symptoms, made the initial problem worse, and severely damaged my immune system.

At the age of twenty-six, I decided to try a more natural approach. My research served me well, and I managed to get off the drugs, but I still had some episodes of breathing difficulty. I was able to control this with herbs and homeopathic remedies, but was disturbed that after all I was doing, this was still happening. Since I started this protocol, I can't even remember the last time I had serious asthma symptoms. I believe the green drinks, not consuming sugar, caffeine (I was truly an addict, convinced that for some people it helped their asthma), or meat, has had a great effect.

However, an even bigger difference is in my mental attitude. Having given up wheat, dairy, and processed foods at the beginning of my search for good health, I felt very deprived. When I was upset, stressed, or otherwise not happy with life, I would eat and eat all those things I knew were bad for me . . . and I would feel good, satisfied. Now my attitude has changed completely. I only want to put into my body things that will really nourish me at a cellular level.

I listen to what my body is saying when it tells me it wants something sweet, and I know now that it needs a little nutrient boost, not a huge slice of chocolate cake. I also take into consideration what is going on emotionally, the power of association, and environment, all of which drive me to eat things that are going to hurt, not heal my body.

Just this past week, I made another breakthrough out of my old thinking pattern. Having had asthma, exercising has already been difficult. My husband had just found a study on exercise-induced asthma and encouraged me to push through the symptoms until the right hormones were released into my body to counteract the wheezing. Well, in our living room, in a very safe way, we tried it, and, lo and behold, it worked! Unbelievable. I have been working out on a Lifecycle every day now for a week and I feel great afterward. I just had to get through that "wall of discomfort."

My husband and I are doing this program together. This has given us an opportunity to really look at what is important to us, where we are going, how we plan to get there, while we are still newlyweds. It has brought us closer together as a family, as we make rather unconventional decisions about the food we eat, how we spend our time and our money on health and ourselves, and just how we journey through the rest of our lives together.

—Diana Y.

It is difficult—indeed, impossible—to say what I gained [during a two-week intensive course at Gary's Florida ranch]. In the process of time, and a deeper internalizing of the Body-Mind-Spirit insights received—these things will become clearer and increasingly real in manifestation. Revelation without manifestation is high-minded soul activity. I want these divine insights to be the bone of my bone and flesh of my flesh I thank you with tears of joy and gratitude (though I "never" cry) for opening this awesome place of beauty and spiritual harmony to those of us who are privileged to come here and make choices.

I saw more things this week and I received just what I came for—but much, much more. I still have a fuzzy, toxic head, but I have focus and motivation and a new sense of who I am, warts and all. I am humbled and delighted by God's ways of revealing ourselves to us. I leave here, reluctantly, with an attitude of gratitude—ready for the next step. I am also leaving with a sense of intuitive awareness that the years to come will be very different and with new consciousness, and the levels of energy revealed that defy our present imaginings. I say yes to whatever my role is in the Divine Awakening. This week has heightened that awareness.

I know now that I am moving toward Divine Health—and that candida is a temporary thing until I learn what it has to teach me.

Again, I thank you and bless you for your gift of self and sharing this holy place.

—Faye Marie L.

I have definitely enjoyed the [anti-aging] protocol. I have lost almost thirty-five pounds. I am not hungry and I feel really strong.

I am much happier and more content with myself and my life in general. I have a positive attitude toward things in general. I have also been gaining more respect from my peers.

—Charlotte

I had symptoms of chronic fatigue syndrome, poor circulation, depression and anxiety. I was sleeping ten to twelve hours a night and was still drowsy during the day. I got sick every few weeks with flulike symptoms.

Now, all of these symptoms are gone. I haven't felt this healthy since I was five!

I have tons of energy during the day. I'm usually in a good mood, and I can do much more because I sleep less.

Friends have asked me to buy "Gary's Green Stuff" for them, and one friend has started on the protocol.

—Maris A.

Since starting with the program last year, I can't begin to imagine my mental outlook and physical ability then and now. To me, the difference is astounding.

Twelve months ago, while starting the program, I felt my first priority was to rid this body of toxins. Many strange things happened, which I shall not enumerate. My physical well-being has improved, but the most wonderful improvement has been my mind-set and intellect.

I have been more humane, open, truthful, and less mean-spirited. One observation: truth has its drawbacks. It is amazing how few people appreciate hearing the truth. They want to be placated, stroked, whether it is the truth or not. Still I will not be as I was.

It is fun to realize that the brain has also become detoxified. The interplay between mind and body is happening to me, although the mind seems to be ahead of the body.

Thank you to the support group and its leaders, Louanne Pennse, and yourself.

—Lorraine V. P.

Weight loss was the first thing I noticed after beginning the program. I lost fifteen pounds and I have been able to keep it off in the time since I completed the program. I am also starting to build muscle from working out three times a week. My self-esteem is higher; I am more confident, and I am no longer intimidated by doctors. I am also motivated to try new things, such as studying a third language and taking dance lessons. I play soccer once a week; I've stopped listening to commercial radio; I don't watch much TV anymore, and I've gotten into reading. When I'm working, I listen to books on tape. Last month I ran a five-mile race. A year ago, I wouldn't consider doing any of it. I worry less; I don't let things get to me. I enjoy my running and walking. I've weeded out all toxic relationships, and finally, I've noticed that I don't get sick as often as I used to and, if I do, it doesn't last as long.

—Dimitrios R.

Participating in Gary Null's anti-aging program has improved my health physically and emotionally. After eliminating dairy foods, sugar, and fried foods from my diet—I was already a vegetarian—my allergies improved and I had fewer colds and better elimination.

I also have had more energy and some weight loss.

The behavior modification aspect of the program has taught me to be more assertive and confident. I am closer to achieving my goals.

—Andrea B.

I had been in a support group for six months. My weight had stabilized and I was getting discouraged. Rather than taking my old path of sabotaging the progress I had made by returning to old ways, I decided to visit Paradise Gardens for a week.

I thought my goal was to lose more weight; however, attending the seminars, watching tapes, and attending your talks made me realize that was a limited goal. If I truly committed to the process unfolding before me, I would have the opportunity to start on the road of being a whole person. The pain of the fragmented, unconscious life I had led was overwhelming, and I now know that the process started in this short week will make the difference between a life lived on the side of mere existance and one which will be lived to its fullest at a high-energy level.

I liked being challenged. Walking six miles to start and increasing the amount every day was something I didn't think I could do, so I stopped thinking and turned the walks into a meditation. I had not thought of this approach before and it has helped me to go farther.

I expect I've never done anything more important in my life.

—Carol N.

Before I began this program, I was stuck in a job I disliked. I was unable to produce anything creative. I am now in the process of getting out of this job—I've already handed in my resignation—and I have made plans to reactivate my creative side.

Before I began the program, I had arthritis that made it impossible for me to walk from time to time. I have no more arthritic pains. The fungus on my right heel disappeared. My hair, which was thinning, is showing accelerated growth. I have practically no ridges on my fingernails and my energy level is up considerably.

Spiritually, I view the future as a good place. My buttons can't be pushed anymore.

I can't give you a straightforward account of the obstacles I have overcome, because I do almost everything in an almost somnambulistic, intuitive way. I do have more inspiring dreams than I used to have, and therefore follow a path that is leading me somewhere, but not in that concrete way.

When I compare myself now to the way I was a year and a half ago, it is that I moved away from fears and doubt toward hope and optimism, and in some respects, my life has taken on a more constructive form.

All your questions gave me an opportunity to deal with issues directly—not my inclination—and therefore, just by thinking of an answer, my life has become redirected and rechanneled.

—Beatrice T.

Many family and friends were surprised to find out I had joined a "detox group." They thought I was already taking very good care of my health and, relative to most people, I was. But I knew there was plenty of room for improvement.

In the eight months since I began this [anti-aging] program, changes are:

- *Physically: I sleep an average of an hour to an hour and a half to two hours less per night and have tons more energy. I am raring to go each morning. I've lost twenty pounds, my skin is smoother, my hair shinier, and my nails stronger. I'm much stronger, with more muscle tone from lots of exercise (power walking, cycling, and Nautilus with some yoga).*
- *Mentally: I have a better perspective overall, am more appreciative, and stop to smell the roses more often.*
- *Work: I am managing two hectic businesses and four employees more calmly and enjoying it. I have lots of ideas of other ventures and I am researching and pursuing some of them, including a book project with a friend that should be fun and will ultimately help people.*
- *Play: I'm taking more time out. It's difficult, but possible, and I'm making it a priority. Also making sure I have plenty of reasons to laugh each day. I love doing things spur of the moment, so I'm ready for action as often as humanly possible.*
- *Relationships: I'm focusing on nontoxic people, detaching with love from the others. I'm finding that many people, including family, friends, and strangers, want to know more about what has me looking, feeling, and acting younger. I find it very gratifying to share what I'm learning.*

—Susan M.

Because of a bladder problem, which had practically taken over my life, I was very limited in my activities. I couldn't make any plans without knowing where the nearest bathroom was in advance. If I walked, it was in a large circle, always leading back to the house within a half hour or so.

With that improving [since beginning to follow the protocol] I can actually visualize a marathon for me in the not-so-distant future, since I expect to continue on this path. I really feel reborn. I think that was actually my biggest hurdle.

I can now travel again, which I had always loved to do and couldn't because it had become such a hassle. I can visit my daughter who lives in California who I seldom see because of constraints on her time at her job and with school.

I was unable to sit through a complete movie without missing the middle or the ending, so I had stopped going. I will again be able to go to museums, musicals and plays, and go to the opera without hopping over people.

I have more energy now and seem to do with less sleep. I start to sing while I'm doing the dishes. Sometimes I don't realize I'm singing until I hear myself. It just comes out, spontaneously, and then I laugh at myself. That's another thing I'm able to do easily—laugh at myself. I don't take myself so seriously as I used to. I was always very sensitive and easily hurt, so I would not stand up for myself to anyone. Now I say what is on my mind. I do challenge people if I feel I am right. That's a big step for me, and a release.

I had feelings of low self-worth, having grown up with criticism and seldom being able to do anything right. Then, when I married, it was just reinforced, and I continued on a downward spiral; that is, until I said, "Enough." I not only turned myself around, but my husband also changed. He is very careful of the things he says and does now, so as not to hurt my feelings— which he admits did not come easily for him.

Uncluttering is an ongoing process. Every day I look to see what I can get rid of. I feel lighter and have opened up some valuable space that was needed. I look forward to doing more of it.

—Mildred L.

I came into the program thinking this would be a good physical change for me. The physical has been the least of the blessings of the program.

That's not to say I haven't noticed any physical changes. I was a confirmed "junk-food junkie": fast-food restaurants, greasy fries and hot dogs, chocolate bars and ice cream. Interestingly, the easiest part of the diet has been the absence of meat. It has become quite a creative and rewarding experience for me to figure out my weekly vegetarian menu. The most difficult thing has been staying away from sugar. That's my everyday challenge.

The first change I saw was very quick. Every autumn, since I was a child, I would develop a terrible bronchial cough. Recently, doctors were treating it like a form of asthma. This cough usually lasted between one and three months. Three days after I started this program, the cough was gone. I attribute this to the absence of dairy foods from my diet.

Other physical benefits: I am only sleeping four and a half to five and a half hours per night and I am rarely tired during the day. Also, a few of my associates says my skin "looks better."

I think the program has become a springboard for me at this time— mentally and physically and even spiritually. It has also been a continual source of discussion, both supportive and adverse. Many, like my father, are amazed I have stuck it out as long as I have. Some, like my mother-in-law, seem to ignore it and insist I eat her store-bought chicken. Many simply don't under-stand this at all, and that too is a great motivator for me to stay with the program.

—Paul A.

My week here [at Paradise Gardens] was both the shortest and longest of my life. Short, because I hated to leave. Long because I have rarely, in my 64½ years, found so much tranquility. Thanks to your teachings I have determined to make a beginning in changing my life. I cannot do it at the pace you suggest, but for my life energy typing, it's a start.

—Bernie P.

For someone with a history of chronic fatigue, committing to a time allotment twice a week to commute to the city was a challenge to me at the start of this program. I also had to adjust to how my family reacted to my lifestyle changes, and I had to get accustomed to the changes in my diet. Physically, the exercise regimen took some getting used to.

I have learned to have a more positive outlook on life, regardless of any negative events that have happened or that will happen. I have learned to control my temper and not make any decisions if I am in an angry state of mind. I will also admit if I make a mistake, even if I risk embarrassment.

I spend more time with my children and am able to remain patient with them, even if they are whining or nagging. I find that I am more courteous on the road, which is important since I spend ten hours a day driving. I know that my positive attitude will lead to total well-being.

Since I began the program, my skin condition [eczema] has improved and my energy seems to be longer-lasting. My senses of taste and smell are im-proved, so that now I desire less sweet and less salty foods. It seems that I have less gray or white hair than before, and I have fewer body aches, and my vision has improved slightly.

Spiritually, I am more willing to help others, even if it inconveniences me. I am also eager to pass on any information that I have learned, if I feel it might benefit the person in need.

I know that respecting others' views and opinions without condemning them is an important part of life. Striving to live guilt-free will open up my mind to new learning experiences.

At first, dealing with my wife's extremely skeptical view of my participating in this study group was hard to overcome. . . . Being that I had adjusted my diet two years prior to joining the study, it hasn't been too hard to work in the few additional changes. Elimination of wheat and sugar was probably the hardest to overcome, but I have kept them out of my diet. My wife is learning how to cook according to my new diet. She is creating some great-tasting dishes. . . .

I feel my health is at about 60 percent now, and I see myself as being closer to 100 percent in a year or less, since I will continue to have a steady desire to do whatever it takes.

—Lou L.

The biggest change I have experienced since beginning this program has come through focus and eliminating toxic people from my life; for being able to say no without feeling guilty. My body requires less sleep, and my elimination is regular.

I have also learned so much more about healing the human body through detoxification. I am truly grateful for this lesson in healing.

—Mutaba H.

Since the beginning of my participation in this program, the following has occurred: increased mental clarity; a better sense of overall calm and relaxation; a much-improved outlook on life; an even broader sense of consciousness and self; less crankiness; less fatigue; improved recall and memory; a much-improved ability to cope with stress; faster and more graceful movement; an improved feeling of mental clarity; overall improvements in my level of energy; clearer skin; clearer nasal passages; less excess mucous; improved resting heart rate; decrease in the amount of sleep needed for rejuvenation; improved workout recovery times; a noticeable increase in lean muscle tissue; improved bowel movements, which are also more regular; less sluggishness; more patience, and a decrease in my tonsil size.

No longer do I have dark shadows under my eyes. There is significant decrease in pain from peripheral neuropathy in both legs and an extremely remarkable decrease in arthritis pain, both resulting from multiple trauma suffered July 7, 1997. The surgeon who operated on my crushed right calcaneus stated that posttraumatic arthritis was inevitable and that I may have to con sider fusion in the future. I haven't gotten sick since I began the program—and that's without a spleen.

I can't thank you enough for the knowledge you've bestowed upon me in any other way than to continue to actualize it. Forever I shall be grateful.

—Patrick H.

Six years ago, I came to a very serious crossroads in my life. I was nutritionally deficient, physically ill, and fatigued—with all the symptoms of Lyme disease—and I had a rotten attitude. After being introduced to Gary's ideas regarding health and fitness, I gradually began to experiment with his concepts and found that I did improve. I learned that I had to take responsibility for myself in every regard and not depend on others to take care of me.

I don't just hand myself over to the professionals anymore, whether it's my physicians or my auto mechanic. I discuss the problem with them and I take the responsibility of making all the final decisions based on my readings and, to a lesser degree, their advice.

I'm feeling much better since I began this journey six years ago and I plan to continue to improve. I'm not looking for shortcuts. I realize I'm in it for the long haul.

—Philip G.

[Since beginning this anti-aging protocol] the cracking in my knuckles from arthritis is gone. My gums, which looked like raw meat for almost four years, are completely healed. My vision has improved somewhat. There definitely is a threshold.

I have an improved relationship with my father, and have gotten rid of some very toxic people—which has made my life much easier. But I have more to go.

I have much more energy. Before, I fell asleep at my desk almost every afternoon.

At some point, a few months after I started the program, I started to feel like I did many years ago, when I was really young. I am much happier. I used to be hungry all the time, really all the time. Now I can go without eating for a long, long time. I'm hardly hungry, even when I sit down to eat. But I eat.

I lost a lot of weight—close to thirty pounds—without effort, and I feel real good about that. I can move about with much more ease. I am very glad all that extra weight is gone.

I am more conscious of my spiritual being. I realize that my spiritual needs have to be taken seriously. I have started to read the Bible again. I pay closer attention to what I am doing and try to be in the present, whatever I am doing. I do the activities for the sake of doing and do not look for rewards or approval. I only look for a happier life. I truly believe that to take care of your spiritual needs first is most important, and everything else will fall into place.

My spiritual and physical being are now at a better level. I am now closer to where I want to be. Thank you very much for your help!

—Sigrid G. E.

Stress is the primary factor in the weight/hypertension problems that prompted me to join the study group.

Through adherence to the protocol, the regenerative powers of my system were tapped. My hair, skin, nails, and overall health improved. A serious problem with heavy menses and anemia, which led to a life-threatening situation, has been alleviated. Although I haven't reached my target weight or controlled my hypertension, I'll regroup and pursue the regimen in a more diligent manner.

This is a life-sustaining protocol. Learning to own my experiences has set me on the path to wellness. Thanks, Gary.

—Trelline G.

Prior to joining Gary's study, I knew that I had some issues, but never realized how serious they really were and how much of an impact they had on my life. The reason I didn't recognize this was because I was too afraid to reach down and examine muself to see it.

I grew up feeling that I was never good enough. I never fit in anywhere and was always the person the class bully beat up. Not having any self-worth or confidence, I became a crowd pleaser. I became whatever anyone wanted me to be just to gain some sort of acceptance. This went on all of my childhood and most of my adult life until I went to Gary's ranch in Florida and started this program, which I have continued since returning home.

This is the area where I made the greatest changes in my life. I look at life from a new perspective, just like I'm starting over again at forty-four!

I was thirty to forty pounds overweight. My blood pressure was 180/110, and my cholesterol was over 290. I drank eighteen cups of coffee a day, never realizing that it was a drug, and I thought Dr. Atkin's high-protein, all-red-meat diet was the answer. Now, my blood pressure is 110/80, a reduction that came without use of drugs. My cholesterol is 240, and I have lost approximately eighteen pounds (after only four months) and would like to lose another eighteen. I no longer use any products with caffeine or sugar. I drink no sodas and eat no red meat. I have reduced my dairy consumption by more than 80 percent and have become a vegetarian—with the occasional exception of fish and chicken.

I feel 100 percent better, and mornings are no longer a problem for me.

I have also started a training program and was accepted to run the New York City Marathon.

—Gary M.

Since I started this program, my health has improved and my emotional wellness is getting along. I have smoother skin and more energy. I gained ten pounds—before, I was underweight. I can lift weights more intensely and my recovery is faster. When I wake up in the morning, I feel clearheaded.

The support group questions have helped me to let go of the past and the people whom I resented. I no longer feel angry and don't waste time brooding over that. I catch myself in the middle of negative thoughts and think of something more helpful instead.

I've let go of the people who don't accept me for who I am. Creating new relationships is still a challenge for me, bring a creative, assertive type, but I'm hopeful. I'm trying to have more fun, to laugh more.

These are the most notable changes . . . so far. Thank you very much for your guidance.

—O. L.

I will say that this program has made me look and feel wonderful. I have unbelievable energy now. I need much less sleep—two hours less a night—and feel better than I did with a full eight hours before I started the protocol. My mind is much clearer and focused. I have always exercised, but now my body is much leaner and my muscles are more defined.

How have I changed physically? My body is much more sensitive now. I can feel the difference when I don't take care of it—miss exercise, eat the wrong foods, or tax it with stress.

I feel the extra energy I have from not overeating and keeping myself clean. I don't get any pains. I was never sickly, but sometimes I might get an ache here or there. Now, I never have anything like that. I always feel great!

I still crave sweets, but now I'm not addicted. I have the willpower to do what is right for myself. Even if I do cheat, it's only eating organic peanut butter and raw honey on organic breads, or unsweetened carob-covered almonds—not anything that is bad for my body.

The biggest change mentally is that I believe in myself more. I look out for my well-being now, and I am learning to say no to people and situations that I should say no to. I am learning how to focus myself and stay unstressed. Sometimes I still become overwhelmed, but now I can calm myself down much easier.

I do not kill myself working now. I know I am human and that I can only do what I am capable of doing. I let the people I do work for know this.

I am making as much time as I can for play. Instead of saying I want to do something or travel somewhere someday, I am planning and doing those things now.

—Marcia D.

Three months before I joined the study I was diagnosed with a melanoma in my right eye. I am legally blind in my left eye, so I was terrified. I was told that it was not small, but not large. My treatment options included removing the eye, radiation—which would leave me blind within five years. Only by probing did I find out that I had the option of doing nothing. The doctor told me that I could "watch it"—but if the cancer grew, it would spread to my liver and I would be dead within a year.

I decided not to just watch it, but instead to do something to be rid of it, or never let it grow.

The first mental challenge was dealing with the authorities. The words of traditional medical doctors were very powerful. The words of Gary Null were also powerful. I needed to become my own authority.

I was also overweight and not taking care of my body. I knew that I was eating poorly. I knew that the cancer was a wakeup call that literally held a gun to my head. I also had migraine headaches, chronic lower back problems, prostate problems, rotator cuff problems in my right shoulder, and arthritis in my right big toe.

Since beginning the protocol, the melanoma has not grown for eight months. The migraines virtually disappeared about two months after changing my diet. I lost thirty-five pounds, and my back problem has shown marked improvement.

Before I began the program, I took a product made of saw palmetto and other herbs for my prostate problems, but it didn't help. Now it works. My body is receptive to healing.

My shoulder is about the same—a minor problem—and my toe is slightly better.

Overall, I just feel better. My energy level varies, but on the whole I am much more energetic, and feel I have a younger body that knows how to heal itself.

—Eugene N.

In the course of the study, I have eliminated dairy, flour, processed food, etc. I have identified and eliminated food allergies. In addition, I've learned and felt the benefits of eating a healthy diet.

I have wonderful skin, and I no longer have colds or sinus problems, which plagued me most of my life. I have more energy, and I no longer experience painful menstrual cramps.

I am able to feel my body processes working. I listen to my body—I never did that before. If I feel any major changes, I am able to identify what the cause was, i.e., sinus headache—I ate something that I was allergic to.

—Nevea V.

My intention [when I started the study group] was to get healthy, to get some energy and gain a feeling of self-motivation back in my life. Well, it happened. I started to let go of things in my life like: I cleaned out my basement. This was a big thing for me, since I had not touched it in fifteen years—I just threw everything away.

I noticed that I was arguing less and less with my wife. I bought her a copy of your book Who Are You Really? *It helped.*

As far as my health is concerned, my energy came back. I started to feel good. My skin became younger-looking, and I began to look at the world differently. Other things started to change also. When I was eighteen years old, as a soccer player, I was kicked on the back of my left leg. That injury turned into varicose veins. Seven months into the protocol, the varicose veins started to shrink. They are now half the size of what they used to be. That is unbelievable. I now need only six or seven hours of sleep a night.

I would say that I have stuck with the protocol 90 percent. Gary, I would love to go to the next level with you. My life is different; my children's lives are different; my wife's life is different. Things are going great, thanks to you.

—Tom G.

I would like to begin by saying thank you for having been the catalyst that is leading to many positive and exciting things in my life. As a result of being in this group, I have seen some specific changes in my physical health and have also developed a far greater awareness of the joy and love in my life and my relationships.

I will start by telling you about the physical changes. I have had two problems that I wanted to try to address differently, since traditional methods were not working. For one, I suffered from headaches for what seems like years. Sometimes, they were just bothersome tension-type headaches, and sometimes they were migraines, close to debilitating.

Since joining the group [eight months earlier] I have been eating a primarily vegetarian diet—including fish; have eliminated caffeine, and, to a large extent, refined sugar; have exercised, and have basically followed the protocol laid out for us. I am happy to be able to say that the frequent tension headaches just don't seem to occur anymore. What this means for me is that I have no need for the Tylenol or ibuprofen that I took regularly—probably on an average of four pills a day for any number of years. The next thing I hope to conquer is the migraines.

I also have had a problem with cold sores. I had an episode a few years ago in which the virus appeared in one of my eyes. Fortunately, my vision wasn't affected, but I did have the cornea scraped, which was a frightening experience.

Since being in the study group and making the nutritional changes, the episodes and severity of cold sores have slowed down, and I have been able to stop taking the antibiotic that was originally recommended. I want to continue working to eliminate them altogether, however.

As I think about the rest of my life to date, I know that I have been very fortunate. I am basically an optimistic person and feel loved and respected in my relationships—this includes in my professional role as well as in my relationship with my husband, our five children, and close friends. I also know that I am effective at what I do. I am an intelligent, supportive woman and have a natural desire to learn new things. And having been in the group has introduced me to many new things that I want to explore. For example, I have enrolled in a fascinating course called *Mind Body Health*, in which I am learning how to practice mindfulness meditation. I am also studying T'ai Chi as a result of having learned about it in our group. But having read Who Are You Really? was probably the most exhilarating experience of all. To be able to understand my own energies and those of the people around me has given me far greater insight and understanding and almost a sense of power or, perhaps better said, empowerment.

—Natalie K.

How have I changed since I began the program six months ago?

- I now exercise six days a week. When I first started walking, it took me thirty minutes to walk a mile. Now I walk a fifteen- to sixteen-minute mile!
- I've lost more than sixty pounds.
- I have eliminated two toxic people in my life.
- I sleep less and better.
- My skin has cleared up.
- I have better bladder control.
- I don't talk on the phone at night anymore, giving me much more free time. Now I do yoga one night and meditate every night.
- I don't gossip or listen to gossip, and I don't engage in negative conversations.
- I am happier.
- I feel joy.
- I am a better healer, a better doctor, a better human being.

With my mental and physical improvement, my patient numbers have increased because of my attitude, and because I am physically stronger, I can see more patients.

Life is good.

—Stacey T.

Before joining the study, I was continually challenged with chronic fatigue. Every day I would be troubled by low energy and other physical symptoms. My adrenal glands were underactive and I was almost constantly under stress. I had hypoglycemia and felt a gnawing hunger until the evening. I was too tired to exercise. I had allergies and sensitivities to many foods and chemicals, and had repeated bouts of sinus infections. My thyroid function was low. I was cold and tired, and I had trouble at night, occasionally waking and not being able to fall asleep again for many hours.

Now I have more energy. Yes! I knew I could, since I had had short episodes of high energy before. I haven't had a sinus infection in ages. I feel a sense of physical integration that I attribute to many things, but especially to T'ai Chi and Chi Gong exercises. My hypoglycemia is practically gone. I don't feel stressed out to the point of being wasted mentally and physically. I wake up earlier and more alert than before.

I trust my body to heal itself. I got rid of my prescription medications.

. . . I see myself as integrating my life more and more in the future, and combining my work with my friends. I feel that keeping healthy, in every way, is not just a personal priority, but it helps in my mission to help others and in my environmental work. I am looking forward to the rest of my life with joy and love!

—Eleanor H.

I would like to share some of the changes I have experienced in the four months since I began this program. Spiritually, I feel as though we, the members, are all one from the same source and receiving the same benefits; for example, breathing the same air, receiving the same sunshine and rain, and desiring the same inner peace.

Emotionally, because of this spiritual awareness, I am able to control my emotions faster. This is due to the fact that I am aware that I can return to the spiritual source for any kind of relief I need. Also, I have discovered that my mental attitude now relaxes my physical body, and I feel less anxiety, less impatience, and more understanding when I interact with my fellow man.

Because of these improvements in my life within such a short time, I must say thanks a lot.

—Samuel N.

The effects your program has had on my life are very powerful. I gave up meat and fowl, sugar and dairy foods soon after starting the program. I had started an exercise program before coming into the study, so I continued it. I gave up drinking twenty-one years ago and smoking ten years ago. Giving up my life-long habit of negative thinking and indulging negative emotions is a different proposition, but I've made real progress with it. I no longer look for the worse parts of a given situation, while ignoring the good. I now find myself feeling very uncomfortable around negative, complaining people, and I quickly get away from them.

I've been putting the program's behavior and attitude modification tech-niques to work in my life as much as possible, and they've been very beneficial. One thing that's been really helpful is the signs and sayings on the mirror. I put a picture of my desired weight goal on my bathroom mirror, on the refrig-erator, and on the dashboard of my car. The effect on my appetite has been tremendous.

I've been very religious about taking the supplements, and judging from the various effects I'm having, they are doing their job.

Some of the changes I've experienced are:

- *Weight loss: 30 percent of goal.*
- *Broke my self-imposed five-mile running barrier for the first time in fifteen years, running eight miles.*
- *I had lost part of my sense of smell five years ago, and it has definitely improved since starting the program.*
- *Increased hair growth and decrease in amount of gray.*
- *Large increase in energy—no more comatose state at 3 P.M. every day.*
- *Increase in self-esteem.*
- *I've begun singing lessons and will perform in a coffeehouse soon.*
- *Took a small comedy part in a church play—something I never would have done before.*
- *Decrease in junk around the house.*
- *Have been reevaluating my priorities and forming some goals for my life.*
- *People tell me that my skin looks better and that I look younger.*

—Rich V.

Following this protocol and answering the questions posed has been the moti-vational force to allow me to achieve the weight loss I wanted and to change my life for the better.

A lot of the questions revived memories of positive attitudes I carried with me twenty years ago, when I had little problem making things happen for me. Over the years, I've lost touch with this reality. It's nice to have it brought back to me and have me working on things from that standpoint.

I am an avid skier and have taught skiing for more than twenty years, full time and part time. Being on the protocol has helped me have the most rewarding season of my career. I've been getting an overwhelming amount of positive feedback from my students. I had the best year of tips received and best lessons taught ever. I was one of twelve out of 270 instructors to receive an award for excellence. I've been relatively injury-free this season. The last four seasons I experienced injuries that lessened my abilities on the slopes for weeks at a time.

I have also decided to retake a high-level certification exam, which I failed when I originally took it fourteen years ago. I feel that my athletic performance has reached the level where I feel comfortable taking it again. I also feel comfortable with the exam being a learning experience, and if I should fail it again, I won't be waiting as long to retake it, but will continue my training and retake it at my earliest convenience.

My level of excitement has increased because of my level of achievement in weight loss, athletic prowess, and positive overall attitude.

I am still working things out and continuing to detoxify my surroundings. I am still a work in progress. I've got a good idea of what changes I must continue to make, and am excited about what these changes will bring to me.

—Marc C.

In the six months since beginning the program, I have changed physically, losing twenty pounds and working out four to five days a week. I have incredible energy and am not tired. I sleep less, but the sleep I get is restful.

Mentally, I am more clear-thinking, making decisions regarding my life and business quicker, as opposed to laboring over them. I have no depression, but a general feeling of grounding and balance. Affirmations work.

Work—love it! I own my own business, an organic vegan home delivery service. Since being a member of the group, I am more organized—no procrastination. Our company has tripled its business. The company has become an extension of my being.

I have much more quality play in my life, and I choose very carefully who I'd like to play with. My time is important. Most important, because work is demanding, I truly enjoy my "playtime." As far as relationships go, once again, time is valuable—which made it easy to shed relationships that were toxic and draining. I moved out of a six-and-a-half-year relationship to a studio apartment that belongs to me—serene, peaceful, and beautiful. I am choosing relationships that are positive.

Although not every day moves gracefully through my life, each day is growing more enjoyable and fun. This support group has helped change my life to a positive, peaceful state of being. A definite catalyst.

—Liz M.

The reason I decided to join the study is a desire to reach my potential spiritually, physically, and emotionally. To achieve this, I must empower myself. The commitment to the program without compromise is a powerful statement. It says that I am making my own choices in my life, and that these choices are positive and affect every aspect. I am in control.

In the past two years, I have been divorced, lost my job, and lost my apartment. The reason that this happened is that I allowed other people to make my decisions for me. Basically, I didn't think enough of myself to express my wants, desires, needs, likes and dislikes, and all the other good stuff that comes along with being a person.

I feel that I have come a long way in the past three months, primarily because of the program. Being in control of my decision of what I will and will not put in my body is empowering. I believe the body is sacred and should be treated as such. It is the temple in which we live.

Physically I do feel more energetic than I did before. Lack of energy was a problem in the past due to my consumption of large amounts of sweets.

Before I was married, I was very spiritual. While I was married, I was less so, due to the demands of being a father, husband, and provider. Now that I am single and possess the solitude necessary for reflection and spiritual growth I am following my path that leads to discovery and wholeness. What I have also discovered is that making positive changes in one aspect of your life leads to positive changes in other areas. Sometimes you don't consciously make positive changes; they just happen, one built upon the other.

—Tom M.

I have changed physically in that I have a lot more energy and I sleep less. I have lost about twenty-five pounds and have a lot more strength and less pain *from fibromyalgia and arthritis. People say my skin looks good and want to know what I am doing—and I tell them. (There are a lot of new Green Stuff users out there!)*

I am mentally clearer and more focused and, as a result, my teaching is better. I am a lot more tolerant and less angry with students and other people, too. I don't let my toxic relatives get to me any more. I even feel that some of my positive energy is rubbing off on them. I have had a lot to deal with in the past six months, including my mother's death and my sister's recent car accident, and I know I wouldn't have been able to cope with this so well without all the changes I have made.

I have a lot more to do in terms of getting rid of years of toxicity and I need to work more on being less angry and more playful.

—Liza S.

It's been approximately twelve weeks since I began your program. My comments will be limited to these twelve weeks; however, please note that I have been following your advice for more than two years, via your radio shows, books and lectures.

During weeks one through six, I felt an unusual amount of fatigue. This was frustrating because I felt it had a negative impact on my exercise program. I work out at a gym at least four times per week. I found myself easily fatigued during my workouts. However, by the seventh week, my strength and endurance returned. In fact, recently I've noticed gains in my strength training—both more weight being lifted and more muscular definition.

Other physical changes I've experienced so far include a cleaner, clearer complexion—friends have also noticed and commented on this—and, unfortunately, an accelerated hair loss.

Probably the most significant emotional change I've experienced is an overall feeling of well-being.

I know the program is helping me physically and the physical improvement makes me feel very good about myself. I've also noticed a great change in my outlook about my work, my friends, and my life. Certain things that seemed so important to me—especially concerning my work—don't have the same importance. . . . I especially feel very aware and alert, and very focused on what's going on around me.

—Chris M.

I would like to thank you, Gary, for your constructive criticism of my power walking, as well as for your encouraging me to compete eventually in this sport. As for my foot problems, I will follow your advice because I trust you. I know I will be cured. I'd like to let you know, Gary, based on my perception, you are a perfect example of mens sana in corpore sana. *You have given me inspiration to strive for the same, although I wonder how far I will get, or when I will feel complete.*

—Rose V.

Before I joined the program, I envisioned myself becoming one of Gary's great success stories, being able to go from one mile running to twenty miles or a marathon's length in a week's time, and being able to prioritize my life in order to work my eight-hour job in eight hours instead of twelve or thirteen, as I have often done in the past.

I tried to compensate for my avoidance of honoring my own belief system as well as compensating for lack of placing my spirituality as my number one priority by taking additional vitamins, supplements, exercise, and helping others.

Now, after my week here, I will continue to raise my vitamins, juices, and exercise, but no longer as a compensation mechanism. I will continue to honor my health with a renewed commitment and vigor to life, because I have humbled myself to God, my higher power, within me. So now I realize that all the problems I had before will still be in there when I return to New Jersey, but I can face them with less fear because I am more of a complete person.

For this I would like to thank Gary Null for his inspiration, insight, and generosity. . . . I hope to repay you every day by providing myself and everyone else in my life with the same love and caring that you have given me, and hopefully it will return to you and your staff tenfold. Thank you.

—Brian B.

I wanted to write you and thank you for helping me find a new direction in life. I went to your ranch in Naples [Florida] as one person and came home another. I have made permanent changes in my life and I feel terrific.

The changes I have gone through are too numerous to list. What I can say is now I feel as if there is nothing I can't do.

Thank you so much again. It is truly wonderful, the way you use your gifts.

—Laura J. G.

My illness had gone undiagnosed for a year and a half and had been debilitating. But this week [at Paradise Gardens] I looked at deeper issues—such as what stands between me and health and well-being.

Your example of how to live with joy, strength, and fierce and unflagging dedication inspires. The best way to express my gratitude will be to heal.

I hope I can return soon and become strong enough, over time, to prevail.

—Nancy A.

I've been "detoxing" for a year now, and my life keeps getting better and better. I almost feel like a child again—the whole world is mine to explore. My life will never be the same.

I also want to thank you for being a wonderful role model in my life. I admire the passion you have for your beliefs and work, your refusal to compromise them, and your dedication to the mastery of each day in your life. You have set the bar very high! Your efforts have made the world and my life better, and I plan to help others grow and improve their lives.

—Mike C.

My spirit is awake for the first time since I was a little girl. I feel as though I have come full circle. . . . I am at last at peace and harmony. Body, mind, and spirit are one.

You have touched so many in my family already. Mike and I have both made life-affirming changes. My father-in-law is beginning to heal. We've made our children healthy again. The effects are endless and go much deeper than mere words can express.

—Gina S.

A new beginning at sixty-seven; what an opportunity for me! I am so grateful to you for showing me how I can do more for myself and others. . . . You have

taught me that there is so much more for me to learn in order to "follow my bliss."

Again, thank you for showing me the way to a healthy body, mind, and spirit.

—Dorothea M.

I began this age-reversing program because I wanted to start living a healthier life. I would start, but go off track. I lacked motivation as well as discipline, but by joining the group, I have become more motivated and disciplined.

I knew exercise was good for my health, but I didn't exercise. By joining the group, I have started to exercise a minimum of three times a week. I now have the motivation to exercise. Since stating this program, I have lost weight and do feel more energetic. The weight loss and high energy I now have is very motivating and I see myself living a healthier life and eating healthier.

—Florence H.

Physically, this program has given me a pathway onto how to extend my lifespan. How to get away from the American diet, how to cope in this society when you are perceived to be different. This program has given me energy, and an overall feeling that my body is much cleaner. It has helped me see that there is another way to live your life.

—David Y.

Before beginning the program, I had had a history of fibrocystic breasts for twenty years. I was underweight and was not exercising at all. I had noticeable hair loss, and I had been taking Synthroid for a history of possible thyroid cancer.

After approximately six months in the program, my fibrocystic breasts have decreased by more than 50 percent, and I have gained two pounds. I am now exercising five to six days a week and I have muscles! My hair loss started to slow down. Also, I have stopped taking Synthroid.

—Yanick D.

*I just improved my body and that helped me feel better emotionally and spiri-
tually. I have learned to give more care for my body in the future.*

—Eva

*Since I started the program, my poor memory and awareness have improved. I
had been full of fear, angry and overreactive, and I felt victimized and had
uncontrolled reactions to very small problems. I am much calmer and happier
now, and shyness, guilt, and low self-esteem are improved. I feel that people
have more respect for me now and that I have more control over many things.*

*Acne is clearing up; my nails look much better now, with the spots on
them going away. Arthritis pain is 70 percent improved and a problem with
dry eyes—I was told by the eye doctor that I would have to take these drops for
the rest of my life—is gone. I am sleeping better and back pain has improved by
30 to 40 percent.*

*I had many allergies—mold, string beans, eggs, grasses, animals, bee pol-
len, and on and on. I was given injections two or three times a week for a year
without getting better. Another allergist told me I am only allergic to yeast.
Nothing seemed to help. I often had trouble breathing, and I had problems
walking into a temple weekends because the air was very toxic with mold.*

*People complimented me that I look ten years younger on a recent trip to
Israel. Several complimented me on my new glasses, but it wasn't the
glasses—it was my new face!*

*I didn't believe that I could have spiritual joy again. I felt a lot older. Now
I believe I can have more joy in general.*

—Moshe M.

*I came into the study detoxing from a twenty-eight-year, progressively abusive
marriage. Drawing on all my resources to get me through—actually having
the source physically removed from the house, restraining order, court appear-
ances, custody hearings for my son.*

*I actually came down with acute myelogenous leukemia during the separa-
tion period. After they got it in remission with chemotherapy, I attended your
lecture on* Who Are You Really? *I approached you for how to get my totally
depleted health back. You said, "Detox," but I had no money to go away for one.*

*The answer to my prayers, literally, came through the radio when you
announced the support group I am now reporting on.*

Mentally I had to pick up the pieces, decide to live healthier, happier, and holier—not than "thou," but by strengthening my faith in God—and building confidence in the derisions and direction that had gotten me this far. Simplifying my life, moving, juicing—these were not options. Survival is where I started.

I had to rebuild my immune system—all my defenses were down. My hair was gone but was growing back. Fingernails, skin, muscles, strength—all weak.

I had never really exercised that regularly. For years I had spurts of energy—perhaps from "toxic relationship drain"—but not consistently. Swimming is something I've always enjoyed—but that was seasonal and sporatic.

Still, I worked thirty hours a week, kept house with three teenagers, cooked, took interior design classes at the Fashion Institute, and did some drapery and design work on the side—before bottoming out.

Coffee got me going in the morning. I ate too much meat and processed food. When I would go out for a walk, it was when I couldn't stand the pressure in the house any longer.

Now I power walk/run three miles at least five times a week—and enjoy it. I do 200 crunches/sit-ups daily, which has made a visible difference. People often comment on how well I look—after cancer, if you're alive, they're surprised, I guess—but it's a boost to keeping up the maintenance protocol.

I could intellectualize how important this study has been to my recovery—but I couldn't seem to do it until Sam, my Hasidic friend in the group, caught up with me on the way to the subway with something important to say: "Patty, you have to thank your ex-husband for freeing you from all the effort and energy it took out of you to keep the marriage going—that now you have all that energy into getting yourself well."

Wow! I couldn't believe that; now I could do it. Amen.

—Patricia B.

PART III

IS IT POSSIBLE TO REVERSE AGING?

One does not evaluate one's own position in terms of what has just been lost, but rather in terms of what remains to work with.

—Robert Grudin, *Time and the Art of Living*

PART 14

IS IT POSSIBLE TO
REVERSE AGING?

4

THEORIES OF AGING

The bottom line: We begin to age the moment we are born. How long the process takes, and how well we do it, depends almost entirely on how well we take care of ourselves.

The human body is a collection of cells—100 trillion by some estimates, but who's counting? The point is, no serious discussion of the aging process can begin without first considering what is taking place at the molecular level as we grow older.

Modern theories of aging generally fall into two camps—damage theories and programmed theories. Damage theories are primarily concerned with the damage that occurs inside the cells over time. Programmed theories center around the idea that aging results in large part from a sort of genetic clock that decides when cells can no longer operate and reproduce at a rate sufficient enough to maintain optimal health. These distinctions are not necessarily mutually exclusive, but they do serve as a useful guide for discussing current thinking on how and why we age the way we do.

DAMAGE THEORIES

While the emphasis and names may vary (e.g., free radical theory, cross-linking theory, radiation theory, DNA repair theory, oxidative stress theory, immune theory, membrane theory, waste accumulation theory, calorie restriction theory, etc.), free radicals lie at the heart of most damage theories of aging.

First identified more than forty years ago by Gerschman, and championed as the key to aging ever since by biochemist Denham Harman of the University of Nebraska, free radicals are molecules with unpaired electrons in their outer shell. Such molecules can wreak havoc on normal cells by attempting to steal an electron from another molecule in order to restore their balance. In doing so they can initiate a destructive cycle that may multiply and quickly spread, destroying healthy cells in the process. This more or less infectious pattern can continue indefinitely.

Free radicals are powerful oxidizing agents that cannot be avoided altogether in that a majority naturally result from many normal reactions in the body involving cellular respiration. While it is required for life and responsible for as much as 95 percent of our molecular energy, oxygen itself is in fact the most prevalent free radical found in the body. Unfortunately, when not kept in check by an adequate supply of antioxidants, which attack them directly and prevent new ones from forming, free radicals can lead to all kinds of degenerative problems such as atherosclerosis, cancer, Alzheimer's disease, cataracts, osteoarthritis, neurological disorders, and immune deficiency.

The free radicals most critical to the aging process include superoxide anion, hydrogen radical, singlet oxygen, hydrogen peroxide, and hypochlorous acid. At the molecular level, they can wage an assault on several fronts, such as damaging immune cells (white blood cells), lysosomes (intracellular particles that contain digestive enzymes), and unsaturated fatty acids (lipid peroxidation), destroying DNA and causing DNA mutations, hardening cell and nuclear membranes, breaking off cell membrane proteins, etc.

The specific site of free radicals is a key factor in determining their degree of danger. Most can be found in the mitochondria, where they cause the least harm. The mitochondria are the cells' chief engines and are surrounded by the cell membranes. These membranes, also a common location for free radicals, are particularly vulnerable because they are composed of unsaturated fatty acids. An interesting aspect is the waste products free radicals leave behind in the wake of their damage to cell membranes. Many cells, particularly heart and nerve cells, accumulate lipofuscin, a yellow pigment, increasingly as they age. Lipofuscin, often referred to as age spots, comes from oxidized fat molecules. Some suggest that eventually the buildup of this molecular trash becomes a burden that damages the cell itself and causes it to stop functioning properly.

Free radicals perhaps do their greatest damage through a process of fusing DNA and protein molecules, referred to as cross-linking. Unlike the other contents of cells, the body cannot produce new strands of DNA. The best it can do is repair them, but not always. In addition to damaging DNA, cross-linking results in the body's essential proteins becoming stiff and therefore unable to function correctly. This process is responsible for many of the symptoms most often associated with aging—cataracts, wrinkles, brittle bones, kidney failure, hardening of the arteries, and immune deficiency. Cross-linking is particularly prevalent in diabetics, as glucose fuels the process, and helps explain why diabetes is a disease recognized for its severe premature aging effects.

In order to combat the dangers of free radicals it is important to identify where they come from. As previously stated, many, if not the majority, of free radicals occur naturally in the body. They are produced as a by-product of normal cellular activity, as well as in response to both psychological and physical stress, an example being excessive exercise. However, free radicals can increasingly be found in our environment in the form of toxic waste, chemicals, pesticides, sunlight, radiation, and cigarette smoke, as well as dietary sources such as coffee, alcohol, fried and barbecued foods, etc. The trick to keeping free radicals under control is to avoid external sources where possible, and to make certain that the body is well supplied with antioxidants to ward off those we cannot.

Most people are familiar with at least some of the benefits attributed to such popular antioxidants as vitamin C, vitamin E, and beta-carotene. The first line of defense against an excess buildup of oxygen at the molecular level consists of three protective enzymes naturally found in the body: superoxide dismutase (SOD), catalase, and glutathione peroxidase.

Free radicals are defeated essentially by being trapped, or isolated, and not allowed to seek out electrons from neighboring cells. Free radicals can then be metabolized and turned into harmless paired oxygen molecules or simply water. Dietary sources of antioxidants (nonenzymatic compounds) can produce similar effects.

While dietary antioxidants such as vitamin C are useful in the fight against free radicals, this is not the only place they are needed in the body. The more antioxidants involved in this fight, the less are available overall. If neither the protective enzymes nor dietary sources of antioxidants can stem the rising tide of free radicals, the cells attempt to destroy them themselves. This burns up vital energy the cells require for more important activities.

While free radicals destroy healthy cells, those cells that are not being destroyed are expending more and more resources both in attempts to keep the free radical onslaught at bay and to clean up and repair the damage that already has been done. Eventually something is going to give. And that something increasingly moves from the molecular level outward, taking the form of heart disease, cancer, diabetes, arthritis, senile dementia, Alzheimer's disease, a weakened immune system, and numerous other ills.

Key to understanding why free radicals are central to damage theories of aging concerns the issue of maintaining oxygen balance within the body. Techniques designed to successfully maintain this delicate balance are at the heart of most natural anti-aging protocols today.

BODY PROGRAMMING THEORIES

Regardless of the interpretation of the causes of aging, there is little debate that excess free radicals are harmful. Those partial to theories that the body is programmed to age in a certain way argue that, while free radicals are clearly an expression of aging at the metabolic level, they alone cannot be a primary cause of it.

Understanding what happens to our bodies (as well as our minds and spirits) as we age is not the same as knowing what triggers the aging process itself. True, free radicals create big trouble, but what allows them to do so much more, say, at age sixty, as opposed to twenty-five?

For some, the answer resides in the genes.

The logic behind programming theories of aging rests on the belief that the body contains a genetic clock that is preset by heredity to begin deteriorating at a given point and time. Central to such theories are results from animal studies involving selected breeding for extended life span and *in vitro* (outside the body) studies show-ing that certain cells stop replicating over time.

Variations on this theme have suggested that the heart has a limited number of potential beats and the immune system generally reaches its greatest strength at puberty, only to gradually decline from then on. While the prospect of a ticking time bomb for self-destruction may bring little solace to the health-conscious individual, there is clearly an element of truth to such thinking, in that all species have a maximum life span and no one lives forever.

The concept of an innate aging clock begs the question of where it is.

Some have argued that it resides specifically in the mitochondrial DNA. Others point to the hypothamalmus, pituitary gland, thymus gland, or pineal gland. Yet it is the work of cell biologist Leonard Hayflick that is not only most responsible for modern programmed theories of aging, but has given rise to the most intriguing idea to date.

In 1961, Hayflick found that human cells, or fibroblasts, while continuing to live, only divide approximately fifty times before ceasing to function correctly. This finite number has come to be known as the Hayflick limit. It is governed by three factors: The first is the maximum life span of the species from which a cell is obtained. Second involves the age of the cell's source, and the third depends on the type of cell itself. An obvious exception to such findings are cancer cells; they never stop dividing. Efforts to explain this apparent contradiction spawned the telomere theory of aging. Developed in the early 1970s, it took hold in 1990 and remains a fertile area of research today.

Telomeres are the protective caps on the ends of chromosomes that carry DNA. With few exceptions, there are forty-six chromosomes on each cell. Every chromosome has two ends with a telomere on each one, which adds up to 92 telomeres per cell. Studies show that a telomere is roughly 5,000 base pairs in length shortly after birth. It is shortened by roughly sixty-five base-pairs with each cell division. Because of this, some researchers argue that the length of telomeres should be considered a biomarker of human cell aging. They note that cells stop dividing when they get too short. This changes their gene expression and results in eventual cell death.

Advocates of the telomere theory suggest that by controlling the activity of telomeres, scientists may both be able to enable some cells critical to the aging process to keep replicating (thus live longer) and prevent others (cancer cells) from doing so. In his book, *Reversing Human Aging*, Dr. Michael Fossel writes:

> Cells have chromosomal "clocks" that determine their life spans. A cell dies when its clock runs down. Cancer cells, on the other hand, continually reset their clocks, allowing themselves to divide forever. If we reset the clock of a normal cell, it lives anew; if we stop the clock of a cancer cell it dies. When we can set the clocks, your cells need not age and cancer can be cured.

It is Fossel's contention that all this may be possible within the next ten years, a case he made in the June 3, 1998, issue of *The Journal of the American Medical Association*. In an article entitled "Telomerase and the Aging Cell: Implications for Human Health," he notes that "recent research has shown that inserting a gene for the protein component of telomerase into aging human cells reextends their telomeres to lengths typical of young cells, and the cells then display all the other identifiable characteristics of young, healthy cells."

Fossel argues that such findings not only suggest that telomeres are the central timing mechanism for cellular aging, but also demonstrate that such a mechanism can be reset, extending their replicative life span, resulting in markers of gene expression typical of younger cells without the hallmarks of malignant transformation.

Taking his case a step farther, he suggests, "It is now possible to explore the fundamental cellular mechanisms underlying human aging and therefore determine the extent to which the major causes of death and disability in aging populations in developed countries—cancer, atherosclerosis, osteoarthritis, macular degeneration, and Alzheimer dementia—are attributable to such fundamental mechanisms. If they are amenable to prevention or treatment by alteration of cellular aging, the clinical implications have few historic precedents."

Fossel's claims are bold, but he is not alone in making them. In a January 16, 1998, article published in *Science*, A. G. Bodnar and colleagues reported on the results of a study in which two telomerase-negative normal human cell types—retinal pigment epithelial cells and foreskin fibroblasts—were transfected with vectors encoding the human telomerase catalytic subunit. At the time of publication, the cells had exceeded the normal life span by twenty divisions, suggesting a causal relationship between telomere shortening and cellular aging.

Designs for telomere inhibitors to fight cancer and inducers to reverse aging are already in the works, and the implications could be profound should they pan out. Still, the theory is not without its critics. One is Hayflick himself, now a faculty member at the University of California at San Francisco Medical School and past president of the Gerontological Society of America. He believes telomeres may be useful for understanding the ultimate limits of life span but do not reveal much about how to directly influence the aging process.

Another is noted molecular biologist Harry Rubin. Rubin has attacked the widely held assumption that there is an intrinsic fixed limit to the number of divisions vertebrate cells can undergo. He argues that studies supporting this idea have been carried out *in vitro* or *ex-vivo* (removed and put back in the body), and it is being placed in these unnatural environments that stops cells from dividing. He takes his critique further, suggesting that results of such studies actually support a more stress-based model of aging, in that it is external factors (putting cells in a foreign culture) that causes a reduction in growth rate, as opposed to any inherited genetic timetable. In other words, it is the cells' inability or failure to successfully adapt to a stressful environment that is most responsible for their failure to replicate, perhaps paralleling conditions created over a lifetime of external assaults to the homeostasis of the body from free radicals and other factors that may produce such damaging effects.

The truth about how and why we age surely involves elements from both the damage and programmed camps. Many of us would like to believe we can exercise absolute control over the speed at which we wear down by implementing proper dietary and lifestyle habits. However, there is simply no denying the fact that the oldest recorded man to date lived to be a mere 120, and most never make it anywhere close.

When measured collectively, human beings, like fruit flies, fall within a generally recognized life span that is, to some degree, genetically determined. The average life expectancy in the United States is approximately seventy-six years. Additionally, the large-scale New England Centenarian Study, in association with Harvard

Medical School, shows that there are approximately forty thousand people over the age of one hundred in the U.S. This translates to 1 centenarian per 10,000 Americans, based on a population of more than 250,000,000. Ninety per cent of these lucky few are women. Similar patterns have been found in other industrialized countries.

We are, however, individuals.

Why can some people run a marathon at age seventy-five while others drop dead from a stroke at forty? Science increasingly suggests that the difference may well involve the daily, personal choices we make concerning how we treat our bodies. Before exploring such choices, it is important to step beyond the cellular level and look more practically at what happens to us as we age in order to understand how to prevent it.

5

THINGS FALL APART: HOW
THE BODY AGES

The obvious endpoint to aging is death.

It is therefore useful to consider mortality rates as a place to start. According to Centers for Disease Control (CDC) statistics for 1996, heart disease, cancer, and stroke continue to be the three leading causes of death in the United States. The estimated rankings based on 1996 data are as follows:

CAUSES OF DEATH
(Based on 1996 Data)

Rank	Disease	Incidence
1	Heart disease	733,834
2	Cancer	544,278
3	Cerebrovascular disease (stroke)	160,431
4	Chronic lung diseases	106,146
5	Accidents	93,874
6	Pneumonia and influenza	82,579
7	Diabetes mellitus	61,559
8	HIV Infection	32,655
9	Suicide	30,862
10	Liver disease	25,135

With respect to the issue of aging, these numbers are telling. What they indicate is that most Americans die of degenerative diseases.

By nature, such conditions develop over a long period of time. They at once seriously influence and are influenced by the aging process. In other words, diabetes can kill you prematurely by accelerating the aging process. You can also develop diabetes as a result of aging too quickly. Throw genetic predispositions into the mix and the question of which comes first is a tricky one.

In his book *How and Why We Age*, Leonard Hayflick presents data obtained from the Baltimore Longitudinal Study of Aging (BLSA). The largest study of its kind ever done, the BLSA began in 1958. Still ongoing, the study makes use of as many as 150 trained research gerontologists whose job it is to examine the physical and mental changes in healthy people as they age. Hayflick summarizes the results to date as follows:

- There is no evidence that a single factor or a single clock regulates the rate of aging in all our organs.
- Because there is a large amount of individual variation, chronological age alone is a poor predictor of performance. Some eighty-year-olds may perform as well as the average fifty-year-old.
- Some things—for example, resting heart rate and personality—do not change with age.
- Some slow losses are not caused by aging but rather diseases, such as arthritis and Alzheimer's disease.
- Some losses are inevitable consequences of aging, unrelated to disease. These physiological changes occur over time as part of the normal aging process; for example, reduction in speed and losses in short-term memory.
- Sudden losses are the result of diseases—especially heart attack and stroke—rather than aging.
- Primary changes can lead to secondary changes. Some normal changes that occur as we age may result from the body's attempts to compensate for some other normal loss. For example, with increasing age, greater cardiac output is required after exercise.
- Lifestyle decisions, notably adoption of a low-cholesterol diet or stopping drinking alcohol or smoking cigarettes, can influence the occurrence or progression of some age-associated diseases. There is no direct effect on the fundamental aging process.

- Longitudinal changes in functions help to distinguish age-associated processes from disease.

Reflecting on such findings, Hayflick writes:

The BLSA tells us that there is no single aging process. A person's rate of aging may vary significantly from what might be predicted from the averages. There is no general pattern of aging applicable to all of our organs. Aging results from the interaction of genetic, environmental, and lifestyle factors. Age changes are highly individualized. The disabilities frequently associated with old age may be caused more by the effects of disease than by aging processes. Chronological age is an unreliable measure of aging—but a proven measure of the passage of time called birthdays and receiving presents.

So be it free radicals, telomeres, or a molecular stew of these and other factors that make us vulnerable over time, the truth is, most people die, if not from specific causes, from a certain pattern of disease. As more than 65 percent of annual American deaths are attributed to heart disease, cancer, and stroke combined, it is worth taking a brief glimpse at each of these gradual killers as part of a general look at how, to paraphrase the poet Yeats,

we fall apart.

HEART DISEASE

The clearest evidence of aging is that which can be seen by the naked eye. Hair loses its pigmentation and becomes gray, or begins to thin and fall out. Fingernails thicken and become brittle. Skin toughens and begins to wrinkle, reducing its sensitivity and making us more susceptible to injury.

Each of these problems is associated with what may perhaps be the most serious change that takes place over time: a reduction in the rate of blood flow throughout the body.

The implications of this are tremendous, not only with respect to this country's perennial leading cause of death, but to a huge number of other, often subtle, conditions, such as impaired memory or lack of sexual arousal. When blood flow is restricted, every system in the body—right down to proper nourishment of the tiniest particles inside our cells—suffers. As many as 60 million Americans currently suffer some sort of heart disease.

The most prevalent form the disease takes is atherosclerosis. The arteries become clogged by an excessive buildup of fats known as plaque. Excess free radicals can convert regular, or *good*, cholesterol, which is required for cell maintenance, into more threatening forms of oxidized, or *bad*, cholesterol—the primary component of plaque. (Hence the strong correlation between heart disease and serum cholesterol levels.)

Plaque develops over time, adhering to the arterial wall and eventually obstructing blood flow. Thus plaque forces the heart to work harder as its blood supply is reduced. This can eventually lead to a full-blown heart attack, as well as stroke, seemingly sudden events that may actually have been decades in the making.

Just as many, if not more, Americans suffer from a condition that, while separate, is intimately linked to heart disease—hypertension. There are two types of hypertension: essential and secondary. More than 90 percent of hypertension cases are diagnosed as essential, meaning the direct cause is not known. Secondary hypertension occurs when endocrine or kidney damage causes a rise in blood pressure. Hypertension is most dangerous due to its potential damage to the heart and blood vessels.

STROKE

Of the total amount of blood pumped by the heart, a quarter of it goes to the brain. Strokes occur when this flow of blood is restricted either due to clots, the rupturing of blood vessels, or a more global obstruction like that associated with atherosclerosis, and thus brain cells die from a lack of oxygen.

Stroke can result in immediate death or severe physical consequences, including limits on the ability to speak, walk, see, talk, and use the hands.

Symptoms associated with stroke depend to a large extent on what areas of the brain are affected. In addition to the number of deaths they cause each year, estimates are more than 2 million

Americans currently suffer from some kind of disability due to strokes.

CANCER

Cancer is a condition in which previously healthy cells mutate and begin to grow out of control. Allowed to continue unchecked, these cancerous cells can rob normal cells of vital nutrients and develop into tumors that can spread throughout the body and eventually overwhelm it.

Almost all cells have the potential to become cancerous. They can function properly one day, turn cancerous the next, and then either be repaired by the immune system or simply be destroyed and replaced. The problem occurs when the immune system malfunctions for whatever reason and cancer cells are allowed to take root and divide.

Cancer can strike anywhere, but is generally divided into five basic types: carcinomas, sarcomas, myelomas, lymphomas, and leukemias.

Most common are carcinomas, which attack the internal organs—prostate and breast, for example—and skin.

Sarcomas are the most deadly and also the most rare, developing in the connective and muscle tissues and hitting the musculoskeletal and lymph systems.

Also rare, myelomas begin in the plasma cells and destroy bone marrow.

Lymphomas are cancers of the lymphatic system, two common examples being Hodgkin's and non-Hodgkin's lymphoma.

Finally, leukemias, unlike the others, take the form of an overproduction of white blood cells rather than tumors, and begin in the tissues of the lymph nodes, spleen, and bone marrow.

Just as some cancers are more common than others, some are also more deadly. For example the incidence of pancreatic cancer in American men is roughly 13,500 new cases per year. Male pancreatic deaths per year are estimated to be approximately 12,000. A similar pattern is seen in women. By contrast, the number of new prostate cancer cases per year is around 165,000. The number of men who actually die from prostate cancer is about 35,000. In women, the ratio with respect to breast cancer is roughly the same.

Much information will be presented on natural approaches concerning how to treat and prevent each of these three diseases, including a host of others. Before doing so, however, it is worth noting additional ways in which some important parts of the body change over time.

THE BRAIN

Aging's most dramatic effects are reserved for the brain. Many people would gladly accept a few less taste buds or a stronger set of reading glasses as a normal consequence of getting older if it was accompanied by a guarantee that their level of mental functioning would not decline. In essence, to experience our ability to think slipping away is to become increasingly estranged from a sense of who we really are.

The brain contains an estimated 100 billion cells and gradually shrinks throughout life, becoming as much as 10 percent smaller by the age of ninety as it was at twenty. It, and an intricate web of peripheral nerves, make up the body's nervous system. Two types of cells—neurons and glial cells—power this system.

Degenerative disorders of the nervous system, such as Alzheimer's disease and other forms of dementia that lead to cognitive deterioration, occur, at least in part, because of the aging of such cells. Glial cells far outnumber neurons and are responsible for protecting them, since neurons generally don't divide and cannot be replaced. The fact that neurons are finite in number also explains why many of the symptoms associated with strokes remain permanent.

Neurons operate via chemical messengers called neurotransmitters. Acetylcholine is considered the most important of these. Others include dopamine, norepinephrine, serotonin, epinephrine, and histamine.

Like neurons themselves, neurotransmitters gradually diminish in number, which limits the ability of neurons to communicate with one another. Neurotransmitters are transmitted between neurons through synapses. These synapses, which connect the neurons, also decline as we age and the less they are used.

THE ENDOCRINE SYSTEM

Home to the cells and tissues responsible for the production of hormones, the endocrine system has factored prominently in many theories and discussions about aging. Hormone levels measurably change over time and directly influence the activity of most cells in the body. Important hormones that have been shown to decrease with age include insulin, growth hormones, thyroid hormones, DHEA, melatonin, testosterone, estrogen, androgens, and aldosterone.

As with free radicals, the question remains whether this is a result of the aging process, an instigator of it, or a combination of the two. Either way, a host of different types of hormone replacement therapies have increasingly made their way into anti-aging protocols. Several of these have produced remarkable benefits and will be discussed in more detail later.

THE IMMUNE SYSTEM

The most notable problem faced by the immune system as we grow older concerns a significant shrinking of the thymus gland, which is responsible for regulating T-cells. While the consequences are many, one of the worst involves the inability to distinguish foreign proteins in the body from minor changes occurring in our normal proteins that have always been there, but are now being altered by age.

Unfortunately, the immune system is often too sensitive for its own good and ends up attacking itself, a process referred to as autoimmunity. Autoimmune conditions include lupus, rheumatoid arthritis, and multiple sclerosis. This, coupled with an overall weakening of the body, can become a great burden on the immune system, making us susceptible to a host of conditions we would normally be able to fend off. These include infections such as pneumonia, not to mention cancer.

THE MUSCULOSKELETAL SYSTEM

In the minds of many, osteoporosis and arthritis are synonymous with aging.

Osteoporosis involves a loss of bone tissue, or density, resulting in weakening of the bones themselves. This occurs for a variety of reasons, including hormonal changes, nutritional deficiencies (such as a failure to absorb enough calcium), and a lack of use from inactivity. Contrary to what you may see in popular media, osteoporosis is not merely a woman's disease. Men also show evidence of bone loss.

Arthritis takes two forms. Osteoarthritis develops when the smooth cartilage surface of the joints connecting bones wears out and becomes inflamed. This might be from overuse or from an inability of cells in this area to replace themselves. Rheumatoid arthritis is an autoimmune disease. The immune system mistakenly identifies its own damaged joint surface cells as the enemy and attacks them. Inflammation worsens and the joint is eventually destroyed.

The primary threat to muscle posed by age is disuse. It's no secret that unused muscle tissues can turn to fat. While cosmetically unpleasant enough, there are more serious problems than sagging triceps and love handles associated with letting such atrophy go unchecked.

Many systems of the body depend on the proper functioning of muscles. Respiration is one. The muscles surrounding the rib cage are directly involved in the ability to breathe deeply. The excretory system is another. Muscles are necessary both for urination and defecation. It is no accident that two of the most common complaints among the elderly are bladder incontinence and constipation.

THE LUNGS

Chronic lung disease is the fourth most prevalent killer in the United States, which is indicative of a weakening of the respiratory system toward the latter stages of life.

The activity of the cilia and elasticity of lung tissue decreases over time, making it more difficult to properly take in oxygen and expel carbon dioxide. This aggravates the critical oxygen balance required for healthy cells.

Add to the equation years of smoking and other environmental insults—secondhand smoke, polluted air, chemical fumes, and the like—and the consequences can be deadly. Symptoms associated with this reduced lung capacity include fatigue, anxiety, and shortness of breath.

THE SKIN AND HAIR

Most skin damage—especially wrinkles and dryness—stems from excess exposure to free radicals and the ultraviolet effects of the sun. This leads to a loss of the protein collagen and an overabundance of another protein, elastin.

Some wrinkles occur as a result of use, such as lines in the face that accentuate common expressions like squinting. Both the outer skin layer, dermis, and inner layer, epidermis, thin with age from a reduction in cells.

Sweat glands either shrink or become damaged over time, which results in reduced perspiration. Evidence of this loss of function lies in the fact that elderly people tend to sweat less.

The elderly become less sensitive to pain as a result of loss of nerve cells in the skin. Also, they are more susceptible to feeling temperature changes, since the number of blood vessels in the skin declines with age as well. The rate of wound healing is commonly reduced for the same reasons.

In most cases, the amount of body hair decreases with age. There are, however, some exceptions. Hair in the nostrils and on the ears and eyebrows may increase just as it is thinning on the scalp. Many women experience unwanted hair growth above the lip and chin as a result of decreased amounts of estrogen at the onset of menopause. Growth patterns of hair also change as we get older, as can color. Because of a reduction in melanin-producing cells in the cortex of the hair, the hair loses its natural color and becomes gray. Like it or not, gray hair has been found to be a reliable indicator of the aging process in general.

Returning to Hayflick and the results from the BSLA, the following is a list of other physical changes that frequently occur with age:

- Increased risk of cavities/periodontal disease
- Metabolism slows/body consumes fewer calories
- Body fat redistribution
- Enlargement of prostate gland
- Decline in visual acuity
- Increased cataract risk
- Interrupted sleep
- Loss of kidney function
- Duller sense of smell
- Progressive hearing loss

6

LIFE EXTENSION TECHNIQUES

I suspect that strategies for prolonging life have been around for as long as human life itself. Yet, despite the plotting, planning, and research—not to mention the wishing, hoping, and dreaming— through the ages, the most dramatic increases have occurred during the past century.

Statistically, this change can be explained by advances in eradicating infectious disease, improved sanitary conditions, and reductions in infant mortality. At least in industrialized countries, fewer people die young than ever before in history. This pushes up the mean with respect to measures of life expectancy. But this is not the entire story. Not only are people merely escaping the fatal childhood diseases of the past, they are also living longer. The maximum human life span may not have changed much over time, but the number of people approaching it continues to rise.

Now, many experts in the field are beginning to think that the science of life extension is on the verge of a paradigm shift. Consider the following passage from Fossel:

> Your life span can be extended by several hundred years. The technical hurdles appear enormous, but so were the ones involved in getting to the moon, building a computer, or sequencing a human gene. These obstacles will be overcome sometime within the next decade.

Granted, intricate concepts like telomeres remain more or less theoretical, but one of the great ironies of the burgeoning science of

135

life extension is that much of it involves practices that are hardly new at all.

EXERCISE

One low-tech way to live longer is to exercise. While it was once widely believed that vigorous exercise was harmful to the body and an obstacle to long life, studies now show the truth is exactly the opposite. Results from dozens of animal and human trials clearly indicate that the old adage "use or lose it" is well founded. In an extensive review of the scientific literature on life extension, Bernarducci and colleagues point out that exercise has historically been thought of as more a modifier of disease than a direct life extender. They cite the results of the well-known Harvard Alumni Health Study involving 17,321 men, however, which suggests that "total energy expenditure and exercise intensity over time is indirectly related to all-cause mortality and independent of disease modification."

DIETARY RESTRICTIONS

Animal studies have consistently shown that reducing the total level of calories consumed can also significantly increase life span. While most of these have been limited to rodents, the implications are clear. We may not be only what we eat, but may well live a lot longer because of how much we don't. Temporarily setting aside the issue of specific dietary nutrients, even more promising are the health-promoting agents increasingly being discovered in foods themselves.

PHYTOCHEMICALS

Phytochemicals, found in edible plants, have been found to exhibit potential benefits in the prevention and treatment of disease. Scientists are only beginning to explore the healing properties of the thousands of natural compounds found only in the foods we eat.

According to the *Journal of the American Dietetic Association*:

It is the position of the American Dietetic Association (ADA) that specific substances in foods (e.g. phytochemicals as naturally occurring components and functional food components) may have a beneficial role in health as part of a varied diet. The Association supports research regarding the health benefits and risks of these substances. Dietetics professionals will continue to work with the food industry and government to ensure that the public has accurate scientific information in this emerging field.

The report goes on to say that phytochemicals are present in many frequently consumed foods, especially fruits, vegetables, grains, legumes, and seeds, as well as in such less common foods as licorice, soy, and green tea. In addition to naturally occurring phytochemicals, scientists are developing what they call functional foods, which consist of any food or food ingredient providing health benefits beyond the traditional nutrients it contains.

Phytochemicals and functional food components have been associated with the prevention and/or treatment of at least three of the leading causes of death in this country—cancer, diabetes, and heart disease—and with the prevention and/or treatment of other medical ailments, including neural tube defects, osteoporosis, abnormal bowel function, and arthritis. Dr. J. F. Potter, professor of epidemiology and director of the University of Minnesota Cancer Prevention Research Unit, has been studying the relationship between diet and cancer for more than fifteen years. Like scientists worldwide, he has found that people whose diets are heavy in fruits and vegetables have lower rates of most cancers. Limonene in citrus fruits, for example, is known to increase the production of enzymes that help the body dispose of potentially carcinogenic substances. Even the National Cancer Institute estimates that one in three cancer deaths are diet related and that eight of ten cancers have a nutritional component.

Phytochemicals have been actively used by pharmaceutical companies in making many of their products. According to a report in *Business Week*, 25 percent of modern pharmaceuticals are derived in some way from plants. The heart medicine digitalis and the cancer drugs vinicistine and taxol are just some examples.

Pharmaceutical companies may soon be motivated to isolate components in foods into pill or supplement form to market the individual elements for their health benefits. However, due to regulatory problems, such companies will have to market naturally occurring components as drugs.

What makes phytochemicals new in the public ranks is their potential health benefits before people get sick, and the saving of both lives and health-care dollars as a direct result of their use. Unfortunately, according to Dr. Stephen L. DeFelic, head of the Foundation for Innovation in Medicine, the field is still in its infancy because of too few large-scale clinical trials focusing on the health benefits of foods. Because phytochemicals cannot be patented, companies are reluctant to finance something that could cost as much as $200 million for the testing and clinical trials required for FDA approved.

Nevertheless, epidemiological evidence and small, closely monitored human trials point to benefits that may well be sleeping giants when it comes to prolonging life. Such is the case with licorice root.

In one USDA study, the extract taken from the licorice root proved to be fifty times sweeter than sugar without promoting tooth decay. It contains prostaglandin inhibitors that may guard against cancer and ulcers, and it is being pursued by many companies that want to use it as a food additive.

In another study, Michael Gould, professor of human oncology at the University of Wisconsin Medical School, has found that *d*-limonene, the major component of orange peel oil, protects rats against breast cancer. In addition to findings such as these, the ADA report notes that well-designed clinical trials indicate the beneficial effects associated with high fruit and vegetable diets cannot be duplicated by nutritional supplementation alone. Clearly, there are more benefits to be had in the healthy foods we eat than are obtained from the most common nutrients often associated with them, such as vitamins C, E, beta-carotene, and niacin.

The material on phytochemical-rich herbs that follows has been obtained from the extensive electronic database assembled by Stephen M. Beckstrom and James A. Duke at the National Germplasm Resources Laboratory, Agriculture Research Service, United States Department of Agriculture. This database is accessible on the World Wide Web at: (http://www.ars-grin.gov/~ngrlsb/).

HEALING PROPERTIES OF PLANTS

Activity	Food Sources
Antiaging	Purslane; Indian Mulberry; Garden Sorrel; Luffa; Da-Zao; Vinespinach; Spinach; Carrot; Nasturtium; Barley; Berro; Roselle; Papaya; Pigweed; Swamp Cabbage; Jew's Mallow; Sweet Potato; Chives; Black Mustard; Bell Pepper.
Antialzheimeran	Brazilnut; Cowage; Dandelion; Soybean; Black Gram; Calabash Gourd; Fenugreek; Shepherd's Purse; Flax; Groundnut; Shagbark Hickory; Ben Nut; Pumpkin; Sunflower; Scotch Pine; Pea; Dang Gui; Lentil; Pignut Hickory.
Antianginal	Lanceleaf Periwinkle; Pignut Hickory; Sharbark; Hickory; Irish Moss; Purslane; Blackbean; Red Cedar; Asparagus; Oats; Cowpea; Ben Nut; Spinach; Purple Tephrosia; Visnaga; Snakeground; Licorice; Black Cherry; Black Gum.
Antianxiety	Pignut Hickory; Shagbark Hickory; Huaco-Mullo; Ramie; Red Cedar; Buffalo Gourd; Texas Colubrina; Tomato; Pigweed; Broccoli; Brigham Tea; Chaff Flower; Wolfberry; Luffa; Spiny Pigweed; American Styrax; Red Clover; Valerian; Angel of Death; Da-Zao.
Antiarrythmic	Lettuce; Asparagus; Purslane; Chinese and Generic Goldthread; Endive; Cowpea; Oats; Black Gram; Radish; Lambsquarter; Pignut Hickory; Chinese Cabbage; Chayote; Dill; Pigweed; Spinach; Cucumber; Huang-Lia; Garland Chrysanthemum.
Antiarthritic	Cantaloupe; English Walnut; Avocado; Camu-camu; Cucumber; Safflower; Apricot; Sunflower; Butternut; Calabash Gourd; Brazilnut; Sesame; Evening Primrose; Pinyon Pine; Marijuana; Canaloupe; Black Cumin; Chilgoza Pine.
Antiatherosclerotic	Camu-camu; Evening Primrose; Broccoli; Pigweed; Tomato; Pignut Hickory; Luffa; Black Currant; Shagbark Hickory; Purslane; Bitter Melon; European Nettle; Black Cherry; Berro; Groundnut; Chinese Cabbage; Broadbean; Spinach; Lambsquarter.

Activity	Food Sources
Antibackache	Nicaraguan Cacao; Cowpea; Black-Cohosh; Asparagus; Spirulina; Yellow Gentian; Ma Huang; Blackbean; Bael de India; Macambo; Pito; Sunflower; Ben Nut; Shepherd's Purse; Okra; High Mallow; Pokeweed; Buchu; Cerraja.
Anticancer	Lemon; Celery; Caraway; Celery; Orange; Cardamom; Fennel; Mandarin; Neroli; Lime; Corn; Bayrum Tree; Mace; Star-Anise; Common Thyme; Sage; Fennel; Cucumber; Carrot; Parsley.
Anticarcinogenic	Mango; Witch Hazel; Asparagus Pea; Emblic; American Dogwood; Pomegranate; Aleppo Oak; Ipecac; Arrow-Poison Tree; Hispid Quabain; Da-Zao; Teak; Ashwagandha; Bogbean; European Squill; Grecian Foxglove; Purslane; Purple Foxglove; Da-Zao.
Anticariogenic	Grape; Copaiba; Lemon; Licorice; Crab's Eye; Lignaloe; Biblical Min; Typical Mountain Mint; Celery; Common Thyme; Wild Bergamot; Tea; Clove; Agrimony; Cubeb; Camphor; African Blue Basil; Coriander; Winter Savory.
Anticataract	Camu-camu; Pansy; Japanese Pagoda Tree; Evening Primrose; Acerola; Campechy; Buckwheat; Sang-Pai-Pi; Onion; Mayapple; Peegee: Strawberry; Sunflower; Bitter Melon; Purging Croton; American Elder.
Anticirrhotic	Licorice; Brazilnut; Crab's Eye; Cowage; Chinese Goldthread; Huang-Lia; Goldenseal; Barberry; Dandelion; Soybean; Black Gram; Calabash Gourd; Couchgrass; Fenugreek; Autumn Crocus; Shepherd's Purse; Huang Po.
Antidepressant	Parsnip; Camu-camu; Acerola; Asparagus; Pignut Hickory; Lettuce; Pigweed; Purslane; Shagbark Hickory; Berro; Lambsquarter; Endive; Spinach; Chinese Cabbage; Broccoli; Cowpea; Huaca-Mullo; Tomato; Chayote; Oats.
Antidiabetic	Chicory; Indian Snakeroot; Common Thyme; Two-Flowered Sandspur; Gobo; Red Clover; Da-Zao; Safflower; Kudzu; Maracuya; Indian Fig; Ramie; Dandelion; Rice Paper Tree; Jack Bean; Burn Mouth Vine; Pyrethrum; Desert Date; Flax; Kudzu.
Antifatigue	Lettuce; Asparagus; Endive; Black Gram; Cowpea; Lambsquarter; Radish; Chayote; Chinese Cabbage; Purslane; Oat;

Activity	Food Sources
	Garland Chrysanthemum; Dill; Dandelion; Pigweed; Cucumber; Kudzu; Spinach; Borage.
Antiglaucomic	Camu-camu; Pansy; Japanese Pagoda Tree; Pumpkin; Acerola; Chinese Foxglove; Buckwheat; Sang-Pai-Pi; Celery; Peegee; Bitter Melon; American Elder; Pokeweed; Parsley; Common Smartweed; Warburghia.
Antihypertensive	Pansy; Japanese Pagoda Tree; Evening Primrose; Endive; Lettuce; Asparagus; Black Gram; Lambsquarter; Cowpea; Radish; Purslane; Chayote; Chinese Cabbage; Oats; Pigweed; Garland Chrysanthemum; Dill; Dandelion; Spinach.
Antihyperthyroid	Guanique; Shagbark Hickory; Pignut Hickory; Black Oak; White Oak; Common Thyme; Northern Red Oak; Blackbean; Lettuce; Grapefruit; Orange; Cabbage; Asparagus; Buckbush; Endive; Shortleaf; Parsley; Red Cedar.
Anti-impotency	Pignut Hickory; Lettuce; Bitter Aloes; Shagbark Hickory; Red Cedar; Chinese Goldthread; Huang-Lia; Generic Goldthread; Asparagus; Sassafras; American Styrax; Black Cherry; Smooth Suman; Spinach; White Oak; Shortleaf Pine; Parsley; American Persimmon; Brussels Sprouts.
Antilupus	Purslane; Wheat; Swamp Cabbage; Indian Mulberry; Nasturtium; Pokeweed; Garland Chrysanthemum; Garden Sorrel; Sensitive Plant; Perejil; Asparagus; Chinese Hibiscus; Da-Zao; Vinespinach; Spinach; Carrot; Barley; Comfrey; Huaco-Mullo.
Antimelanomic	Grape; Lemon; Himalayan Mayapple; Wild Bergamot; Ajwan; Common Thyme; Asparagus Pea; Nude Mountain Mint; Horsemint; Small-Flowered Oregano; American Dogwood; Tonka Bean; Winter Savory; Portuguese Thyme; Agbo; Waldmeister; Autumn Crocus; Mayapple; Creeping Thyme; Da-Zao.
Antiosteoarthritic	Camu-camu; Bitter Melon; Emblic; Bell Pepper; Cayenne; Horseradish; Cashew; English Walnut; Vinespinach; Guava; Sallow Thorn; Berro; Garden Sorrel; Chaya; Calamansi; Broccoli; Black Currant; Cassava.

Activity	Food Sources
Antioxidant	Parsnip; Pawpaw; Red Mangrove; Camu-camu; Rowan Berry; Pansy; Japanese Pagoda Tree; Arbutus; Date Palm; Pomengranate; Emblic; Canaigre; Vanilla; Babul; Carrot; Licorice; Gum Ghatti; Coffee; Water Chestnut.
Antiparkinsonian	Camu-camu; Acerola; Broadbean; Ben Nut; Sunflower; Buffalo Gourd; Cowage; Berro; Asparagus; Black Cumin; Blackbean; Spinach; Chaya; Asparagus Pea; Jew's Mallow; Soybean; Vinespinach; Swamp Cabbage; Pigweed.
Antirheumatic	Sunflower; Licorice; Lemon; White Willow; Crab's Eye; Ajwan; Nude Mountain Mint; Horsemint; Common Thyme; Cornmint; Wild Bergamot; Evening Primrose; Sunflower; Winter Savory; Ben Nut; Autumn Crocus; Asparagus Pea; Yellow Gentian.
Antischizophrenic	Indian Snakeroot; Licorice; Celandine; Gaunique; Fenugreek; Shagbark Hickory; Avocado; Ajwan; Pea; Spiny Pigweed; Pea; American Ginseng; Pignut Hickory; Wheat; Potato; Barley; Rice; Sesame; Soybean; Black Oak.
Antistress	Parsnip; Parsley; Fenugreek; Mace; Chinese Ginseng; Black Nightshade; Perilla; Carrot; Eleuthero Ginseng; Purslane; Air Potato; Parsley; Indian Snakeroot; Indian Mulberry; Nasturtium; Pokeweed; Garland Chrysanthemum.
Antitumor	Lemon; Indian Snakeroot; Common Thyme; Celery; Two-Flowered Sandspur; Red Clover; Da-Zao; Safflower; Kudzu; Maracuya; Indian Fig; Ramie; Rice Paper Tree; Jack Bean; Copaiba; Evening Primrose; Burn Mouth Vine; Pyrethrum; Desert Date.
Cancer-preventive	Avocado; Safflower; Celery; Khasi Pine; Apricot; Cantaloupe; Common Thyme; Lemon; English Walnut; Marshmallow; Chilgoza Pine; Brazilnut; Karaya; Watermelon; Buffalo Gourd; Indian Snakeroot; Evening Primrose; Cucumber.
Cardiotonic	Tea; Guarana; Chinese Goldthread; Generic Goldthread; Black Pepper; Ouabain; Huang-Lia; Coffee; Goldenseal; Bloodroot; Cacao; Abata Cola; Yoko; Genipap; Mate; Horse Chestnut; Barberry; Ma Huang; Clove; Cayenne.

Activity	Food Sources
Hypoglycemic	Evening Primrose; Tea; Chinese Goldthread; Sanchi Ginseng; Gaurana; Greek Sage; Huang-Lia; Onion; Goldenseal; Physic Nut; Mayapple; Coffee; Oleander; Rosemary; Periwinkle; Tonka Bean; Garlic; Cinnamon; Barberry.
Hypotensive	Indian Snakeroot; Common Thyme; Two-Flowered Sandspur; Parsnip; Red Clover; Da-Zao; Ramie; Camu-camu; Safflower; Kudzu; Maracuya; Indian Fig; Evening Primrose; Burn Mouth Vine; Rice Paper Tree; Jack Bean; Pyrethrum; Desert Date; Flax; Kudzu.
Immunostimulant	Chicory; Gobo; Elecampane; Dandelion; Licorice; Coneflower; Costus; Leopard's-Bane; Crab's Eye; Coffee; Mugwort; Chinese Goldthread; Generic Goldthread; Java-Olive; Huang-Lia; Goldenseal; Beet; Malangra; Lambsquarter.

SMART DRUGS

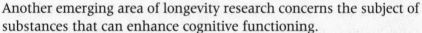

Another emerging area of longevity research concerns the subject of substances that can enhance cognitive functioning.

In their 1990 book, *Smart Drugs & Nutrients: How to Improve Your Memory and Increase Your Intelligence Using the Latest Discoveries in Neuroscience*, Dr. Ward Dean and John Morgethaler described a host of pharmaceuticals—vitamins, herbs, and hormones—that have been found to do just that. Due to the strong interest in their work, the same authors followed up three years later with an updated version under the name *Smart Drugs II*.

Similar material has been published that focuses more broadly on life extension. Smart drugs generally fall into seven classes: vasodilators, nootropics, neurotransmitter modulators/replacements, nerve growth factors, essential nutrients, aluminum chelators, and miscellaneous substances. The following is a list of some examples, accompanied by brief descriptions.

Adranifil (Olmifon)

Adranifil, a member of the eugregorics class of drugs, acts on parts of the brain responsible for depression and declining alertness associated with aging. In addition to its chief ability, which is to increase alertness, studies have shown adranifil may have direct anti-aging effects on the brain and be of help in the treatment of Alzheimer's disease. Other positive effects that have been reported following adranifil use include improvements in memory, clarity of thought, sleep, fatigue, self-esteem, and attitude.

While such effects resemble those of caffeine, the benefits of adranifil have proven to be much more long-lasting, while not being accompanied by problems of tolerance.

Ideal dosage ranges from two to four tablets per day. Contraindications include epilepsy, kidney or liver damage, pregnancy, tranquilizer or antipsychotic medication use.

Aminoguanidine

Aminoguanidine is a new anti-aging drug that is best used to prevent the aging process rather than as a treatment once the debilitating effects of aging have occurred. Its primary action is to stop the cross-linking of proteins, which leads directly to aging damage that cannot be reversed. This cross-linking process is particularly prevalent in diabetics, as it feeds off glucose.

Aminoguanidine works by linking itself with substances that can cause cross-links, hence keeping cross-links from starting and possibly preventing the onset of such aging-related conditions as senile cataracts, thickening of the arteries, kidney failure, thinning bones, osteoarthritis, and especially skin wrinkles. Cross-linking can alter every protein in the body, resulting in steady deterioration.

Aminoguanidine can interfere with this process, which makes it a promising new anti-aging therapy. The ideal dose is approximately 300 mg twice per day.

Biostim

First used in France fifteen years ago, biostim's chief anti-aging benefit is that of enhancing the immune system as it gradually diminishes over time. Widely used against chronic bronchitis, which is a leading cause of death among hospital patients and a problem that hits the elderly especially hard, biostim is also often used to boost the weakened state of immunity in cancer patients. Studies show that it is capable of fighting off numerous types of infection.

One placebo-controlled study involving three hundred elderly patients found that three months' treatment with biostim significantly reduced the rate of lung infections for up to one year. For prime effects, two biostim tablets should be taken per day for the first eight days of the treatment course, followed by three weeks off. This course should be repeated twice more, with only one tablet per day. Contraindications include any autoimmune diseases; children and pregnant or lactating women should not take biostim.

Bromocriptine

Bromocriptine has been found to improve memory by acting on the dopaminergic system of the brain. Also, it may play an important role in other conditions associated with aging, notably Parkinson's disease and hypertension. In this study, bromocriptine was administered in dosages of from 2.5 mg to 8 mg per day over a period of eight weeks.

Doses of 1.25 to 2.5 mg per day have been shown to be effective in improving sleep patterns, and in improving symptoms associated with restless leg syndrome. Bromocriptine has exhibited anticancer activity in patients with advanced breast cancer, and may be useful in treating depression, as well as low sex drive in males.

Centrophenoxine

Studies show that centrophenoxine can be effective against age-induced brain damage, including stroke. Results of animal trials indicate long-term use of centrophenoxine can decrease lipofuscin in brain and cells; reverse the buildup of mineral potassium in brain cells, attack free radical–induced aging damage, and improve learning ability.

Centrophenoxine has been shown to be effective against mental deterioration and to improve memory in the healthy elderly as well as dementia patients. Contraindications include convulsive disorders; patients with severe high blood pressure and pregnant and lactating women should not take centrophenoxine.

Deaner/DMAE

Deaner was pulled from the U.S. market by the FDA in 1983 under the reasoning that, while safe, it was not effective for its approved purpose, which was the treatment of hyperactive children. The drug is still available in Europe.

Deaner stimulates the central nervous system, and studies suggest it can counter deterioration in cognitive function associated with aging, and help fight fatigue and depression. Exactly how this is achieved is not certain, but researchers have found that deaner raises phosphatidylcholine levels in the brain.

The active factor in deaner, DMAE, is available in other forms and is increasingly used as a nutritional supplement. DMAE has been shown capable of increasing mood, memory and learning capacity, and life span in animal studies.

Ideal deaner dosage varies, with the most common approximating 400 mg per day, beginning with lower levels and working up. DMAE dosages range between 500 mg to 1000 mg per day.

Dilantin

Dilantin (phenytoin or diphenylhydantoin) is approved only for treatment of epilepsy in the U.S. but is perhaps most noted for its effects on depression, as championed by celebrity financier Jack Dreyfus.

Dilantin has been claimed to benefit more than a hundred additional conditions, including the ability to learn, long-term memory, verbal performance, obesity, motion sickness, wound healing, alcoholism, and drug addiction. Animals studies have shown that dilantin can reduce tumor incidence, prolong life span, and prolong reproductive period.

The suggested dose for dilantin ranges between 25 to 50 mg per day in nonepileptics.

Hydergine

Hydergine is available only by prescription in the United States, having been approved by the FDA as a treatment for senile dementia. Generically, hydergine is also known as egroloid mesylates and dihydrogenated ergot alkaloids.

This drug is an extract of ergot, which is a fungus found on rye. Its chief action is that of increasing oxygen to the brain. Hydergine has proven effective in the treatment of Alzheimer's disease. Results of one double-blind, placebo-controlled study found that the long-term administration of ergoloid mesylates had beneficial effects with respect to aging-related symptoms such as tiredness and dizziness and led to improvements in measures of intelligence among healthy, elderly subjects.

A review of twenty-six other studies involving the clinical effects of hydergine on numerous conditions associated with aging showed therapeutic benefits with respect to cognitive dysfunctions, mood depression, and subjective scores of overall well-being. Doses of 12 mg per day significantly enhanced cognitive function in healthy young volunteers.

In stroke patients suffering from mental disturbances, doses of 6 mg per day had beneficial effects. Hydergine has exhibited anti-aging effects in the brains of rats. Oral hydergine produced significant improvements in symptoms of sleep disturbance, agitation, and depression in patients suffering from alcohol-related encephalopathy. Hydergine protected against alcohol-induced effects of aging in mice as well.

In a study of nursing home patients, the administration of hydergine over a period of twenty-four weeks led to significant improvements in symptoms of senile mental deterioration. Doses of 6 mg per day of hydergine taken over a period of twelve weeks led to significant improvements in memory among elderly outpatients suffering from mild memory impairment. Daily intravenous infusion of 3 mg co-dergocrine mesylate ("hydergine") for a fourteen-day period produced significant improvements in symptoms associated with multi-infarct dementia, including cognitive dysfunction, depression, fatigue, and withdrawal in elderly patients. Results of additional animal and human studies point to the potential benefits of hydergine in the treatment of elderly patients suffering from mental impairment. The administration of hydergine/nifedipine (pontuc) had significant anti-hypertensive effects in elderly patients with isolated systolic hypertension. Patients treated with co-dergocrine experienced significant reductions in platelet deposition relative to controls, suggesting it may be useful in preventing mural thrombus formation, transient ischemic attacks, and atherosclerosis. Hydergine taken at doses of 3 to 6 mg per day produced benefits in 55 percent of patients suffering from bronchial asthma, with 25 percent reporting significant improvement. In a study of patients suffering from problems on the cochlear compartment and/or vestibular level that clinically manifested by perceptive hypoacusia, tinnitus, and rotatory vertigo, treatment with hydergine doses of 30 drops three time per day, totaling 4.5 mg/day, over a period between thirty and ninty days led to a global improvement in vertigo symptoms among 93.7 percent of patients. A 57.1 percent improvement was seen in tinnitus symptoms and there was 20 percent improvement with respect to hypoacusia. A single oral dose of 2 mg of hydergine exhibited PRL inhibitory activity and proved effective in treating hyperprolactinemic anovulatory patients. In general, the ideal dose of hydergine is approximately 10 mg per day.

KH3

KH3 is a popular drug the world over due to its chief anti-aging ingredient—procaine. Procaine acts on cell membranes by increasing the rate of oxygen consumption; hence its antioxidant effects.

Studies suggest KH3 may be beneficial with respect to memory and mental focus by increasing blood circulation in the brain. One placebo-controlled study involving elderly subjects found that five months' worth of KH3 treatment significantly improved memory. Three others produced similar results. Patients suffering from hearing loss taking two KH3 capsules per day experienced improvements in hearing and general feelings of well-being.

In a study of fifty elderly patients with high blood pressure, KH3 was able to lower blood pressure and decrease reliance on blood-pressure-lowering drugs. KH3 has improved muscle strength and symptoms of incontinence in healthy elderly subjects as well. A recommended course of treatment consists of one to two capsules of KH3 at breakfast over a period of five months. Children, pregnant and lactating women, and those allergic to procaine should not use KH3.

Nimodipine

Nimodipine is a calcium-channel blocker licensed in the U.S. for treatment of hemorrhagic stroke. Like many smart drugs, the potential benefits of nimodipine far exceed those for which it has been approved by the FDA. Nimodipine increases blood flow to the brain, which makes it a good drug not only for stroke, but for conditions such as epilepsy, anxiety, dementia, and Alzheimer's as well.

An Italian study on the effects of aging on the brain found that the administration of 90 mg per day of nimodipine to elderly patients led to improved mental performance in 70 percent of those taking the drug. Animal studies have produced similar results, while also showing that nimodipine can reduce stress-related illnesses and prevent seizures either induced by ischemia or alcohol and opiate withdrawal.

Contraindications for nimodipine use include other calcium-channel blockers, high doses of dilantin, and pregnancy. Doses range from 60 mg every four hours to treat subarachnoid hemor-rrhage to 90 mg per day for Alzheimer's. In healthy people look-ing to improve cognitive performance, a dose of 30 mg per day is suggested.

Oxiracetam

Oxiracetam is a piracetam analog that animal studies indicate can improve learning and memory. Similar results were obtained with respect to improved memory in a group of elderly patients suf-fering from dementia. Another study of patients suffering from de-mentia found that the administration of 800 mg of oxiracetam twice a day over a period of twelve weeks significantly improved memory and concentration.

When taken together with piracetam at doses of 6000 mg per day over a two-month period by human subjects, oxiracetam pro-duced beneficial results against psychosomatic and neurologic symptoms, and also gave evidence of an ability to reduce platelet aggregation. The best doses of oxiracetam have been shown to range between 1200 to 2400 mg per day.

Permixon

Permixon holds great promise as an alternative to surgery for men suffering from problems of the prostate.

In one study, men with enlarged prostates received 320 mg per day of permixon over a period of thirty days. Results showed sig-nificant improvements relative to controls with respect to symptoms including night urination, pain during urination, urine flow rate, and urine retention following urination.

Piracetam

Piracetam is considered one of the strongest nootropic drugs studied. A large body of research points to its potential as a cognitive enhancer and intelligence booster, which has made it one of the premier smart drugs widely available today. Piracetam has exhibited anti-aging effects in mice with respect to deficits of the central muscarinic cholinergic receptor function, and was shown to improve age-related diminished driving skills by upwards of 80 percent in a study of elderly drivers.

Studies have also proven piracetam effective in the treatment of a host of cognitive disorders and improves cognitive function in general. It increases the flow of information between brain hemispheres, which has been linked to enhanced creativity. Results of one twelve-week trial showed that the administration of either 2.4 or 4.8 g per day of piracetam to elderly psychiatric patients with mild diffuse cerebral impairment led to general improvements, particularly with respect to socialization, cooperation, and alertness. Significant improvements were also found with respect to memory performance and IQ scores.

The intravenous administration of 6 g b.i.d. of piracetam over a period of two weeks led to significant improvements in most cortical areas of Alzheimer's patients. Doses of 9 g per day to a group of twelve Alzheimer's patients and 2.4 g per day in sixteen patients with mild senile dementia led to increases in alertness among patients in both groups. The combined administration of 1600 mg three times daily of piracetam and 400 mg three times daily of pentoxifylline led to improvements in psychointellectual performance in elderly patients suffering from recent onset of slight to moderate mental deterioration. A single dose of 2400 mg of piracetam exhibited antihypoxidotic effects in healthy males.

The combined administration of 200 mg of oral viloxazine and 9 g of oral piracetam per day over a period of three months led to improvements in elderly outpatients suffering from depression. Piracetam proved effective in the treatment of alcoholic patients hospitalized due to acute withdrawal syndrome, and improved brain injury in rats following long-term alcohol exposure and withdrawal.

Another study found that piracetam treatment improved cognitive functions, including short-term memory and concentration, in alcoholic patients suffering from organic mental disorder. Several studies have indicated that piracetam may be helpful for dyslexics. In one, doses of 3300 mg per day taken over a period of twelve weeks significantly increased reading speed and number of words written in a timed period among a group of dyslexic boys between the ages of eight and thirteen. Dyslexic children between the ages of seven and a half and thirteen years old who were treated with piracetam experienced significantly improved reading ability and comprehension scores relative to controls.

Another study followed sixteen dyslexic children through adulthood and then compared them to fourteen healthy students during a twenty-one-day period of piracetam treatment. Results showed significant increases in verbal learning among dyslexics (15 percent) and students (8.6 percent).

Mycoclonus patients treated with 8–9 g per day of oral piracetam experienced significant benefits with no side effects. The administration of up to 10 g per day of piracetam to three patients suffering from progressive myoclonus epilepsy led to the elimination of photoparoxysmal responses in each. In a study of sixty myoclonus patients treated with piracetam, results showed the drug to be effective with respect to gait ataxia, handwriting, motivation, sleep trouble, attention deficit, depression, and convulsions.

A pilot study found that piracetam proved extremely effective with respect to the pursuit of tracking among five of five vertigo patients receiving the drug. Piracetam coupled with ergotoxin proved significantly effective in alleviating symptoms associated with vertigo in vertigo patients and those suffering from related symptoms. The combination of piracetam and dihydroergocristine in fifty-five vertiginous patients administered over a period of three months had beneficial effects.

Results of another double-blind, placebo-controlled study showed that piracetam significantly reduced symptoms associated with vertigo in patients suffering from the condition. The administration of piracetam had beneficial effects with respect to clinical improvement of acute circulatory insufficiency and an analgesic effect in myocardial infarct patients. Piracetam proved effective in controlling spasticity in eight of sixteen cerebral palsy patients. Intravenous doses of 30 mg/kg bw (ten–twelve injections per course) of piracetam had beneficial immune enhancing effects on patients suffering from chronic bronchitis. The intravenous administration of 10 g per day of piracetam diluted in a 250-ml saline solution over a period of three days led to improvements in six out of nine patients suffering from sudden hearing loss.

Piracetam can prevent the onset of neuropathic pain syndrome, and improve visuomotor reaction time and accuracy in Parkinson's patients. The administration of 4800 mg per day of piracetam over a period of eight weeks to patients with postconcussional syndrome significantly reduced symptoms associated with the condition, including fatigue, sweating, vertigo, headache, reduced alertness, and intense sweating. Doses of 8 g per day of piracetam proved beneficial in the treatment of patients suffering from primary as well as secondary Raynaud's syndrome. Piracetam can be helpful against sickle cell disease. It has exhibited antiulcer activity in rats.

Treatment with piracetam had beneficial effects on the depth of consciousness and psychic function in patients suffering from acute viral neuroinfections. One hundred brain tumor patients administered piracetam were able to maintain near normal consciousness postoperatively to a degree significantly greater than controls.

Piracetam has exhibited antihypoxic effects in that it inhibited free-radical lipid peroxidation, retarded the consumption of oxygen in liver mitochondria and enhanced hemoglobin oxygen-binding properties. Other conditions for which the drug has shown promise include burns, diabetes, hypoxia, stroke, goiter, sleep disturbance, cardiovascular disease, stress, mental fatigue, and epilepsy. Suggested doses can go as high 4,800 mg per day split into three separate doses. Like all pharmaceutical drugs, piracetam has side effects. You must consult your physician to weigh the benefits against the side effects before using it.

Pyroglutamate (PCA)

Pyroglutamate is an amino acid found in fruits, vegetables, meat, and dairy products that studies indicate may be a powerful booster of cognitive ability. Results of animal studies show pyroglutamate can improve learning and memory, as well as produce anti-anxiety effects.

Additional human studies have shown pyroglutamate can be helpful against alcohol-induced memory loss, in patients suffering from multi-infarct dementia, and in elderly patients with verbal memory decline. Pyroglutamate has been used successfully against alcoholism, senility, and mental retardation in Italy. The recommended dose for pyroglutamate ranges between 500 to 1000 mg per day.

Rulid (Roxithromycin)

Rulid, a powerful antibiotic developed in France, has been used to treat a variety of infections, including those of the lungs (including pneumonia and bronchitis); ear, nose, and throat; urinary tract; skin; genitals, etc.

The suggested doses of Rulid is 150 mg taken twice per day before meals over a period not to exceed ten days.

Vasopressin

Vasopressin is a peptide hormone stimulated by acetylcholine that is intricately involved in the process of memory and has shown high promise in the treatment of memory loss and learning problems when taken synthetically as a supplement

The only form of vasopressin that is presently available in the U.S. is diapid, a nasal spray used to treat excessive urination in diabetics.

Vincamine

An extract of periwinkle, vincamine works by increasing blood flow to and enhancing oxygen usage by the brain.

It has been used against a host of different conditions, including depression, memory loss, high blood pressure, vertigo, poor mental focus, and hearing problems. Studies also indicate it may be effective against alcohol-induced brain damage and in patients suffering from Alzheimer's. Suggested dosage is 30 mg taken every twelve hours.

Vinpocetine

Vinpocetine is a smart drug that works primarily by enhancing the utilization of oxygen by and increasing blood flow to the brain. Due to these effects, it has been shown to significantly improve memory in healthy subjects.

Results of another study involving 800 patients with various eye problems showed a 71 percent rate of improvement. Vinpocetine proved most effective against dry macular degeneration. It is also capable of improving blood flow to the inner ear and has thus been used effectively against such problems as cochleovestibiluar neuritis and presbyacusis. Viopocetine can alleviate symptoms associated with menopause as well. Suggested dosage is one to two 5mg tablets taken three times daily.

See also the reports on acetyl-l-arnitine, choline, deprenyl, DHEA, ginkgo biloba, ginseng, melatonin, and phosphatidylserine in the sections on nutrients and herbs.

NUTRIENTS

❖

The verdict is in on the case for nutrition as a life extender. The sheer volume of peer review studies supporting the link between diet and good health is clear and convincing evidence for those willing to take the time to look.

Data continues to support the use of supplements as well. The days when anyone could seriously question the value of things like vitamin C are over. The more important issue now and for the future is to specifically determine which nutrients do what, and at what doses. The material that follows is based on the most up-to-date information available.

Acetyl-L-carnitine

Acetyl-L-carnitine (ALC) is a powerful anti-aging nutrient that studies increasingly show can benefit patients suffering from a host of aging-related conditions.

Specific to the aging process itself, ALC at doses of 1500 mg to 2 g per day administered to elderly patients with mild mental impairments proved to be beneficial against cognitive and emotional-affective mental impairment. Supplemental ALC has improved diminished walking capacity in the elderly. Numerous other animal studies point to similar direct anti-aging effects of ALC.

No disease is more associated with the negative effects of aging than Alzheimer's. ALC has been found to be particularly beneficial to patients suffering from this condition. In one study, 2.5 g per day of acetyl levocarnitine hypochloride administered for three months, followed by 3 g for three months on mild to moderately demented Alzheimer's patients showed those receiving the treatment experienced significantly less deterioration in timed cancellation tasks and digit span.

In another, 2 g of acetyl-L-carnitine per day for twenty-four weeks had beneficial short-term memory effects on patients with Alzheimer's-type dementia. ALC has proven to be effective against dementia in non-Alzheimer's patients as well.

Loss of neurological function and control is a common problem associated with aging. The administration of either 1 or 2 g per day for seven days of acetyl-L-carnitine has led to improvements in H response, sleep stages, and spindling activity in Parkinson's disease patients. Doses of 3 g per day coupled with 50 mg of methylprednis-olone for two weeks led to significant functional recovery of the nerves in patients suffering from idiopathic facial paralysis.

Animals studies point to ALC's capacity to improve neurological function as well.

Evidence exists suggesting ALC may possess anticancer activity. The same is true with heart disease. One study found that 3 mg per day of acetyl-L-carnitine administered intravenously to five patients undergoing aortic reconstructive surgery prior to ischemia induction had positive effects on the amelioration of human skeletal muscle damage induced by ischemia-reperfusion. A number of animal stud-ies also point to the usefulness of ALC in treating diabetes.

Stroke victims have also benefited from supplemental ALC. Re-sults from one study showed that acetyl-L-carnitine had significant positive effects on memory and cognitive performance tasks in el-derly patients with cerebrovascular insufficiency. Intravenous ad-ministration of 1.5 g of acetyl-L-carnitine led to improvements in cerebral blood flow in cerebrovasular disease patients who had suf-fered from a stroke at least six months prior to treatment. Another study showed that intravenous administration of 1500 mg of acetyl-L-carnitine had beneficial effects on four out of ten patients suffer-ing from brain ischemia.

Other conditions ALC holds promise for include depression, chronic fatigue syndrome, AIDS, cognitive dysfunction associated with alcoholism, amenorrhea, and Down's syndrome.

With respect to depression, the administration of 3 g per day of acetyl-L-carnitine for thirty–sixty days significantly reduced the severity of symptoms in senile patients between the ages of sixty and eighty. Supplementation with 1500 mg per day of acetyl-L-carnitine led to significant improvements in patients between the ages of seventy and eighty suffering from symptoms of depression.

Another study showed the administration of acetyl-L-carnitine to be significantly effective relative to controls in reducing depressive symptoms among elderly patients hospitalized for depression.

Suggested doses of acetyl-L-carnitine range from 1000 to 2000 mg per day.

Acidophilus

Lactobacillus acidophilus is a fermented bacteria found in the vagina, mouth, and small intestine, and is directly involved in the digestion of milk sugar. Colon cancer patients administered Lactobacillus acidophilus fermented milk have experienced a significant increase in numbers of intestinal lactobacilli and dietary calcium intake, while also showing decreasing trends in levels of both soluble faecal bile acids and faecal bacterial enzymes, both being colon cancer risk factors.

Results of *in vitro* studies have found that lactobacilli and other lactic acid bacteria can absorb cooked food mutagens. Human studies have demonstrated that Lactobacillus acidophilus consumption can significantly reduce mutagen excretion following fried meat consumption. Multibacterial combinations of Lactobacillus acidophilus (10(9)) and Bifidobacterium bifidum (10(9)) administered to elderly patients with bowel disorders have proven effective with respect to restoration of duodenal bacterial flora and subsidence of clinical symptoms.

Another study concluded that the administration of six capsules of live lyophilized Lactobacillus acidophilus (10(9) CFU/ml) per day produced significant relief of symptoms in elderly patients suffering from bowel disorders involving symptoms of diarrhea, abdominal pain, and meteorism.

In postmenopausal women, local treatment with vaginal tablets containing 0.03 mg of estriol provided total restoration of the vaginal environment while simultaneous implantation of Lactobacillus acidophilus restored an acid vaginal milieu. Studies also show it can be highly beneficial in patients suffering from vaginitis. Lactobacillus acidophilus has exhibited immune enhancing, cardioprotective and anticancer effects in animals studies.

Alpha-carotene

When combined with other natural carotenoids, alpha-carotene has been shown to inhibit the formation of colon cancer in rats.

Another study concluded that alpha-carotene obtained from palm oil was even more effective than beta-carotene in preventing the onset of liver and lung cancer in mice.

Alpha-carotene has been shown to be up to ten times more effective than beta-carotene in inhibiting the proliferation of human cancer cells *in vitro*. It has exhibited chemopreventive effects against oil-induced skin tumors in mice as well.

Alpha-Lipoic Acid

Alpha-lipoic acid is an important antioxidant that has been shown to boost the power of other antioxidants as well, including glutathione and vitamin E. Results from numerous studies point to the efficacy of alpha-lipoic acid in the treatment of diabetes.

In one, the administration of 600 mg of alpha-lipoic acid over a period of three months led to improvements in symptoms of distal symmetric neuropathy in patients suffering from long-term diabetic late syndrome. Another showed that 1000 mg of alpha-lipoic acid significantly increased insulin, stimulating glucose disposal in NIDDM patients. Intravenous administration of 600 mg per day of alpha-lipoic acid over a period of three weeks reduced symptoms associated with diabetic peripheral neuropathy in NIDDM patients. Patients suffering from diabetic neuropathy have also improved following the oral intake of alpha-lipoic acid at doses of either 2×50 mg or 2×100 mg per day.

Additional studies suggest alpha-lipoic acid may have benefits for stroke victims, protect against cardiac ischemia/reperfusion injury, prevent cataracts, help prevent cancer, and improve memory. Doses of 0.15 g per day of lipoic acid for one month have had positive effects in patients with stages I and II open-angle glaucoma. It has also exhibited anti-HIV activity both *in vitro* and *in visto*.

Ascorbyl Palmitate

Ascorbyl palmitate is a lipid soluble derivative of ascorbic acid that studies have shown can significantly inhibit colon cancer in rats.

Betaine

Results from a host of studies indicate that betaine is capable of exhibiting anticonvulsive activity, osmoprotective effects, protecting rats against alcohol-induced liver damage, useful in the treatment of homocystinuria and neurological impairment.

BHT

A common antioxidant food additive to prevent spoilage in packaging, BHT (butylated hydroxytoluene) has been shown to extend life span in mice and has exhibited superoxide scavenger (anti-aging) effects *in vitro*. Studies have indicated, however, that some people may have adverse reactions to BHT when used as an additive.

Bifidus

Bifidus (bifidobacterium bifidum) are abundant in the large intestine, and can also be found in lower levels in the smaller intestine and vagina. Proper digestion and absorption of nutrients plays a critical role in the aging process

These bacteria are believed to decline with age, and thus supplemental use of bifidus may be directly involved with aging in this respect. A host of peer review studies support the use of bifidus in the treatment of bowel and gastric disorders, including ulcer and diarrhea, which can often disrupt digestion and lead to larger health problems.

Bifidus may be effective in preventing the risk of cancer and also helps to strengthen the immune system. In one controlled study involving twelve healthy subjects, researchers found that 500 ml per day of Bifodium longum–enriched yogurt and 5 g of lactulose/L led to stability of the human fecal flora, a marker for colon cancer risk.

Another study concluded that bifidobacterium bifidus proved to be useful in the treatment of women suffering from epithelial cancer. Animal experiments have demonstrated bifidus can inhibit the development of liver, colon, and mammary tumors. Bifidus has also exhibited anti-cancer activity *in vitro*. With respect to immune enhancement, the regular intake of Bifidobacterium bifidum and Lactobacillus acidophilus has been proven to modulate immunological and inflammatory responses in human subjects. Similar findings have been obtained in studies involving mice.

Biotin

A B-complex vitamin, regular use of biotin has been linked to improvements in patients suffering from diabetes, and can help counter the problem of brittle nails often associated with aging. In diabetic patients experiencing symptoms of peripheral neuropathy, high doses of biotin administered over a period of one to two years led to improvements within four to eight weeks of the start of treatment. Animal experiments have shown that biotin can improve glucose and insulin tolerance as well as reduce hepatic phosphoenolpyruvate carboxykinase in diabetic mice. Biotin has also been linked to improvements in nondiabetic patients suffering from different neurological disorders.

Daily biotin supplementation over a period of six months has been proven effective in treating brittle nails. One case study reported on a young women with adult-onset myoclonus, ataxia, hearing loss, seizures, hemianopia, and hemiparesis who was treated with large doses of biotin and showed favorable results. Biotin has also improved skin conditions in dogs.

Borage Oil

Borage oil can be beneficial in the treatment of patients suffering from atopic dermatitis and has been shown to help reduce blood pressure in hypertensive rats.

Boron

Boron is a trace mineral that is primarily obtained through fruits and vegetables. Daily intake of 6 mg per day of boron has been shown to produce significant improvement in patients suffering from arthritis. Boron supplementation can also enhance cognitive performance and brain function, and has exhibited anti-HIV protease activity.

Calcium

The role of calcium in both the prevention and treatment of osteoporosis is well documented in the scientific literature. Results of one double-blind, placebo-controlled study that examined the effects of 1000 mg per day of calcium in combination with 50,000 IU per week of vitamin D on the effects of corticosteroid-induced osteoporosis showed treatment could help prevent early bone loss in the spine of such subjects.

Another looked at the effects of increased exercise and dietary calcium in women who had been postmenopausal for longer than ten years. Results showed that calcium supplementation in the form of either 1 g per night in tablets or 1 g per night in milk powder led to bone loss cessation over a period of two years. Such effects were increased when combined with exercise. Calcium supplementation can improve the bone mass of postmenopausal women using estrogen replacement therapy and with a low intake of dietary intake calcium.

Findings from a three-year study showed that supplementation with 1.2 g of calcium and 800 IU of vitamin D_3 reduced the number of hip fractures and other nonvertebral fractures among ambulatory women living in nursing homes by 23 percent.

In addition to its role in countering the problems associated with bone loss, high calcium intake may be effective in the treatment of such unrelated diseases as arterial hypertension, nephrolithiasis, colon cancer, etc.

Choline

Supplemental choline alfoscerate treatment is capable of counteracting various anatomical changes of the rat hippocampus associated with aging. Additional animal studies point to its cardioprotective activity, potential benefits for stroke victims, and positive effects on memory.

In humans, choline has also been shown to improve symptoms associated with stroke when administered at intravenous doses of 1000 mg per day over a period of two weeks. Elderly patients have reported relief from a host of neurological conditions such as dizziness, cephalea, insomnia, depression, and poor memory following supplementation with a 6-ml-per-day dose.

Head injury patients have experienced benefits from choline, as have those suffering from hemiplegia, hepatic steatosis, and seizures. Tarkive dyskinesia is another disorder where choline treatment has proven highly effective, with dosage ranging from approximately 500 to 1200 mg per day.

Chromium

Chromium is an important micronutrient that has been reported capable of dramatically increasing the life span of rodents. In humans, chromium is most noted for its beneficial effects in patients suffering from diabetes. One review article of fifteen controlled studies on the relationship between supplemental chromium compounds and impaired glucose tolerance found a pattern of improvement in efficiency of insulin or the blood lipid profile of subjects treated with chromium.

Another study concluded that the administration of 200 micrograms of chromium in healthy subjects significantly reduced ninety-minute glucose concentrations and fasting glucose concentrations. Doses of 200 micrograms of chromium alleviated hypoglycemic symptoms and significantly increased minimum serum glucose levels seen two to four hours after a glucose load in female hypoglycemic patients. Significant improvements in insulin binding to red blood cells and insulin receptor number were seen as well.

In elderly patients, oral glucose tolerance curves decreased from 60 to 120 minutes with the 60-minute values being significantly reduced following supplementation over a period of twelve weeks. Patients with clinical symptoms of hypoglycemia have shown a reduced negative part of the glucose tolerance curve and improvements in chilliness, trembling, emotional instability, and disorientation following treatment with 125 micrograms of chromium per day for three months.

Supplemental chromium picolinate administered for two months produced a significant reduction in serum triglycerides in patients suffering from noninsulin dependent diabetes. Chromium has exhibited similar antidiabetic acivity in studies involving rats.

Heart disease is another area where chromium has shown positive effects. Results of one double-blind, placebo-controlled study showed that atherosclerosis patients treated with 250 micrograms of chromium for seven to sixteen months experienced lower serum triglycerides relative to controls. Supplementation with 600 mcg per day of chromium over a period of two months has produced beneficial increases in HDL cholesterol levels among men on beta-blockers. Doses of 200 micrograms of chromium chloride and 100 mg of nicotinic acid per day over a period of several months can reduce serum cholesterol levels.

Treatment of Turner's syndrome patients with 30 g of brewer's yeast containing 50 micgrograms of chromium per day for eight weeks produced a reduction in cholesterol and/or triglyceride levels and an increase in high-density lipoprotein cholesterol as well.

Citrus Bioflavonoids

Studies indicate that citrus bioflavonoids such as nobiletin and tangeretin are likely involved in cancer chemoprevention.

Cod Liver Oil

Numerous studies have pointed to the benefits of cod liver oil in the prevention of heart disease. In one Norwegian trial, healthy men who received 20 ml per day for three weeks exhibited beneficial effects with respect to serum lipids and platelets, which can decrease the tendency to thrombosis.

Another study found that the daily administration of 25 ml of cod liver oil for eight weeks in healthy subjects significantly reduced mean thromboxane B_2 levels in both men and women.

Cod liver oil administered over a period of six weeks has also been shown to significantly reduce neutrophil chemotaxis toward both chemoattractants and monocyte chemotaxis toward N-FMLP in healthy men. In addition to its benefits concerning the heart, supplemental cod liver oil may help alleviate musculoskeletal pain in patients suffering from musculoskeletal disease as well.

Coenzyme Q_{10}

Coenzyme Q_{10} is an important part of the metabolic process. It is involved in the energy process and can be synthesized in the body. Studies show that CoQ_{10} holds major promise in the treatment of a wide variety of degenerative diseases, including AIDS, diabetes, stroke, cancer, and especially heart disease.

One study examined the effects of 150 mg per of CoQ_{10} for four weeks on exercise performance in middle-aged, stable angina pectoris patients. Results indicated CoQ_{10} to be an effective and safe treatment. Another study determined that 30–60 mg per day of CoQ_{10} administered orally for six days preoperatively significantly increased heart tolerance to ischemia during aortic clamping.

Elective coronary artery bypass patients pretreated with 150 mg per day of CoQ_{10} for seven days prior to surgery showed a significantly lower incidence of ventricular arrhythmias during the recovery period than controls. Patients pretreated with CoQ_{10} in another study had less left arterial pressure, a decreased incidence of low cardiac output, a wider pulse pressure, and a better preserved right and left ventricular myocardial ultrastructure relative to controls.

One patient with mitochondrial encephalomyopathy and cyto-chrome-c oxidase deficiency who took high doses of CoQ_{10} for two years experienced a decrease in abnormal elevation of the serum lactate per pyruvate ratio and the increased concentration of serum lactate plus pyruvate induced by exercise. Results also showed that CoQ_{10} improved impaired central and peripheral nerve conductivities. Pretreatment with 5 mg/kg administered intravenously of CoQ_{10} was effective in the prevention of left ventricular depression in early reperfusion and in minimizing myocardial cellular injury during coronary artery bypass grafting followed by reperfusion.

Patients suffering from symptoms commonly preceding congestive heart failure showed that the administration of CoQ_{10} led to improvement in all patients, high blood pressure reduction in 80 percent, improved diastolic function in all; reduction in myocardial thickness in 53 percent of hypertensives and 36 percent of the combined prolapse and fatigue syndrome groups; and reduction in fractional shortening in those high at control and an increase in those initially low.

Intake of 2 mg/kg per day of CoQ_{10} coupled with conventional therapy in chronic congestive heart failure patients significantly decreased hospitalization rates for heart failure worsening and complication incidence. The administration of 50 mg per day of CoQ_{10} for four weeks combined with conventional therapy led to improvements in dyspnea at rest, exertional dyspnea, palpitation, cyanosis, hepatomegaly, pulmonary rates, ankle edema, heart rate, and both systolic and diastolic blood pressure in patients with chronic heart failure. CoQ_{10} administered in doses of 60 mg per day for two months reduced blood viscosity in patients with ischemic heart disease.

Another study examined the effects of 100 mg per day of CoQ_{10} for two months on dilated cardiomyopathy patients and found that CoQ_{10} deficiency could be reversed through supplementation, and that CoQ_{10} treatment may be effective when coupled with conventional treatment in patients with chronic cardiac failure.

Doses of 100 mg of CoQ_{10} per day administered orally can be an effective treatment for chronic cardiomyopathy and advanced chronic heart failure. When CoQ_{10} was administered to nineteen chronic myocardial disease patients, results showed that eighteen experienced improved activity tolerance with replacement therapy and also found significant improvements among patients in stroke volume measured by impedance cardiography, and ejection fractions calculated from systolic time intervals.

The administration of 3.0–3.4 mg per day (average) of CoQ_{10} was effective against cardiac dysfunction in patients with mitral valve prolapse and improved stress-induced cardiac dysfunction. Results of many animal studies support the role of CoQ_{10} in the prevention and treatment of heart disease.

In the case of cancer, one review article has noted 390 mg per day of CoQ_{10} proved effective in three breast cancer patients monitored over a three- to five-year period. Another study of breast cancer patients treated with 90 mg of CoQ_{10}, in addition to other antioxidants and fatty acids, showed partial tumor regression. CoQ_{10} administered intravenously at doses of 1 mg/kg per day have prevented adriamycin and dauborubicin-induced side effects in malignant lymphoma patients, including alopecia, fever, nausea and vomiting, diarrhea, and stomatitis. Results from animal studies point to the anticancer effects of CoQ_{10} as well.

In addition to the conditions already noted, CoQ_{10} can boost immune response when administered alone or in combination with vitamin B_6. The administration of 120 to 150 mg of CoQ_{10} per day has led to an improvement in abnormal metabolism of pyruvate and NADH oxidation in the skeletal muscle of Kearns-Sayre Syndrome patients. CoQ_{10} also decreased the concentration of CSF protein and CSF lactate/pyruvate ratio, while improvements were seen in neurologic symptoms and ECG abnormalities as well. Pretreatment with CoQ_{10} can inhibit liver damage in mice.

Chronic lung disease patients have experienced positive results following the oral administration of 90 mg per day of CoQ_{10} for eight weeks. Animal studies also indicate CoQ_{10} can be effective in the treatment of hearing loss and muscle injury.

Conjugated Linoleic Acid

Studies indicate that linoleic acid may hold promise for patients suffering from multiple sclerosis. The anticancer activity of conjugated linoleic acid has been well established both *in vitro* and from results of animal studies involving rats and mice. In addition, it has significantly reduced LDL cholesterol and triglyceride levels in rabbits.

Deprenyl

Deprenyl works on the brain by enhancing activity in the dopa-mine-rich region known as the substantia nigra. The drug was first introduced by a Hungarian researcher as an alternative to L-dopa treatment for Parkinson's due to the debilitating side effects some-times associated with L-dopa. Following years of positive study re-sults, recent large-scale British research, however, has raised serious questions about the efficacy and safety of deprenyl itself when com-bined with L-dopa.

The earlier work on deprenyl and Parkinson's did find the drug to be effective in many cases. For example, the intake of 10 mg per day of deprenyl delayed the onset of disability associated with early, untreated Parkinson's disease in study.

In another, the same dose prolonged the beneficial effects of levodopa and was effective against mild "on-off" disabilities in pa-tients suffering from idiopathic Parkinson's disease. Twelve months of treatment with 10 mg per day by patients suffering from mild stages of Parkinson's disease cut the risk of further progression to a stage requiring L-dopa therapy by half. The administration of 5 mg per day of deprenyl for a period of four weeks reduced dependence on levodopa in Parkinson's patients.

A study involving forty-eight patients with Parkinson's disease found that the addition of deprenyl to previous levodopa plus decar-boxylase-inhibitor therapy proved beneficial with respect to mild on-off phenomena and end-of-dose akinesia. The administration of 5–10 mg of deprenyl over a period of one to three months signifi-cantly decreased L-dopa–induced fluctuations in disease severity in twenty-six of forty-five Parkinson's patients studied. Early adminis-tration of 10 mg per day of deprenyl delayed the need for L-dopa therapy and disease progression in patients suffering from Parkin-son's disease. The administration of 5 mg b.i.d of deprenyl over a period of six weeks exhibited moderately beneficial effects in Par-kinson's patients with symptoms fluctuations. Doses of 5 to10 mg of deprenyl cut the need for levedopa by 20–50 percent in patients suffering from Parkinson's disease. Doses of 20 mg per day had sig-nificant beneficial effects in patients suffering from idiopathic Par-kinson's disease and reduced their dependence on L-dopa by an average of 30 percent. The addition of deprenyl to normal Madopar therapy led to improvements of disability, prolongation of life expectancy, and a reduction of Madopar-induced side effects in patients suffering from Parkinson's disease. While opinion is now mixed in light of the new findings from more long-term follow-up trials, many researchers still believe deprenyl can be an effective therapy for Parkinson's, but at much lower doses, perhaps no higher than 10 mg per week rather than per day, and alone rather than in combination with L-dopa.

In addition to its use with Parkinson's patients, deprenyl has been the subject of a fair amount of studies in other areas related to aging as well. Results have indicated that it can significantly prolong the life span, enhance cognitive function, prevent oxidative damage, and reduce the expression of some microantomical changes of the brain in aging rats. It can also improve spatial memory in aged dogs. Deprenyl has exhibited good results in studies on Alzheimer's disease.

Results of one indicated that the addition of 5 mg b.i.d of oral l-deprenyl to the normal treatment of Alzheimer's patients taking tacrine or physostigmine over a period of four weeks led to significant improvement. Another found that the administration of l-deprenyl over a period of six months led to significant improvements of memory and learning skills in patients suffering from Alzheimer's. Doses of 10 mg per day of l-deprenyl over a period of six months led to significant improvements of cognitive function in patients suffering from dementia of the Alzheimer's type. Three to six months treatment with (-)deprenyl produced significant improvements in elderly females patients suffering from senile dementia of Alzheimer type. Intake of 10 mg per day significantly improved episodic memory, sustained consciousness, and performance on complex learning tasks in patients also suffering from dementia of the Alzheimer's type. Deprenyl exhibited long-lasting aphrodisiac effects on male rats. It can also significantly reduce the incidence of mammary and pituitary tumors in rats.

The administration of 20 mg per day of l-deprenyl or greater over a period of six weeks had beneficial effects in patients suffering from atypical depression. Doses of 30 mg per day or more of (-)-deprenyl for a minimum of six weeks exhibited superior antidepressant effects in depressed outpatients relative to controls. The combination of 5–10 mg per day of l-deprenyl and 250 mg per day of l-phenylalanine administered either orally or intravenously to patients suffering from unipolar depression showed beneficial antidepressive effects in 90 percent of outpatients and 80.5 percent of inpatients. L-deprenyl exhibited anticonvulsant effects against different kinds of seizure in mice, suggesting it may be effective in the treatment of epilepsy. The combined administration of fluoxetine and l-deprenyl proved effective in the case of a nineteen-year-old female Hunting-ton's disease patient who experienced significant affective, behav-ioral, and motoric improvements following treatment. L-deprenyl is useful as a prophylactic treatment for brain tissue in rats when administered prior to hypoxia/ischemia. An average daily dose of 8.1 mg of deprenyl taken over a period of approximately seven months was an effective, side-effect-free treatment for attention deficit asso-ciated with Tourette's syndrome in children ranging in age from six- to eighteen years old. The intraperitoneal and intracerebroventricu-lar administration of l-deprenyl also significantly attenuated re-straint stress-induced gastric ulcers in rats.

Suggested dosage for deprenyl varies according to age, but the approximate range falls between 5 to 10 mg per day.

DHEA

DHEA (dehydroepiandrosterone) is a steroid hormone produced by the adrenal glands that has been linked directly to the aging process, as well as numerous conditions associated with it. The amount of DHEA in the body steadily declines over time, which has prompted many researchers to suggest that DHEA levels should be considered a biomarker for aging.

Studies involving older individuals indicate that DHEA pos-sesses beneficial effects with respect to muscle strength, immune function, and overall quality of life. One placebo-controlled cross-over trial gave nightly doses of DHEA at 50 mg to thirteen men and seventeen women between forty and seventy years of age over a six-month period. DHEA and DHEA sulfate serum levels were restored to those found in young adults within two weeks of the DHEA re-placement and were sustained throughout the three months of the study. There was a two-fold increase in serum levels of androgens (androstenedione, testosterone, and dehydrotestosterone) with only a small rise in adrostenedione in men. Insulinlike growth factor-1 decreased significantly, and insulin growth factor binding protein-1 decreased significantly for both genders. This was associated with a remarkable increase in physical and psychological well-being for the majority of men and women with change in libido. Significantly lower levels of serum DHEA-S have been found in elderly Japanese patients suffering from Alzheimer's and/or cerebrovascular dementia relative to age-matched healthy controls. DHEA can be effective against amnesia associated with dementia, and in maintaining the function of neuronal cells that may reduce progress toward Alzheimer's.

Results of a double-blind, placebo-controlled study examining the effects of a 500-mg oral dose of DHEA on the sleep stages, sleep stage–specific electroencephalogram (EEG) power spectra, and concurrent hormone secretion in ten healthy young male subjects showed that DHEA significantly increased REM sleep relative to controls, with no changes seen in the other sleep variables. Previous studies have shown REM sleep to be involved in memory storage; thus these findings point to a benefit of DHEA in age-related dementia. The administration of 30–90 mg of DHEA per day over a period of four weeks led to significant improvements in middle-aged and elderly patients suffering from symptoms of depression and impaired memory performance.

Another study showed a positive correlation between DHEA levels and improvements in depressive symptoms among patients suffering from unipolar depression. DHEA has also improved memory in mice.

Inverse associations have been noted between DHEA levels and death from any cause, particularly death from cardiovascular disease in men over age fifty. DHEA has exhibited anticancer activity in rats and mice. High doses have shown modest reductions on viral load in patients infected with HIV. An inverse association between DHEA levels and increased HIV progression was seen in a study of patients with CD4 counts below 300. Supplemental DHEA to levels greater than 400 mg/dl increased survival in such patients. The administration of DHEA at doses of 300–600 mg p.o. b.i.d. for twenty-eight days, following a thirty-day washout period of antivirals, significantly decreased viral load in HIV-positive patients with CD4 counts above 50 and below 300. An average oral dose of 75 mg qd of DHEA coupled with standard antiviral treatment given to patients infected with HIV led to significant increases in CD4 and CD8 counts. DHEA can inhibit *in vitro* HIV replication, and it has been shown that high-risk homosexual males who were HIV-negative had significantly higher DHEA levels than age-matched HIV-positive males. DHEA reduced the number of lupus flares in a study of fifty patients when taken over a three–twelve month period. DHEA had therapeutic effects on diabetic mice by producing a rapid remission of hyperglycemia, a preservation of beta-cell structure and function, and an increased insulin sensitivity as measured by glucose tolerance tests. Treatment with DHEA effectively countered defects in influenza immunity associated with aging in older mice.

DHEA has exhibited anti-obesity effects in mice, and can modify food selection in rats leading them to consume diets low in fat. DHEA taken four times daily led to a substantially mean body fat reduction of 31 percent after twenty-eight days. No changes occurred in overall weight, and LDL levels also fell by 7.5 percent. DHEA can stimulate the activity of T-cells, B-cells, and macrophages, thus strengthening the immune system. In a study of mice infected with encephalitis, DHEA was able to significantly slow the rate of disease onset and mortality. Topical use of DHEA has proven effective in restoring immune function in burned mice. DHEA can significantly reduced the risk of atherosclerosis in rabbits. Low DHEA levels have been associated with the risk of acute heart attacks, coronary heart disease, and myocardial infarction. DHEA has been found to benefit symptoms associated with menopause and lupus, and enhance the efficacy of vaccination against influenza in the elderly as well.

Common DHEA doses range from 50 to 2500 mg per day. Contraindications include prostate cancer and benign prostatic hypertrophy.

Folic Acid

Folic acid (vitamin B_4) deficiency is a common vitamin deficiency around the world and has been linked to osteoporosis. When administered at weekly doses of either 5 mg or 27.5 mg folic acid can protect against methotrexate toxicity in rheumatoid arthritis patients without effecting the efficacy of the drug. Studies also indicate folic acid at daily doses of either 2.5 mg or 10 mg over a six-week period can reduce normal and increase plasma homocysteine concentrations in myocardial infarction patients. The administration of 250 mg per day of vitamin B_6 and 5 mg of folic acid for six weeks normalized homocysteine metabolism in young patients with arterial occlusive disease. Reductions in the risk of cardiovascular disease in patients with chronic renal insufficiency have been reported following the administration of 5 mg of folic acid per day for an average of fifteen days. Dialysis patients administered 300 mg of pyridoxine and 5 mg of folic acid per day have experienced a reduction in the risk of cardiovascular disease as well. Supplemental folic acid has also produced positive results in patients suffering myelopathy associated with macrotic anemia, in cervical dysplasia patients when taken at 10 mg per day for three months, in patients suffering from gingivital inflammations at doses of 4 mg per day for one month, those with chronic renal failure at 10 mg per day for three months, and in multiple sclerosis patients at doses of 200–300 mcg per day. Doses of 400 mcg every other day for sixteen weeks had positive effects on zinc homeostasis in men. Animal studies suggest folic acid may also be beneficial in the fight against cancer.

Daily intake of 6400 micrograms of folate plus 20 micrograms cobalamin over a period of two months has produced beneficial effects in patients with idiopathic osteoarthritis. When combined with vitamin B_{12}, folate has been shown to reduce cellular atypia squamous metaplasia in heavy smokers over a period of one year.

Other studies indicate supplemental folate may be helpful in the treatment of various behavioral disorders associated with aging. Folate levels in the brain are believed to decrease with time, leading researchers to suggest that folate therapy could reverse symptoms related to declining cognitive performance and mood status. Additionally, an inverse correlation between serum folate levels and the risk of fatal coronary heart disease has been documented in studies involving both men and women.

Glutathione

Glutathione is made up of glutamic acid, glycine, and cysteine—all three amino acids. Significant positive associations have been shown between blood glutathione levels and a host of biomedical/psychological traits among the elderly, including fewer illnesses, higher levels of self-rated health, lower cholesterol, lower body mass index, and lower blood pressures.

Those suffering from arthritis, diabetes, or heart disease showed significantly lower glutathione levels than those without disease.

Authors of another study examining blood glutathione levels have concluded that physical health and longevity are closely related. Results of population-based, case-control study found an inverse correlation between dietary glutathione intake and the relative risk of oral cancer.

Supplemental glutathione at doses of 1.5 g/m2 in 100 mL of normal saline solution over a fifteen-minute period immediately prior to cisplatin exposure and at a dose of 600 mg by intramuscular injection on days two to five has proven to be effective in the prevention of cisplatin-induced neuropathy without reducing the efficacy of chemotherapeutic drugs in patients with advanced gastric cancer. When a dose of 3 g/m2 of glutathione was added to treatment with 100 mg/m2 of cisplatin every twenty-one days, ovarian cancer patients were able to withstand more cisplatin cycles and their overall quality of life was improved, including symptoms of depression, emesis, and neurotoxicity. The intravenous administration of 2.5–5 g in 100–200 ml of normal saline of glutathione over fifteen minutes prior to cisplatin treatment has been shown to be an effective means of enhancing the drugs efficacy in patients with ovarian cancer. Glutathione administered at 5 g per day to patients suffering from hepatocellular carcinoma had beneficial effects in women, but not in men. Results from animal studies support the use of glutathione as a cancer therapy.

In addition to its direct anti-aging and chemopreventive effects, studies show glutathione can be useful in the treatment of a host of other conditions. One is liver damage. Glutathione is central to the protection against oxygen radical injury following brief periods of total hepatic ischemia in rats. Intravenous administration of high doses of glutathione for two weeks has led to significant improvements of the enzyme patterns in the livers of chronic alcoholics, and has significantly improved the rate of various hepatic tests in patients with chronic steatosic liver disease. In men suffering from infertility, 600 mg per day of glutathione taken for two months significantly improved sperm motility patterns. Glutathione has also inhibited the replication of HIV-1 and Herpes-1 *in vitro*. Intravenous injection of 1.5 g/kg of glutathione reduced decreases in local cerebral glucose utilization in rats induced by a neurotoxic and blocked neuronal loss in hippocampal CA1 and CA3 regions and prevented the development of hippocampal edema. Glutathione has reduced and/or diminished the severity of sugar cataractogenesis in the rat lens, offered protection against oxidative injury in the human retinal pigment epithelium, reduced and/or prevented shock-induced behavioral depression in mice, prevented diabetic neuropathy in diabetic rats, protected against oxidative inactivation of alveolar inflammatory cells in an *in vitro* model of emphysema due to smoking, reduced cisplatin-induced neurotoxicity/neuropathy in rats, protected against gastric mucosal injury both in humans and in rats, protected rats from radiation injury of the parotid glands, significantly delayed the appearance of scurvy in ascorbate-deficient guinea pigs, and enhanced T-cell activity *in vitro*. Animal studies also indicate glutathione can produce cardioprotective and antioxidant effects.

Hesperidin

Hesperidin is a citrus bioflavonoid found in orange peel. Animal studies point to the efficacy of hesperidin as both a chemopreventive agent and a promising treatment for high blood pressure and cholesterol. Results of one double-blind, placebo-controlled study involving human patients with symptomatic capillary fragility showed significant improvement following intake of a veno-active flavonoid fraction consisting of 90 percent micronized diosmin and 10 percent hesperidin for six weeks. Hesperidin has also been shown to possess signficant analgesic and anti-inflammatory effects.

Human Growth Hormone

Results of one double-blind, placebo-controlled study showed that the administration of recombinant human growth hormone over a period of twenty-six weeks at doses of 0.013–0.026 U/kg per day taken at bedtime to patients with adult-onset growth hormone deficiency led to improvements in body composition, fat distribution, bone and mineral metabolism, and psychiatric symptoms. Another study of twenty patients with adult-onset growth hormone deficiency who received doses of IU/m2 per day over a period of one year produced similar results.

Studies have shown that growth hormone therapy at doses of 0.6 and 1.2 IU per day can increased serum insulinlike growth factors-I to normal ranges following twelve weeks of treatment in growth-hormone-deficient adults. Low-dose, long-term GH therapy can prolong life expectancy in mice.

Inositol

Inositol niacinate administered at doses of 1.2 g three times per day over a period of four to six weeks has produced beneficial results in patients suffering from ischemic ulcers due to chronic arterial occlusion. Inositol hexasulfate taken intravenously can produce anticoagulant effects. Depressed patients have experienced significant improvements following 12 g per day of inositol over a period of one month. Three months' worth of supplemental inositol at 6 g per day has proven effective against diabetic polyneuropathy. Results from numerous animal studies indicate inositol possesses strong anticancer properties as well.

Iodine

The best sources of dietary iodine, an essential mineral, can be found in seafood and iodized salt. Many people experience symptoms of thyroid dysfunction as they age, such as weight gain, lack of energy, poor mood, etc. Iodine has been shown to inhibit thyroid cell growth *in vitro* and in animal models. When applied in the form of a topical cream, povidone-iodine's antibacterial, antifungal, and antiviral effects have been well established in the scientific literature. Topical iodine has also been shown to be a useful treatment for wound healing.

Iron

Doses of 105 mg per day of supplemental iron taken orally over a period of six weeks has been shown to be effective in the treatment of elderly patients suffering from iron deficiency anemia.

For normal supplements, smaller doses are advised. Too much can contribute to heart disease.

L-dopa

One of the most documented changes in the body associated with aging is the loss of dopamine levels in the brain. L-dopa is an amino acid nutrient available by prescription that is converted into dopamine in the brain. L-dopa's primary use has been in the treatment of Parkinson's disease.

One double-blind study concluded that the administration of levodopa alone or coupled with a stable dose of amantadine had a beneficial effects in Parkinson's patients lasting three years or more. The visual contrast sensitivity of Parkinson's patients improved to near normal levels following treatment with L-dopa. Low doses of levodopa administered on alternate days proved beneficial in patients with early Parkinson's disease and produced fewer side effects than when taken daily.

Parkinson's patients administered daily doses of levodopa beginning at a mean of 662.5 mg five times per week and then changing to a mean of 800 mg three times a week after the first year of treatment experienced improved measures of rigidity, tremor, and bradykinesia. The oral administration of levodopa led to improvements in swallowing abnormalities among patients suffering from Parkinson's.

Parkinson's patients receiving intravenous levodopa experienced reductions in anxiety and elevated mood. Results of another study found that the administration of L-dopa to Parkinson's patients provided its greatest level of benefit after a treatment period of three years. Intake of 100 mg of L-dopa plus decarboxylase inhibitor had blood pressure lowering effects on patients with Parkinson's disease. Intravenous L-dopa significantly improved cerebral blood flow problems in patients with idiopathic Parkinson's disease. L-dopa can also significantly improve color discrimination in Parkinson's patients.

While only approved by the FDA for use against Parkinson's, research suggests L-dopa may have a far broader range of therapeutic effects. Clinical and experimental studies have shown a high therapeutic activity of L-dopa in combination with more conventional therapies in the treatment of myocardial infarction patients. Combining L-dopa to more conventional therapies had positive effects on heart patients suffering from severe dysfunction of the left ventricle when administered over a period of three months. The administration of 250 mg per day of L-dopa over a period of six months proved to be a useful treatment in patients suffering from early stages of presenile dementia. One gram per day of L-dopa reduced the intensity of involuntary movements in patients suffering from

tardive dyskinesia. Treatment with low-dose L-dopa had significantly beneficial effects over a period of five years with respect to
dystonia and insomnia without dyskinesia. L-dopa can be effective
in controlling periodic movements in sleep in patients suffering
from narcolepsy. Two weeks of L-dopa treatment improved vigilance
levels in patients suffering from narcolepsy. L-dopa has had beneficial effects in patients suffering from craniocerebral trauma. It can
be of benefit in patients suffering from bipolar affective disorders.

In a study of twenty-five patients with pathological laughing
and/or crying, treatment with either levodopa or amantadine hydrochloride treatment produced significant improvements in ten patients. L-dopa improved symptoms of extrapyramidal dysfunction,
including rigidity, stiffness, ambulation difficulties, shuffling gait,
dysarthria, drooling, swallowing dysfunction, hypomimetic, inex-
pressive faces, and bradykinesia in children between the ages of four
through thirteen years infected with HIV-1.

The short-term administration of L-dopa had positive effects on
women suffering from amenorrhea-galactorrhea syndrome. The administration of 500 mg of L-dopa per day leading up to 500 mg three
times per day over a period of six months accelerated the rate of
healing in patients suffering from long bone fractures. One case report of a thiry-year-old woman with acute hepatic failure in the fifth
month of pregnancy showed a significant improvement in levels of
both consciousness and electroencephalogram following L-dopa
therapy. A week of daily levodopa administration improved visual
acuity in 70 percent of the amblyopia patients examined. One study
revealed a significant improvement in visual acuity due to visual
loss from nonarteritic anterior ischemic neuropathy among patients
receiving low-dose levodopa and carbidopa over a period of twelve
weeks. The administration of L-dopa significantly improved the
death rate of patients suffering from measles encephalitis. L-dopa
administered in doses ranging between 500 mg to 750 mg per day
for two months exhibited stimulatory effects on spermatogenesis in
males suffering from primary sterility. L-dopa treatment exhibited
beneficial effects in patients suffering from duodenal ulcer, and in
those experiencing restless leg syndrome. The administration of up
to 1250 mg per day of L-dopa over a period of six weeks produced
significant improvements in patients suffering from schizophrenia.

One study showed that treatment with L-dopa produced an immediate significant improvement in an eight-year-old boy suffering from walking difficulties caused by Segawa-syndrome-related dystonia. L-dopa has proven useful in patients suffering from torsion dystonia. In mice, L-dopa has been shown capable of extending the life span as much as 50 percent.

Lycopene

Lycopene is a carotenoid and powerful antioxidant (stronger than beta carotene) that gives tomatoes as well other fruits such as watermelon, pink grapefruit, papaya, and guava their red color. While lycopene is the most abundant carotenoid in the human blood and tissues, it is not produced naturally in the body and thus must be obtained through dietary sources.

Recent studies point to the growing interest in lycopene and its potential for promoting health, particularly with respect to heart disease and cancer. A six-year study of 48,000 male health professionals conducted by Harvard Medical School found that the consumption of tomato products more than twice per week reduced prostate cancer risk by 35 percent. Results of a large human case-control study found that the consumption of foods containing lycopene, found primarily in tomatoes and tomato products, may contribute to a reduced risk of myocardial infarction. Another study showed dietary supplementation with lycopene can lower concentrations of plasma LDL cholesterol. Lycopene has exhibited anticancer effects both *in vitro* and in studies involving animals.

MEA

The first experiments of Denham Harman, previously noted as the father of the free radical theory of aging, tested the ability of several drugs, including BHT and MEA (2-mercaptoethylamine), to extend lifespan in mice. Such experiments produced an extension of approximately 20 percent. Future studies involving MEA produced extensions as high as 30 to 50 percent. MEA, a synthetic antioxidant and sulfur containing radiation protector, has been shown to increase the lifespan of WI-38 cells in vitro by 6.5 percent. Results from additional studies indicate MEA may be capable of inhibiting the replication of HIV *in vitro* as well. Consistent with the free radical theory of aging, MEA's most noted activity is that of protecting DNA against the harmful effects of irradiation associated with cancer treatments.

Melatonin

The pineal hormone melatonin is best known for its role in promoting sleep. While the number of studies continue to increase concerning its potential in this area, new research also suggests it may have a much wider array of potential benefits.

The aging process is one such area, with data indicating that melatonin may delay the effects of aging by attenuating negative effects associated with free radical–induced neuronal damage. Melatonin has been shown to be a potent free radical scavenger that acts as a primary nonenzymatic antioxidative defense against the destruction caused by hydroxyl free radicals. Hence, melatonin can slow the rate of aging and the time of onset of age-related diseases. Animal studies support such findings.

Melatonin may also act directly against some of the key degenerative diseases associated with aging, most notably cancer. One study found that 10 mg per day of oral melatonin administered to patients with metastatic non-small cell lung cancer at 8 P.M. produced beneficial effects and was well tolerated when coupled with neuroimmunotherapeutic therapy. Doses of 20 mg per day of melatonin combined with tamoxifen induced objective tumor regressions in metastatic breast cancer patients. Low dose IL-2 coupled with 50 mg of melatonin per day beginning seven days prior to IL-2 therapy proved to be an effective treatment for advanced digestive tract tumors. In another study, 22 renal cell carcinoma patients were monitored for the effect of a twelve-month regimen of three mega units of intramuscular human lymphoblastoid interferon three times weekly and 10 mg per day of oral melatonin. Results showed seven remissions and disease stablizations.

Melatonin can improve quality of life and survival time in brain metastases patients. Treatment with 20 mg per day of intramuscular melatonin in cancer patients with metastatic bold tumor followed up with 10 oral mg per day in patients experiencing remission indicated that melatonin had beneficial effects in such patients with respect to PS and quality of life. Doses of 20 mg per day of oral melatonin may be a factor involved in the treatment of chemotherapy-induced myelodysplatic syndrome in cancer patients. Melatonin offers protection against interleukin-2, and the two agents synergize in their anti-cancer effects. In forty advanced melanoma patients treated with daily doses of oral melatonin ranging from 5 mg/m2 to

700 mg/m2, results showed partial responses in six patients and stable disease in six others after five weeks of follow-up.

Results from animal studies indicate melatonin has cardioprotective, anti-diabetic, anti-glucocorticoid, anti-convulsant, anti-cataract, and immunoenhancing effects; improves adrenal function; can reduce the severity of colitis, seizures, brain injury, and gastric lesions; delayed disease onset and death due to viral encephalitis. Melatonin has also exhibited cytoprotective and antioxidant activity *in vitro*.

The ideal dose of melatonin varies widely across individuals, but experts believe 3 to 10 mg taken at night will produce positive effects in most people.

Molybdenum

Molybdenum is an essential trace mineral required for the activity of several enzymes that is obtained through dietary sources such as legumes, dark green leafy vegetables, buckwheat, barley, oats, and sunflower seeds. The highest concentrations in the body can be found in the liver, kidneys, adrenal gland, skin, and bones. Estimates of the minimum dietary requirement range between 25mg and 75 mg per day.

Animal studies indicate that molybdenum can significantly reduce the incidence of tumors associated with esophageal, mammary, and forestomach cancer. Similar results have been seen *in vitro*. Findings from one Japanese study showed an inverse correlation between molybdenum levels and rates of rectal cancer mortality in women. Magnesium molybdate administered in doses of 0.06–0.2 g Mo has been used as a treatment against anemia and appetite booster. Epidemiological studies in the Europe and U.S. suggest molybdenum may have cariostatic effects.

NAC

N-acetyl-l-cysteine is a proven cancer fighter in animal studies and *in vitro*, and has shown great promise across a number of other degenerative conditions. Heart disease is one where studies support the use of NAC. The administration of 150 mg/kg-1 of NAC has significantly increased cardiac output and reduced systemic vascular resistance in patients requiring hemodynamic monitoring due to sepsis syndrome. Results of another study found that the intravenous administration of 2 g of NAC over fifteen minutes followed by 5 mg/kg/hr coupled with intravenous isosorbide denitrate led to partial prevention of anti-anginal effect tolerance often associated with isosorbide treatment alone in anginal patients.

The intravenous administration of 100 mg/kg of NAC potentiated nitroglycerin-induced vasodilater effects in patients undergoing cardiac catheterization for chest pain investigation. Acute myocardial infarction patients who were treated with 15 g of intravenous NAC over a twenty-four-hour period coupled with intravenous nitroglycerin showed significant reductions in levels of oxidative controls relative to controls.

Results also showed a trend toward improved preservation of the left ventricular function as well as more rapid reperfusion. Pretreatment of cardiac risk patients with the 150 mg/kg NAC onVO2 showed that NAC worked to preserve VO2, oxygen delivery, CI, LVSWI, and PvaCO2 during brief hyperoxia and prevented clinical signs of myocardial ischemia. The combination of intravenous NAC (5g six hourly) and nitroglycerine in unstable angina pectoris patients augments nitroglycerine's clinical benefits primarily by decreased acute myocardial infarction incidence. Large doses of NAC increased exercise capacity in isosorbide-5-mononitrate-treated angina pectoris patients. A bolus of 100 mg/kg of NAC followed by a continuos infusion of 20mg/kg in the bypass circuit on oxidative response of neutrophils during cardiopulmonary bypass in adult patients showed significantly lower levels of oxidative burst response of neutrophils among those receiving the NAC than controls throughout the bypass.

Diabetes is another disease that can both accelerate the aging process and result from it, where studies suggest NAC may be of value. AIDS is a disease involving immune system failure that also causes the body to age prematurely and where NAC can help counter such effects. Studies indicate NAC may also produce positive effects on such problems as adult respiratory distress syndrome, chronic bronchitis, middle ear infections, gallstones, hepatitis, liver damage, lung damage, muscle fatigue, stroke, Sjogren's syndrome, brain injury, COPD, cutaneous inflammation, and glutathione deficiency.

Olive Oil

Olive oil has been shown to be effective against arthritis, cancer, and heart disease; three of the most common conditions associated with aging. With respect to cancer, one study demonstrated a significant inverse association between olive oil and the risk of breast cancer in a large trial of Greek women. Results of another recognized a similar pattern with women in Italy. The same correlation has also been seen in Spanish women. Supplementation with 50 g per day of olive oil over a period of two weeks has proven capable of modifying LDL lipid composition and enriching the lipoprotein with oleic acid and sitosterol in healthy males.

Another study indicated that natural antioxidants found in the extra-virgin olive oil prevalent in Mediterranean diets are involved in inhibiting the formation of cytotoxic products and delaying atherosclerotic damage.

Omega Fatty Acids

Omega fatty acids are found in many kinds of fish and various oils, including flaxseed oil, linseed oil, and evening primrose oil. Numerous studies have shown clinical benefits following ingestion of n-3 fatty acids in patients suffering from rheumatoid arthritis. One found that the oral intake of 2.6 g per day of omega-3 fatty acids by rheumatoid arthritis patients over a period of twelve months led to significant improvements in symptoms associated with the disease. Omega fatty acids may also be useful in the treatment and prevention of cancer.

Supplementation with arginine, RNA, and omega-3 fatty acids in the early postoperative time period have improved postoperative immunologic responses in patients undergoing surgery for gastroinestinal cancer. Daily supplementation with omega-3 fatty acids (fish oil containing 4 g of eicosapentaenoic acid and 3.6 g of docosahexaenoic acid) over a period of twelve weeks had chemopreventive effects in patients suffering from sporadic adenomatous colorectal polyps. The consumption of 18 g of fish oil per day over a period of forty days significantly increased T-helper/T-suppresser cell ratio in cancer patients with solid tumors.

Heart disease is another area where omega fatty acid supplementation has produced positive effects. One study showed that small doses of oral omega-3 fatty acids had significant positive effects on platelet activity when administered over a period of six weeks in hyperlipidemic patients with preexisting, established atherothrombotic disorders. The consumption of a fish oil diet containing 24 g of omega-3 fatty acids per day for gout weekly by healthy subjects reduced LDL plasma levels relative to controls. The oral administration of high levels of omega-3 fatty acids dramatically reduced VLDL triglyceride levels associated with a high-carbohydrate diet in healthy subjects.

Daily ingestion of low levels of marine fish oil (900 mg f omega-3 fatty acids) over a period of thirty days had positive effects on clotting and lipid profiles in healthy male subjects. Daily supplementation with omega-3 fatty acids over a period of four weeks had antihypertensive and hypotriglyceridaemic effects in hypertensive patients taking either beta blockers or diuretics for the disease.

Diabetics have also experienced benefits from omega fatty acids. One study found that short-term daily supplementation with omega-3 fatty acids (5.4 g eicosapentaenoic acid and 2.3 g docosahexaenoic acid) over a period of four weeks led to positive changes with respect to vascular risk factors common to type 1 insulin-dependent diabetics.

Supplementation with 3 g of the omega 3 fatty acids eicosapentaenoic and docosahexaenoic acid per day over a period of eight weeks led to an increase of the membrane phospholipid unsaturation and the sphingomyelin content in noninsulin-dependent patients. Supplemental omega-3 fatty acids have also exhibited inhibitory effects against the onset of experimental diabetic cardiomyopathy in diabetic rats.

PABA

PABA (Para-Aminobenzoic Acid) is a member of the B vitamin group and part of the folic acid molecule. Dietary sources of PABA include eggs, liver, wheat germ, whole grains, rice, and brewers yeast. PABA is perhaps most noted for its protective effects against skin damage, making it a widely used ingredient in suntan lotions. The administration of PABA has been shown to inhibit the development of skin tumors in mice exposed to ultraviolet light. When combined with alcohol and used in the form of a sunscreen, results from one study also showed PABA reduced the incidence of skin cancer in an eleven-year old patient with pigmentosum. PABA is also often used as a blood tonic, antiobiotic, intestinal cleanser, stress reducer, and to reverse gray hair and stimulate hair growth. It has exhibited anti-herpes in animal studies as well. There is no current RDA for

PABA, however. A suggested dose ranges between 30 to 100 mg per day.

Pantothenic Acid

Pantothenic acid (vitamin B_5) has demonstrated significant anticancer and cardioprotective effects in vitro.

Results of one case study also indicated that large doses of pantothenic acid can improve myocardial growth and function, neutrophil cell count, hypocholesterolaemia and hyperuricaemia. Daily doses of 300 and 600 mg of calcium pantothemate and 90 mg and 180 mg of pantethein taken for three to four weeks had positive immunomodulatory action in hepatitis patients. Pantothenic acid can protect against liver damage in rats as well.

Phosphatidylserine

A phospholipid component of brain cell membranes, phosphatidylserine has exhibited direct anti-aging effects in animal studies. One has indicated it can improve the release of acetylccholine in aging rats. Another showed that the administration of phosphatidylserine balanced age-altered enzymatic functions in rats.

Phosphatidylserine administered to aging rats can restore acetylcholine by maintaining a sufficient level in the cortical slices, and decrease the number of seizures due to spontaneous EEG bursts by 65 percent and the length of seizure duration by 70 percent. The administration of phosphatidylserine to rats led to a reduction in decreases in acetylcholine release due to age by influencing mechanism of stimulus-secretion coupling.

Alzheimer's disease and senile patients have also experienced benefits following treatment with phosphatidylserine. Doses of 400 mg per day led to significant, short-term neuropsychological improvements in such patients relative to controls. The administration of 300 mg per day for eight weeks led to significant clinical improvements in patients with mild primary degenerative dementia. In another study, Alzheimer's patients received 100 mg per day of bovine cortex phosphatidylserine for twelve weeks. Results showed the treatment improved several cognitive measures relative to controls. Animal trials have produced similar results.

Phosphatidylserine has promise for cancer and heart disease as well. Bovine cortex phosphatidylserine has significantly reduced experimental autoimmune encephalomyelitis in mice, while not inhibiting effector T-cells. Another study found that parental administration of liposomes containing the aminophospholipids phosphatidylserine and phosphatidylethanolamine is an efficient mode to decrease the endotoxin-induced production of tumor necrosis factor in mice and rabbits.

The intravenous administration of 30 to 60 mg of phosphatidyl serine emulsion has led to a rapid reduction in blood coagulation activity in a dose-dependent manner.

Animal studies indicate phosphatidylserine can have positive immune enhancing effects and reduce the clinical severity and mortality in allergic neuritis. Schizophrenia and epilepsy patients have benefited from phosphatidylserine. Stress is another condition that phostphatidylserine can help. The administration of 800 mg per day of phosphatidylserine for ten days on neuroendocrine responses to physical stress in healthy males found it counteracted activation of the hypothalamo-pituitary-adrenal axis induced by stress. Pretreatment of healthy males with doses of 50 and 75 mg per day of brain cortex–derived phosphatidlyserine produced a significant blunting of the ACTH and cortisol responses to physical stress.

Phosphatidylserine should not be taken with anticoagulant medication. The suggested dose is 100 to 200 mg taken orally twice per day, or 100 to 250 mg per day intravenously.

Potassium

In additional to its potential benefits for diabetics, supplemental potassium is widely recognized in the scientific literature as a useful treatment for heart disease. One study found that 80 mmol per day of potassium led to a decline in systolic and diastolic blood pressure among middle-aged African-Americans on a low-potassium diet. Moderate restriction of dietary sodium coupled with 60 mmol per day of supplemental potassium for two months led to the reduction of supine blood pressure in patients with moderate to mild essential hypertension.

Supplementation with 60 mmol per day of potassium chloride for six weeks ameliorated diuretic-induced hypokalemia and led to a decrease in blood pressure in hypertension patients. Potassium supplementation at 60 mmol per day showed a significant reduction in the orthostatic fall in systolic blood pressure and supine blood pressure and control phases in elderly patients with symptomatic idiopathic postural hypotension. Potassium has significantly reduced systolic blood pressure in healthy, normotensive children. Doses of 2 mg per day of supplemental potassium hydrochloride or a combination of 2 g per day of potassium hydrochloride and 1000 mg per day of magnesium hydroxide added to twenty-four weeks of diuretic therapy after the eighth week suppressed ventricular ectopic activity in mild hypertensives.

Another study compared the effects of 64 mmol per day of supplemental potassium with 10 mg per day of bendrofulazide in black patients suffering from untreated hypertension. Results showed the two treatments to be equally effective in reducing diastolic blood pressure over a twenty-eight-week period, with those receiving potassium exhibiting fewer side effects. Essential hypertension patients who received either a low-sodium diet, high-sodium diet, or high-sodium diet combined with KCl supplementation showed that blood pressure increased during NaCl loading and decreased during KCl supplementation. A study of untreated essential hypertensive patients who received 64 mmol KCl or placebo during two four-week periods found that by the fourth week of the potassium supplementation period, significant reductions were seen in diastolic blood pressure.

A meta-analysis involving nineteen clinical trials found that oral potassium supplements significantly lower systolic and diastolic blood pressure, with the strongest effects seen in patients with high blood pressure. A mild hypotensive effect following high potassium intake (72 mmol/day) coupled with moderate sodium restriction over a period of six weeks was found in young patients with hypertension. Daily supplementation with 65 mmol of potassium chloride salt over a six-week period significantly reduced systolic and diastolic blood pressure in hypertensive black females. Potassium chloride given at doses of 60 mmol per day reduced twenty-four-hour ambulatory blood pressure in untreated elderly hypertensives after a period of four weeks. And 100 mmol per day of supplemental potassium administered over a period of ten days can modify noradrenergic blood pressure regulation in hypertensives.

Hypertensive patients experienced reductions in blood pressure following long-term but not short-term supplementation with potassium. Intravenous potassium chloride administered at doses of

0.5 meq/kg over a two-hour period were effective and without side effects in pediatric postoperative cardiac patients as well.

Pycnogenol

Pycnogenol is an extremely powerful antioxidant consisting of the bioflavanoid proanthocyanidin that can be extracted from pine bark and grape seeds. Studied since the 1950s, many have suggested pycnogenol may be the most potent antioxidant yet discovered, far surpassing even vitamin E and vitamin C in strength. Peer review studies indicate it is indeed a proven free radical scavenger and antioxident that has been shown to exhibit anticancer activity. Supplementation with 150 mg per day can have beneficial effects on capillary resistance disorders in human diabetic and hypertension patients. Results from another human study showed that the administration of 4 tablets containing 50 mg of procyanidolic oligomers per day for 5 weeks had significant beneficial effects relative to controls with respect to various conditions associated with light vision. Pycnogenol has been found to protect vascular endothelial cells from oxidant injury *in vitro*, and exhibited immune enhancing activity in mice.

Quercetin

Several studies have documented the anticancer activity of the bioflavonoid quercetin *in vitro*, while results from animal trials demonstrate cardioprotective and antidiabetic effects as well. Intravenous administration of quercetin and tocopherol acetate for seven days has been found to enhance normalization of clinical indices and restoration of the immune homeostasis in patients suffering from Flexner's dysentery. Quercetive taken three hours prior to acute systemic hypoxia combined with hyperthermia at doses of 100 mg/kg prevented drastic activation of lipid peroxidation and arachidonic acid metabolism. Animal studies suggest quercetin can inhibit gastric ulcers.

Rutin

Results from animal studies indicate that rutin, another bioflavonoid, can suppress tumors associated with colon cancer and delay the development of hypercholesterinemia and peroxidation syndrome, as well as aortal atherosclerotic affection. Rutin has exhibited antioxidant and free radical scavenging activity *in vitro*, and provided protection against gastric injury in rats. Additionally, rutin improves the absorption of vitamin C, promotes circulation, and is a popular remedy for a host of different conditions such as bruises, muscle pain, high cholesterol, cirrhosis, rheumatic disorders, cataracts, hemorrhoids, constipation, and stress. Dietary sources of rutin include the white area under the skin of citrus fruits, white core of green peppers, rose hips, prunes, cherries, apricots, rhubarb, lemongrass, mint, chamomile, and buckwheat.

S-Adenodylmethionine (SAMe)

SAMe (S-Adenosylmethionine) is a nontoxic, natural metablite of methionine, an amino acid, which has received a great deal of recent attention for its potential anti-aging effects.

SAMe can be found in most tissues of the body and is necessary for the proper utilization of melatonin. Clinical trials involving more than 22,000 osteoarthritis patients between the years of 1982 and 1987 support the efficacy and tolerability of SAMe in treating those suffering from the disease. SAMe administered over a period of twenty-four months in patients with osteoarthritis of the knee, hip, and spine at doses of 600 mg daily for the first two weeks and 400 mg per day thereafter proved clinically effective, and improved feelings of depression often associated with the disease as well.

A study involving 20,641 patients with osteoarthritis of the knee, hip, and spine found ademetionine tablets administered over a period of eight weeks showed good effectiveness in 71 percent of patients, moderate effectiveness in 21 percent, and poor in 9 percent. Patients with osteoarthritis of the knee, hip, and/or spine who received either 1,200 mg of S-adenosylmethionine (SAMe) per day or 1,200 mg of ibuprofen per day or 150 mg of indomethacin per day over a period of four weeks experienced an alleviating of symptoms, including morning stiffness, pain at rest, pain on motion, crepitus, swelling, and limitation of motion of the affected joints. In a double-blind, placebo-controlled study, patients with unilateral knee osteoarthritis received either 1,200 mg of SAMe per day or 20 mg per day of oral piroxicam over a period of eighty-four days. Both treatments produced significant improvements in total pain scores after being administered for twenty-eight days.

A similar trial involving 734 subjects compared the efficacy of

1,200 mg per day of SAMe with 750 mg per day of naproxen in the treatment of osteoarthritis of the hip, knee, spine, and hand, and showed both drugs proved more effective than controls. SAMe also was significantly more tolerable than naproxen. Intramuscular administration of SAMe had chondoprotective effects in rabbits with surgical-induced osteoarthritis. Intake of 30 mg of SAMe intravenously twice a day over a two-week period had significant anti-inflammatory effects and no side effects in osteoarthrosis patients. Patients with hip and/or knee osteoarthritis who received either 1,200 mg of SAMe per day or 1,200 mg of ibuprofen per day over a period of thirty days found SAMe was more effective in alleviating symptoms associated with disease than ibuprofen. Intramuscular administration of SAMe had protective effects in rabbits with experimental-induced degenerative arthropathy of the knee. Weekly intra-articular doses of SAMe significantly reduced the severity of experimentally induced osteoarthritis in rats.

SAMe has been shown to be especially effective against depression. One study showed seven of nine patients receiving treatment with SAMe for depression experienced improvement or total remission of symptoms. Another found oral administration of SAMe proved to be an effective and quick-acting antidepressant in patients suffering from major depression. When compared with oral imipramine, the intravenous administration of SAMe for two weeks was significantly more effective in patients suffering from depression. SAMe has also been shown to be superior to tricylic antidepressants and desipramine. The parental administration of 400 mg of SAMe over a period 15 days remitted depressive symptoms in patients suffering from depression. The oral administration of 1,600 mg per day of SAMe over a month period significantly improved depressive symptoms in postmenopausal female patients suffering from major depression. SAMe has been shown to be an effective treatment for management of primary fibromyalgia mainly due to its ability to improve the patient's depressive state and reduce the number of trigger points. Oral doses of 800 mg per day of SAMe led to improvements with respect to pain, fatigue, morning stiffness, and mood in patients suffering from primary fibromyalgia.

Numerous studies point to the ability of SAMe to counter the effects of liver damage. The administration of 30 mg of SAMe six times per day coupled with 6000 gamma per day of vitamin B_{12} produced significant improvements of biochemical parameters in patients with hepatic cirrhosis or various chronic hepatites. In another study, patients suffering from hepatic cirrhosis were intravenously treated for a period of thirty days with 150 mg per day SAMe and 2000 gamma per day of vitamin B_{12}, or with vitamin B_{12} alone. Results showed significant improvements in the groups of patients receiving the combined treatment only.

The intravenous administration of two daily doses of 15 mg of SAMe over a period of twenty days led to significant improvement in patients hospitalized for chronic hepatitis. Four daily doses of 15 mg administered over a month had significant beneficial effects in hepatitic cirrhosis patients. Intravenous doses of 30–45 mg per day of SAMe over a period of 30–60 days led to significant improvements in patients suffering from cirrhosis of the liver and other chronic hepatites. The short-term administration of 1600 mg per day of SAMe had significant clinical benefits in patients suffering from intrahepatic cholestasis relative to controls.

Pregnant women suffering from intrahepatic cholestasis who received SAMe at intravenous doses of 800 mg per day exhibited significantly lower levels of total bile acids, serum conjugated bilirubin, and aminotransferases than controls. Such patients showed significant decreases in pruritus as well. Oral intake of 30 mg of SAMe four to five times per day had significant beneficial effects on liver function in nine brothers suffering from Wilson's Disease. Several studies have indicated that SAMe can prevent the development of liver cancer in rats.

SAMe has exerted anti-inflammatory activity in the inhibiting of oedema and pleurisy in rats. The administration of SAMe protected against energy failure in cerebral ischemia of rats while also increasing recovery time. SAMe administered at daily doses of between 800 and 1200 mg has proven to be equally as effective as naproxen in the treatment of patients suffering from activated gonarthrosis, with both drugs showing significant improvement across all parameters studied. SAMe has been determined to be effective in countering lead poisoning in both rodent and human studies. Intake of 800 mg per day of SAMe over a period of three months increased basal mobility of spermatozoa in six out of ten male infertility cases treated. SAMe administered at doses of 800 mg per day worked as a physiological antidote against estrogen hepatobiliary toxicity in women with prior intrahepatic cholestasis of pregnancy. SAMe can also alleviate pain in patients suffering from migraines.

The suggested dose for SAMe falls between the range of 800 and 1600 mg per day.

Selenium

Selenium is an essential trace mineral and important antioxidant that has been found to work synergistically with vitamin E. One study has determined that supplemental beta-carotene and selenium enhanced the immune function among a group of healthy elderly subjects. Supplemental selenium has also restored cell proliferation defects associated with aging in mice by increasing the number of high-affinity IL-2 receptors. Results of dozens of animal and *in vitro* studies have pointed to the role of selenium in helping to prevent and treat cancer. Another showed an inverse association between selenium status and the risk of lung cancer in a large-scale, three-year trial of Dutch men and women between the ages of fifty-five and sixty-nine.

One review article has cited numerous epidemiological studies indicating a significant inverse association between selenium intake and the risk of cancer in humans.

Selenium may also play a role in preventing heart disease and diabetes. One study showed that when sodium selenite was added to the drinking water of rats for four weeks, they experienced protective effects against experimentally induced cardiac ischemia and reperfusion. Selenium and vitamin E administered together protected rabbits against heart muscle changes associated with a high-fat diet. Selenium supplementation reduced adriamycin-induced cardiotoxicity in isolated rat hearts undergoing a sequence of ischemia/reperfusion. Combined supplementation with selenium and vitamin E has protected the kidneys from glumerular lesions in diabetic rats. Supplemental selenium has exhibited insulinlike effects in diabetic mice. It has decreased elevated serum glucose levels in experimentally induced diabetic rats as well.

Immune function can also be improved by selenium. One study found that three months of selenium supplementation at thrice weekly doses of 500 micrograms followed by three months at 200 micrograms improved T-cell response to phytohaemoagglution and significant progressive increase in delayed-type hypersensitivity in haemodialysis patients. Another showed that supplementation with 200 micrograms of selenium per day for two to four months led to enhanced immune response in patients suffering from short-bowel syndrome. Other conditions selenium has shown to benefit include Keshan disease, kidney damage, lupus, poor mood, myotonic dystrophy, ulcers, and dental cavities.

Superoxide Dismutase (SOD)

Superoxide dismutase is an antioxidant enzyme that can counter damaging free-radical effects at the cellular level. Research indicates SOD can also be useful against many specific conditions directly. One study has shown that recombinant human superoxide dismutase exhibited inhibitory effects on the articular cartilage tissue damage associated with osteoarthritis. Others have shown that superoxide dismutase produced significant benefits for those suffering from osteoarthritis as well. Results of another study showed that treatment with CuZn superoxide dismutase significantly improved clinical symptoms associated with Behcet's syndrome.

Superoxide radicals have inhibited vasogenic brain edema onset following brain injury. The administration of SOD reduced the severity of bronchopulmonary dysplasia in infants suffering from respiratory distress syndrome. Superoxide dismutase was effective in reducing radio-induced cystitis in patients suffering from bladder cancer. Pretreatment with SOD or allopurinol attenuated ischemia and reperfusion-induced cochlear damage in rats. Fanconi anaemia patients who received 25 mg/kg per day of human SOD for two weeks experienced a reduction of lymphocyte chromosomal aberrations induced by diepoxybutane. Mice treated with SOD at the late period of influenza infection increased survival rates by between 30 and 50 percent.

The intravenous administration of SOD normalized systemic circulation and vascular permeability of gastric mucosa while also preventing stress-induced gastric injury in rats. Superoxide dismutase enhanced the life span of rats exposed to hemorrhagic shock. Treatment with SOD reduced motor dysfunction and spinal infarcts a week following ischemia in rabbits. Superoxide dismutase has exhibited significant protective effects against kidney damage induced by ischemia and reperfusion in dogs and rats. Glycosulated SOD derivates, galactosylated and mannosylated, prevented ischemia/reperfusion-induced liver damage in rats. Superoxide dismutase has protected against lung damage in numerous animal trials. The administration of 3000 mg per day of intravenous recombinant human SOD administered over a period of five days following multiple injuries attenuated multiple organ failure with respect to cardiovascular and pulmonary functions in human patients. Superoxide dismutase protected against muscle and neuronal injury induced by ischemia/reperfusion in rats. Superoxide dismutase exhibited beneficial effects in patients suffering from plastic penile induration. A single intratracheal dose of recombinant human SOD had protective effects against lung injury in preterm infants suffering from respiratory distress syndrome. Topical superoxide dismutase is an effective treatment against burn-induced skin lesions in human patients. The administration of human recombinant SOD protected against ischemic neuronal damage in gerbils. Intra-articular injection of superoxide dismutase was an effective treatment for TMJ patients not responsive to traditional therapy.

Superoxide dismutase has exhibited protective effects against intestinal ulcers in rats and bladder ulcers in female patients. The intravenous administration of 1000 units per kg of polyethylene glycol-conjugated SOD within six hours of injury was an effective treatment for patients suffering from burns. It has exhibited burn healing effects in animal trials. A host of animal studies also point to the potential of SOD in the prevention and treatment of heart disease.

Trimethylglycine
Results from several Russian studies have shown that trimethylglycine can protect against experimentally induced atherosclerosis in rabbits.

Vitamin A/Beta-carotene
Vitamin A and beta-carotene, a precursor to vitamin A, are powerful antioxidants intimately involved in the aging process and conditions associated with it. Both are abundant in green leafy vegetables and other fruits and vegetables, including carrots, sweet potatoes, yams, apricots, and melons. Beta-carotene administered by itself and in combination with selenium has been shown to enhance natural killer cell activity in elderly subjects. Results of an-

other study found that the median life span of the common housefly could be increased by up to 17.5 percent following an increase in dietary vitamin A to adequate from inadequate levels during the various stages of development.

Beta-carotene supplementation at doses of 30 mg per day or more for two months significantly enhanced immune reaction in elderly volunteers. Alzheimer's patients have been found to have significantly lower plasma levels of vitamin E and vitamin A than controls. Inverse associations have also been noted between serum concentrations and dietary levels of beta-carotene and the risk of development of cataracts. Rats with experimentally induced arthritis experienced a toxicity-free decrease in clinical disease following the oral administration of retinoids, suggesting retinoids should be considered as possible therapeutic agents in treating rheumatoid arthritis. Combined supplementation with 2.4 mg of retinol and 60 mg of elemental iron has been shown to reverse anemia in pregnant women. High doses of vitamin A and vitamin E have halted the progression of symptoms associated with abetalipoproteinemia.

Treatment of thirty acne vulgaris patients with 0.025 percent vitamin A acid in gel form for twelve weeks reduced the amount of papules, pustules, and comedones in twenty-five of the patients. Retinol, in doses of 300,000 IU and 400,000 IU in women and men, respectively, has been found to be a safe and effective treatment for acne as well.

Vitamin injections have been effective in children with chronic cholestasis. Three months of oral beta-carotene supplementation effectively normalized excess lipid peroxidation in vitamin A deficient cystic fibrosis patients. Darier's disease patients receiving $1 \times 10 (6)$ IU of oral vitamin A daily for fourteen days experienced a 50 percent to 80 percent improvement in skin lesions. Supplemental beta-carotene combined with other antioxidants has exhibited antidiabetic effects in rats.

Among erythropoietic protoporphyria patients, 84 percent treated with 180 mg/day of oral beta-carotene showed a threefold increase in their ability to tolerate sunlight. Similar effects were seen in mice. Treatment with either a 100,000 IU or 200,000 IU dose of vitamin A was effective against Bitot's spots in Indonesian children. Long-term oral therapy with daily doses of 18,000 IE retinol, 70 mg

L-cystine, and 700 mg gelatin led to an improvement of diffuse hair loss relative to controls.

Treatment with vitamins A and E for 28–48 days improved symptoms in forty middle-aged to elderly patients affected by presbycusis (hearing loss). Topical treatment of primary herpetic keratitis with 0.25 percent of retinoic acid significantly reduced the severity of epithelial lesions in rabbits. Topical instillation of retinoic acid into the eyes of rabbits at the same dose also reduced the rate of incorporation of thymide into DNA by 27 percent. Patients with congenital ichthyosiform erythroderma have benefited from treatment with oral retinoic acid. Vitamin A supplementation for two weeks had positive effects on experimentally induced intestinal anastomosis in rabbits. Megadoses of oral vitamin A have proven effective against lesions associated with Kyrle's disease. Systemic lupus erythematosus patients treated with 100,000 IU daily of vitamin A for two weeks experienced an enhancement of antibody-dependent cell-mediated cytotoxicity, natural killer cell activity and blastogenic response to plant mitogens and interleukin-2.

Mortality rates were significantly reduced in children aged four to twenty-four months hospitalized from measles following supplementation with vitamin A. Another study showed that oral supplementation with 400,000 IU vitamin A led to a reduction or morbidity and mortality in children hospitalized with measles. Data showed that children taking vitamin A had significantly faster recovery times with respect to pneumonia and diarrhea, they had less croup, spent less time in the hospital, and had a death rate during hospitalization of half that of controls. Mortality and susceptibility to infection and diarrhea have been shown to be greater in vitamin A deficient children, particularly with respect to measles. Studies have shown vitamin A–supplementation reduced mortality and complications resulting from measles, and that supplementation with vitamin A could reduce the rate of childhood mortality by a mean of 35 percent and the rate of childhood mortality from measles specifically by a minimum of 50 percent, with researchers estimating that vitamin A supplementation of deficient children could prevent as many as 1–3-million death each year worldwide. Vitamin A can be effective in the treatment of menorrhagia.

It has been successful as a topical agent among patients suffering from plantar warts, and against papillomas in rabbits. High doses of corticosteroids and vitamin A have produced clinical recovery in patients suffering from pneumonia. Supplementation with 15,000 IU per day of vitamin A proved to have beneficial effects on the course of retinitis pigementosa. Oral vitamin A administered to mice prevents stress-induced immunological disorders: depression of antibody-forming cell production, decrease in natural killer cell activity, and T-lymphocyte mitogenic response. Data have also demonstrated that vitamin A prevents the development of thymus atrophy, lymphopenia and depression of phagocytic activity of peritoneal macrophages. Vitamin A has significantly reduced the incidence and size of stress-induced ulcer formation in rats and duodenal ulcers in human patients. A decrease in beta-carotene levels along with other antioxidants can alter the local immune response in women, creating disturbances in vaginal flora, candida overgrowth, and vaginal candidiasis development. Patients with primary biliary cirrhosis who received supplementation with 25,000 to 50,000 IU of vitamin A per day for four to twelve weeks experienced normalization of serum vitamin A levels and subsequent significant improvements in dark adaptation. Vitamin A has protected against liver damage in animals as well. Vitamin A was an effective agent for reversing the inhibition of cell-mediated immunity in burned mice. Rabbits with corneal epithelial wounds treated with 0.1 percent alltransretinoic acid three times per day experienced a 21 percent increase in the healing rate relative to controls. Treatment five times a day resulted in an increase of 35 percent. Supplemental retinyl acetate, beta-carotene, or in some cases all-trans-retinoic acid effectively enhanced wound healing in rats. Additional studies point to the wound healing effects of vitamin A as well. Supplemental vitamin A has been shown to benefit patients suffering from xerophthalmia, and children and adults suffering from varying degrees of blindness. Vitamin A supplementation has led to a reduction in the incidence of both diarrhea and respiratory disease in children.

Vitamin A intake has reduced childhood mortality rates in developing countries as well, including children born to mothers infected with HIV. Vitamin A deficiency has been linked to suppressed immunologic status and clinical outcomes in patients infected with HIV, and an increased rate of mother-to-child transmission of HIV. Supplementation with 180 mg per day of beta-carotene for four weeks significantly increased CD4 counts in HIV-infected patients.

Supplementation with 60 mg of beta-carotene per day increased immune status in AIDS patients. In one pilot study, ten patients infected with HIV who had just discontinued use of either AZT or DDI received one session of whole body hyperthermia with a noninvasive procedure at forty-two degrees Celsius core temperature for one hour, and subsequently supplemented with 120 mg per day of beta-carotene. Results showed the treatment was tolerated well by all patients aside from one who died within four months. The remaining nine experienced an HIV burden diminution, clinical improvement and amelioration of laboratory data, and reported subjective improvements in overall quality of life. Another study examined the effects of 30 mg per day of beta-carotene for four months on the lymphocytes of eleven AIDS patients. Results showed significant increases in the number of cells with NK markers and markers of activation after three months. High-dietary vitamin A was associated with a retarded death rate in mice infected with LP-BM5 murine leukemia, an AIDS-like condition, relative to controls. ARC patients supplemented with beta-carotene experienced a decrease in the progress toward AIDS, as well as recoveries from asthenia, fever, nocturnal sweating, diarrhea, and weight loss.

Numerous studies have shown an inverse association between vitamin A and/or beta carotene levels and the risk of cancer. Others have noted that supplemental vitamin A and beta-carotene can also produce positive results. One showed that 60 mg of vitamin A a week for six months produced a total remission of leukoplakias in 57 percent of the betal quid tobacco chewing fishermen from India examined. A reduction of micronucleated cells was seen in 96 percent of the subjects. Doses of 2.2 mmol per week of beta-carotene produced remission of leukoplakia in 14.8 percent and a reduction of micronucleated cells in 98 percent. The formation of new leukoplakia was completely suppressed by vitamin A and repressed by 50 percent as a result of beta-carotene with six months. Withdrawal of either beta-carotene or vitamin A supplementation resulted in the reappearance of leukoplakias and an increase in the frequency of micronuclei in oral mucosa. Lower doses of both agents prolonged the effect of the original treatment by a minimum of eight additional months. Another study reported results of a large trial of locally applied beta-trans retinoic acid that showed it to be an effective agent in reversing moderate cases of cervical intraepithelial neoplasia.

Presupplementation with beta-carotene (30 mg per day) can prevent beta-carotene depletion in the skin caused by ultraviolet radiation and in turn extend the prevention of free radical damage due to such radiation. High intake of beta-carotene may protect women against developing ovarian cancer. Patients undergoing endoscopic removal of polyps who received a combination of 30,000 U of vitamin A, 70 mg of vitamin E, and 1 g of vitamin C daily showed a significantly lower level of polyp reappearance relative to those receiving 20–40 g per day of lactulose or no treatment at all. Beta-carotene has proved to be an important dietary variable in improving survival in breast cancer patients. Supplementation with the effects of 30 mg of oral beta-carotene per day for six months on twenty male patients who had previously undergone resection of colonic adenocarcinoma inhibited mucosal ornithine decarboxylase activity by 44 percent after two weeks of beta-carotene administration and 57 percent after nine weeks, remaining low for up to six months following discontinuation of this protocol.

Smokeless tobacco use, and oral lesion patients who received 30 mg per day of beta-carotene experienced a dramatic improvement of the oral mucosa. More than half of patients with premalignant lesions of the oral cavity who were given daily doses of 30 mg of beta-carotene, 1000 mg of ascorbic acid, and 800 IU of alpha tocopherol for nine months experienced either partial or complete clinical resolution of their oral lesion. The administration of beta-carotene in doses of 30 mg per day had marked protective activity against oral premalignancy. Daily oral administration of 300,000 IU of vitamin A for twelve months significantly reduced the number of tobacco related new primary tumors in lung cancer patients relative to controls.

Supplementation with vitamins A, C, and E in patients with colorectal adenomas six months after complete polypectomy lead to a reduction in abnormalities in cell kinetics that may indicate a precancerous condition. In the cases of two cutaneous metastatic melanoma patients who were treated topically with beta-all-trans-retinoic acid, one experienced a complete regression of the treated lesions, while the other experienced partial regression. Three months' worth of supplementing the diet of 40 rural Filipino betel chewers with sealed capsules of retinol (100 000 IU/week) and beta-carotene (300 000 IU/week) was associated with a threefold decrease in the mean proportion of cells with micronuclei inside the cheek pouch.

Male patients with metastastic unresectable squamous cell carcinoma of the lung who were treated with up to seven treatment courses of either 13-cis vitamin A acid or vitamin A palmitate over a period of sixty weeks experienced significant immune potentiating effects. Supplementation with beta-carotene–rich foods can counteract the cancer causing-effects of smoke from cigarettes by maintaining vitamin A levels in smokers. Doses of 100,000 IU per day of vitamin A for two weeks produced an enhancement of antibody-dependent cell-mediated cytotoxicity, natural killer cell activity and blastogenic response to plant mitogens in patients with chronic lymphocytic leukemia.

Retinoic acid has been shown to be an effective treatment for chemically induced tumors. In one particular study, its use resulted in either complete or partial bladder papilloma regression in thirty-three patients. Daily supplementation of gastric mucosa patients with 20 mg of beta-carotene for three weeks produced a significant decrease of ornithine decarboxylase activity, which has been associated with cell proliferation and tumor promotion. Supplementation with 180 mg per week of beta-carotene and beta-carotene combined with 100,000 IU of vitamin A per week led to the remission and inhibition of new oral leukoplakia in subjects who chewed tobacco-containing betel quids on a daily basis.

Beta-carotene supplementation (180 mg/week, given twice weekly in six capsules of 30 mg each) proved to be an efficient inhibitor of exfoliated cells with micronuclei in the oral mucosa of smokeless tobacco chewers not already deficient in vitamin A. Vitamin A has exhibited protective effects against lung cancer in males and bladder cancer in both sexes. Local application of vitamin A acid had beneficial effects on women with moderate cervical dysplasia.

Benign breast disease patients orally administered 150,000 IU of vitamin A per day experienced complete or partial remissions and marked pain reductions. Animal studies point to the anti-cancer effects of vitamin A and beta-carotene. Similar results have been seen *in vitro*.

As with cancer, studies show an inverse association between

plasma levels of vitamins A and beta-carotene and the risk of heart disease. Supplementation has also produced direct results. In one study, patients undergoing carotid endarterectomy who were pre-treated with low-dose, oral beta-carotene experienced a fifty-fold increase in their plaque beta-carotene level, and the plaque from beta-carotene–treated patients had higher carotenoid levels and higher absorption compared with controls. The administration of 2 microM of beta-carotene proved more potent than 40 microM of alpha-tocopherol in inhibiting LDL oxidation and thus could be a key factor in atherosclerosis prevention. Animal trials support such findings.

Vitamin B$_1$

Vitamin B$_1$ (thiamine) is a powerful antioxidant. Supplementation with 100 mg per day of vitamin B$_1$ over a twelve-week period has been shown to elicit positive effects in patients suffering from Alzheimer's disease. Vitamin B$_1$ is also a proven fatigue fighter. Results of one double-blind, placebo-controlled study examining the effects of 10 mg of thiamin per day on healthy elderly Irish women showed that the women receiving thiamin had significant increases in energy intake, appetite, body weight, and general well-being.

Fatigue and daytime sleep were also decreased by supplementation. Daily supplementation with 200 mg of vitamin B$_1$ has been shown to improve left ventricular function in congestive heart failure patients. Patients suffering from pulmonary and myocardial insufficiency have benefited from postoperative vitamin B$_1$ injections (50 mg/kg). Results of another study demonstrated a single dose of thiamin produced significant protective effects in patients with ischemic heart damage. Dogs administered high doses of vitamin B$_1$ have experienced significant cardiovascular protection as well.

Thiamine has exhibited anti-HIV activity *in vitro*. In epileptics, it has produced improvements in neuropsychological functions, including visuo-spatial analysis, visuo-motor speed, and verbal abstracting ability. It has had cholinomimemetic effects on the central nervous system of healthy young adults. Another study involving two middle-aged patients who developed severe metabolic acidosis following abdominal surgery found that two 400 mg doses of thiamine immediately eliminated the lactic acidosis in both patients. Thiamine administered in doses of 50 mg per capita per day for thirty days significantly reduced blood glucose levels in patients with liver cirrhosis. Supplementation with 200 mg per day of thiamine over a one-week period restored levels of thiamine pyrophosphate, an essential co-factor in intermediary metabolism, to normal levels in chronic liver disease patients. Vitamin B_1 can improve conditions of seasonal ataxia. Thiamine administration following surgery prevented decreased blood corticosteroid levels during the postoperative period in patients subjected to herniotomy or appendectomy under local anesthesia.

Vitamin B_2

Results from animal and *in vitro* studies point to the efficacy of vitamin B_2 (riboflavin) in inhibiting the risk of cancer and heart disease. Supplemental vitamin B_2 has also been shown to be useful in the treatment of geriatric depression. Vitamin B_2 has exhibited antibacterial effects in mice and antistroke potential in rats. Two review articles have noted its antioxidant activity. Migraine patients receiving 40 mg of riboflavin in a single oral dose for at least three months have shown significant improvement following treatment. Riboflavin deficiency is known to induce cataract formation in animals.

Vitamin B_6

Vitamin B_6 (pyridoxine) is central to the body's manufacture of neurotransmitters, which are crucial to proper mental functioning. Vitamin B_6 supplementation has improved memory in healthy elderly men when administered in doses of 20 mg pyridoxine HCL per day for three months. The normalization of vitamin B_6 levels in HIV-infected patients suffering from a deficiency led to significant improvements in CD4 cell number as well as other functional parameters of immunity. Oral administration of vitamin B_6 at doses of 180 mg per day coupled with 40 mg of iron for twenty weeks led to significant improvements in hemodialysis patients. The administration of 200 mg per day of pyridoxine for five months led to significant improvement in children suffering from bronchial asthma. Vitamin B_6 treatment has proven effective in the treatment of autistic children. High vitamin B_6 intake suppressed the development of experimentally induced tumors in mice by regulating PLP growth or by immune enhancement.

Pyridoxine can regulate human melanoma cells *in vitro*. Tumor necrosis factor coupled with pyridoxine may be a more effective cancer treatment than the administration of tumor necrosis factor by itself. Vitamin B$_6$ can kill hepatoma cells *in vitro* and may be an effective antineoplastic agent. Six weeks' worth of treatment with 250 mg of vitamin B$_6$ and 5 mg of folic acid in patients with mild hyperhomocystinemia and cardiovascular disease normalized postload homocysteine concentration in 92 percent of patients, and fasting homoscyteimenia was normalized in 91 percent.

Patients taking vitamin B$_6$ for carpal tunnel syndrome and other degenerative diseases exhibited a risk of developing acute cardiac chest pain or myocardial infarction, which was less than patients who had not taken vitamin B$_6$. Results also showed a life span eight years longer among elderly patients who died from myocardial infarction relative to those who had not taken vitamin B$_6$. Vitamin B$_6$ has also been highly useful against carpal tunnel syndrome itself. Supplementation with 100 mg of vitamin B$_6$ per day corrected deficiencies in patients suffering from carpal tunnel syndrome as well as produced improvements in symptoms associated with the condition. A twelve-year study found that 68 percent of a group of 494 patients treated with 100 mg per day of vitamin B$_6$ experienced improvement in symptoms associated with carpal tunnel syndrome. Carpal tunnel syndrome patients have experienced benefits from treatment with 150 mg of pyridoxine per day for three months, despite having no initial deficiencies in the vitamin. A twelve-week treatment with vitamin B$_6$ proved to be effective in four patients suffering from carpal tunnel syndrome.

Cariogenic diets supplemented with vitamin B$_6$ and zinc led to a reduction in the number of dental carries in rats relative to controls. Gestational diabetes can be caused by increased xanthurenic-acid synthesis during pregnancy and vitamin B$_6$ supplementation can normalize the production of xanthurenic-acid by restoring tryptophan metabolism and thus improve oral glucose tolerance in such patients. Pyridoxine and methlyphenidate were more effective than controls in reducing symptoms associated with hyperkinesis in six patients. Male patients undergoing hemodialysis who received supplemental pyridoxine hydrochloride at doses of 50 mg per over a three- to five-week period experienced improvement in numerous parameters of immune function following the treatment. Vitamin

B_6 has also improved symptoms associated with PMS, pregnancy-induced nausea and vomiting, and primary hyperoxaluria.

Vitamin B_{12}

Vitamin B_{12} (cyanocobalamin) has been shown to exhibit anti-tumor effects and enhance cognitive performance in mice. *In vitro* studies point to its immune-enhancing activity on human T-cells. Vitamin B_{12} also appears to be useful in the treatment of patients suffering from Alzheimer's disease. Supplementation with 250 mcg/ml has signicantly improved cognitive function in HIV-infected patients. It can produce benefits in pernicious anemia patients. Two elderly patients deficient in vitamin B_{12} and suffering low immunoglobulin levels experienced a return to normal of such levels following supplementation with vitamin B_{12}. Results of another study found that supplementation with vitamin B_{12} led to marked improvements in outpatients suffering from recurrent aphthous initially deficient in vitamin B_{12}. Smokers of twenty years or more with metaplasia on one or more sputnam samples were given 10 mg of folate coupled with 500 micrograms of vitamin B_{12} for four months, which led to significant reductions of atypia. Vitamin B_{12} supplements have the potential to reverse some of the negative effects of chronic exposure to nitro oxide inhalation common to dental settings. Subjects with normal vitamin B_{12} levels who received supplements via injection scored better on the MMPI relative to subjects not receiving the supplements. Supplemental B_{12} has produced positive effects in hepatitis patients. Chronic multiple sclerosis patients taking 600 mcg of vitamin B_{12} every day for six months showed improvement in both abnormalities of the visual and brainstem auditory–evoked potentials relative to controls. Vitamin B_{12} supplementation at doses of 3 mg per day may advance human circadian rhythms by increasing circadian clock light sensitivity in healthy subjects. Additional studies highlight the ability of vitamin B_{12} to improve sleep as well.

Vitamin C

Vitamin C (ascorbic acid) is a water-soluble vitamin and essential antioxidant found in many fruits and vegetables. An insufficient intake of antioxidants has been linked to a higher risk of cancer and many other forms of degenerative diseases. One large study has demonstrated a significant relationship between low vitamin C intake and higher risks of heart disease mortality and overall mortality over the following ten-year time period. Additional studies have noted connections between vitamin C and other antioxidants and cataracts. Vitamin C has also been shown to be essential as a scavenger of free radicals, which is important in collagen formation, and hormone and neurotransmitter synthesis.

Additional research has examined the effects of ascorbic acid on cell proliferation and collagen expression in dermal fibroblasts from young children (ages three–eight) and the elderly (ages seventy-eight–ninety-three). The presence of ascorbic acid in both age groups resulted in a faster rate of cell proliferation and reached higher densities than controls. Collagen biosynthesis was found to be inversely related to age, while the stimulation by ascorbic acid appeared to be age independent. Beta-carotene (15–30 mg/day), vitamin E (15 mg/day), and vitamin C (30 mg/day) have all been shown to produce an increase of singlet oxygen protection of erythrocytes of subjects after just fifteen days of treatment. Significant positive correlations have been found between dietary ascorbic acid and HDLC, the intake of carbohydrates and protein and total fat in subjects over sixty-five. Significant negative correlations were found between dietary ascorbic acid and LDLC and LDLC/HDLC, suggesting a preventive role of ascorbic acid in atherogenic diseases. Another study has found that high vitamin C serum concentrations have resulted in lower blood glucose response in subjects of all ages. A similar relationship was found between vitamin E consumption and serum.

Daily ingestion of less than 100 mg of ascorbic acid resulted in the highest number of nonspecific clinical signs and symptoms. Daily ingestion of 200 mg or more of ascorbic acid resulted in the least for all ages. Those who ingested the most vitamin C (fifty years of age or older) were clinically similar to the forty-year-olds who ingested the least. Elderly lymphocytes cultured in the presence of 10 micrograms/ml of vitamin C and pre-incubated overnight, resulted in mitogen-stimulated lymphocyte proliferation, which was similar to that from younger controls without vitamin C in culture. Oral ingestion of 2 g of vitamin C daily on certain *in vitro* and *in vivo* immunologic parameters in the elderly has also been examined and proved to be beneficial. These results coupled with related findings in the study point to vitamin C as a potentially effective agent in enhancing immune functions in the elderly. Patients with age-related diseases such as diabetes, arthritis, vascular disease and hypertension have experienced positive results following treatment with metal chelator EDTA and antioxidants such as vitamin C, E, beta-carotene, selenium, zinc, and chromium.

Arthritis patients have benefited from supplemental vitamin C, with animal models supporting such findings. Patients suffering from cataracts have also found relief from treatment with vitamin C. Low vitamin C intake and consuming less than 3.5 servings of fruits and vegetables per day were found to be associated with an increased risk of cortical cataracts. Ascorbate significantly prevented selenite-induced cataracts in rats as well. Vitamin C may also be related to asthma. Studies show that vitamin C intake in the general population correlates with the incidence of asthma. Asthma symptoms in adults have been shown to decrease following vitamin C supplementation. Standard anti-asthma chemoprophylaxis (SAC) supplemented with 1 g of ascorbic acid (Redoxon) daily experienced less severe and fewer asthma attacks when ascorbic acid was given as a single daily dose for a six-month period. It significantly improved polymorphonuclear leucocyte (PMNL) motility and decreased antistreptolysin O (ASO) levels in children with bronchial asthma.

Another study of 124 patients with bronchial asthma found that 96.8 percent were deficient in ascorbic acid. Treatment that did not include vitamin C was ineffective. Administering doses of 275–300 mg of vitamin C, in combination with other vitamins, over many days proved more successful.

Approximately 35 percent of reproductive-age women in the United States consume less than 30 mg of vitamin C, while 68 percent consume less than 88 mg. Vitamin C is an independent risk factor for cervical dysplasia when other variables such as age and sexual activity are controlled. Research indicates vitamin C can decrease the duration of the common cold. Increasing vitamin C intake can benefit patients with active or inactive Crohn's disease, and improve adrenal function.

A 10 percent ascorbic acid solution can improve dermatitis. Synthetic ascorbic acid solution decreased symptoms in 74 percent of patients suffering from perennial allergic rhinitis. Another study found that 2 g of vitamin C administered to patients with allergic rhinititis produced significant positive effects one hour after treatment. Ascorbic acid can counter the effects of alcohol toxicity. Oral administration of 1 g per day of ascorbic acid for three days has produced antihistamine effects. Doses of 2 g per day had similar results in smokers. Ascorbic acid can also induce antipsychotic effects. Doses of 8 g/70 kg/day of ascorbic acid added to autistic treatment over a thirty-week period led to a reduction in symptom severity. The administration of ascorbic acid and alphatocopherol significantly improved neutrophil (PMN) locomotroy defect in patients suffering from blunt trauma. Ascorbic acid has exhibited anticandida activity *in vitro*. A study of men between twenty and thirty-five years old found that heavy smokers who consumed more than 200 mg/d of supplemental ascorbic acid experienced improvements in sperm quality relative to fertility.

Additional research supports such findings with respect to the role of vitamin C in promoting fertility. Studies indicate vitamin C may be effective against hepatitis, herpes, fatigue liver disease, Menkes disease, neutrophil dysfunction, obesity, ocular inflammation, opiate addiction, Paget's disease, pancreatitis, schizophrenia, sickle cell anemia, stress, stroke, sunburn, tetanus, glaucoma, glutathione deficiency, HTLV-I associated myelopathy, respiratory infections, cognitive impairment, retinal light damage, and symptoms associated with menopause. Research also indicates ascorbic acid aerosol in a dose of approximately 1 mg a puff up to a maximum of 300 mg/day could be an effective and novel way to stop smoking. Gingival bleeding has been linked to vitamin C deficiencies.

Parkinson's disease is another age-related condition that can be helped by vitamin C. The same is true of diabetes. One study found that 2 g per day of ascorbic acid taken for two weeks delayed the insulin response to a glucose challenge in nonglycemic adults and subsequently prolonged the postprandial hyperglycemia. Supplements of 100–600 mg per day of vitamin C daily taken for fifty-eight days were effective in decreasing the accumulation of sorbitol 2 in the erythrocytes of young insulin-dependent diabetics. Vitamin C has also been shown to be beneficial in the healing of various wounds. Doses between 500 to 3,000 mg a day have produced results in patients recovering from surgery, decubital ulcers, leg ulcers, and other unspecified injuries.

The immune system is another area where vitamin C plays a central role. Normal adult volunteers who ingested 2 to 3 g of ascorbate daily experienced enhanced neutrophil motility to a chemotactic stimulus of endotoxin-activated authologous serum. Stimulation of lymphocyte transformation to phytohaemagglutinin and concanavalin A was also detected in volunteers after the ingestion of 2 and 3 g of daily ascorbate.

Dietary supplementation with vitamins A, C, and E resulted in improved cell-mediated immune function indicated by significant increases in the total number of T-cells, T4 subsets, T4 to T8 ratio, and the proliferation of lymphocytes in response to phytohaemagagglutinin. Ascorbate acid inhibits human natural killer cell activity in a dose-dependent manner while not effecting effector/target cell binding or interferon or interlekin-2-induced increases of NK activity. AIDS is a disease of immune failure. Vitamin C has proven capable of combating its deadly effects on several fronts, including the suppression of HIV directly. Researchers have argued that doses as large as 50–200 g per twenty-four hours of ascorbate can suppress AIDS symptoms and reduce secondary infections.

No two areas have received as much attention in the scientific literature concerning vitamin C as its relations to cancer and heart disease. With respect to cancer, the evidence suggests deficiencies in vitamin C can be a risk factor for developing it, while vitamin C supplementation may be a useful therapy against the disease. Well over one hundred studies have been done on the role of vitamin C in cancer prevention, with most finding statistically significant effects. Protective effects have been shown for cancers of the pancreas, oral cavity, stomach, esophagus, cervix, rectum, breast, and lung. Results of one Latin American study found that vitamin C significantly decreased the risk of invasive cervical cancer, as was the case with beta-carotene and other carotenoids. Vitamin C supplement use was shown to be inversely related to bladder and colon cancer in women in an eight-year follow-up study beginning in 1981 of 11,580 residents of a retirement community initially free from cancer. Doses of 3 g per day have reduced polyp area in the treatment of patients suffering from large bowel adenomas over a nine-month period. One study involving patients with acute nonlymphocytic leukemia found that the numbers of leukemic bone marrow cell colonies grown in culture were decreased 21 percent of control in 7/28 patients by adding 0.3 mg of L-ascorbic acid to the culture medium. Concentrations of L-ascorbic acid as low as 0.1 milliM were capable of suppressing the leukemic cell colony in cultures of both leukemic and normal marrow cells. In another study, eighty-one patients with premalignant lesions of the oral cavity were given 30 mg of beta-carotene, 1000 mg of ascorbic acid, and 800 IU of alphatocopherol daily for nine months. The test concluded that 55.6 percent experienced either complete or partial clinical resolution of their lesions.

Plasma vitamin C has been found to reduce the risk of cancer by 60 percent in a trial of 117 cervical cancer patients. Patients with oral leukoplakia who were administered 30 mg of beta-carotene, 1000 mg of ascorbic acid, and 800 IU of alphatocopherol per day for nine months experienced either partial or complete clinical resolution of their oral lesions. Lung cancer and bladder cancer patients treated with doses of 5 g per day of ascorbic acid experienced a correction in low haematic levels of vitamin C and an increase in defense reactions against these types of cancer. Vitamin C supplementation decreased gastric mucosal DNA damage in cancer patients, which suggests that it may provide a protective role against the onset of gastric cancer. Treatment of sixty-two high-risk patients for gastric cancer with 1 g of ascorbic acid taken four times a day for four weeks found that ascorbic acid given in high doses can reduce the intragastric formation of nitrite and N-nitroso compounds. Two sets of Japanese clinical trials involving the use of supplemental ascorbate to treat terminal cancer patients showed the average survival time of high ascorbate patients was 246 days, compared to 43 days for low ascorbate patients in the first trial, and high ascorbate patients surviving an average of 115 days compared to 48 days for those in the low ascorbate group in the second trial. A comparative study of normal and malignant conditions in humans and in mice found that serum levels of vitamin C were lower in all human malignant cases relative to controls. With respect to mice, results showed that vitamin C and vitamin A supplementation administered at the start of tumor development reduced both tumor take and rate of growth and prolonged host survival relative to controls.

Another trial compared 294 incurable patients treated with supplemental ascorbate with 1532 untreated patients who served as controls over a 4.5-year period. The median survival time of the ascorbate group was 343 days, compared to 180 days for the controls. Postoperative treatment of ninety-five stomach cancer patients with vitamins C, E, and A has led to a decreased rate of postoperative complications from 30.9 percent to 1.9 percent. Results from animal studies support the anti-cancer effects of vitamin C. *In vitro* experiments do as well.

On the heart disease front, vitamin C is increasingly being recognized for its potential benefits. Men possessing low antioxidant status supplemented with 600 mg of ascorbic acid, 300 mg of alpha-tocopherol, 27 mg of beta-carotene, and 75 mg of selenium daily experienced reductions in lipid peroxidation, platelet aggregation, platelet production of thromboxone A2, and platelet activation *in vivo*. Another study showed that six weeks of ascorbic acid supplementation lowered pulse and systolic pressure in patients suffering from borderline hypertension.

A randomized trial of eighty-one patients with coronary artery disease determined that both unstable patients as well as patients with stable coronary artery disease requiring coronary artery bypass grafting benefited from treatment with vitamin E, vitamin C, and perioperative allopurinol. The treatment of idopathic thrombocytopenic purpura with ascorbate was successful in seven out of eleven patients, improving both the intravascular survival of platelets as well as platelet count. Vitamin C and vitamin E supplementation for ten days prior to donating blood resulted in a significant decrease in lipid peroxidation in stored red cells in both irradiated and non-irradiated samples relative to controls.

Research shows that LDL is protected against atherogenic modification by vitamin C due to ascorbic acid's free scavenging, which keeps aqueous oxidants from oxidizing LDL, and that stable modification of LDL by DHA or decomposition products thereof imparts increased resistance to metal ion-dependent oxidation. Intravenous infusion of 2 g of ascorbic acid in ten healthy volunteers resulted in a reduction of malondialdehyde concentrations and platelet aggregation inhibition. Patients with a history of myocardial infarction that were treated with 2 g of vitamin C daily experienced an increase of approximately 96 percent in serum ascorbate acid, while their fibrinolytic activity increased by 45 percent and platelet adhesive index decreased by 27 percent. A 12 percent drop was seen in their serum cholesterol level, beta lipoproteins were reduced significantly, and an increase occurred in the alpha fraction.

Similar results were seen in a second placebo-controlled group of acute myocardial infarction patients given 2 g daily of vitamin C for twenty days. Fibrinolytic activity rose 62.5 percent and serum ascorbic acid 94 percent after forty days. Doses of 1 g of vitamin C were shown to prevent platelet adhesiveness and platelet aggregation induced by feeding healthy males 75 g of butter. The administration of 1 g of vitamin C every eight hours over ten days in coronary artery disease patients significantly reduced platelet adhesiveness and platelet aggregation as well. Systolic blood pressure has been inversely associated with serum ascorbic acid levels in healthy adults between the ages of thirty and thirty-nine. Increases in ascorbic acid levels decreased the prevalence of hypertension. Subjects given 500 mg per day of vitamin C experienced significant reductions in body fat, systolic blood pressure, and pulse, and a significant increase in high density lipoprotein relative to controls.

Healthy young people randomly administered 1 g of ascorbic acid experienced a subsequent significant 16 percent fall in serum cholesterol within two months. A group of healthy older people recorded a 14 percent fall following a similar supplement within 6–12. Patients undergoing cardiopulmonary bypass who received 250 mg/kg of ascorbic acid experienced a decrease of lipid peroxidation in the cell membrane and protected the myocardium from ischemia-repurfusion injury during and after the operation by removing radicals.

Vitamin D

Vitamin D is a fat-soluble vitamin that stimulates calcium absorption, and the efficacy of vitamin D in preventing bone loss is well established. Results of numerous studies indicate that doses ranging from 400 to 15,000 IU of vitamin D per day can significantly reduce the rate of bone loss and bone fracture in women. Doses of 1 microgram per day of vitamin D have been shown to reduce blood pressure in hypercalcemic patients. Vitamin D may also be effective against cancer. Results of one nineteen-year-long study of 1954 Chicago men showed that an intake of greater than 3.75 micrograms per day of vitamin D was associated with a 50 percent reduction of colorectal cancer. Another large study found that moderately elevated concentrations of 25-hydroxyvitamin D ranging in dosage from 65–100 nmol/L showed even stronger association with reduction in incidence of the disease among a population of 25,620 individuals. Vitamin D has been noted as a potential treatment for prostate cancer. Additional findings support the anti-cancer activity of vitamin D both *in vitro* and in animal models.

Supplementation with 1000 IU per day of vitamin D over a period of one year prevented bone loss in Crohn's disease patients. It has produced dramatic improvements in postmenopausal women suffering from severe migraines. Low levels of vitamin D in patients with nephrotic syndrome were normalized following long-term supplementation with daily doses of 25 micrograms of vitamin D_3 per os. Two review articles have cited studies showing the efficacy of vitamin D_3 analogs in providing significant improvements of psoriatic lesions. Vitamin D has also produced healing in patients suffering from rickets.

Vitamin E

Vitamin E (alpha-tocopherol) can be found in eggs, wheat germ, green leafy vegetables, and various oils. Like vitamin C, vitamin E is a powerful antioxidant central to combating the aging process at both the cellular level and in the context of preventing and treating many degenerative conditions associated with it. Vitamin E is an essential nutrient, in that it is not synthesized in the body, and protects cells membranes from free-radical reactions.

One study of men older than fifty-five showed that supplemental vitamin E at doses of 800 IU over a period of forty-eight days protected against oxidative stress produced by vigorous exercise. Results of similar studies support such findings. A trial involving thirty-two healthy subjects over the age of sixty has shown that the administration of 800 mg per day of vitamin E for one month enhanced immune function relative to controls. Rats fed a diet enriched with sodium selenite and alphatocopherol experienced a reduction in the production of lipid peroxides in the serum and liver, thus inhibiting the aging process. Vitamin E in combination with manntiol, and dexamethasone have exhibited significant cerebral protective effects in dogs. Vitamin E–enriched lipoproteins have been shown to increase neuron longevity *in vitro*.

Vitamin E inhibits amyloid beta protein–induced cell death, a key factor in Alzheimer's disease; and has been shown to protect against oxidative damage caused by gene coding of superoxide dismutase on chromosome 21 resulting in excess activity of the enzyme, again suggesting its potential as a preventive approach to Alzheimer's. Levels of vitamin E have been reported to be twice as high in the midbrain of Alzheimer's patients and Alzheimer's patients with signs of Parkinson's disease relative to controls. Animal studies have also exhibited promise for the treatment of Alzheimer's disease. Inverse associations have been noted in the literature between serum levels of vitamin E and the risk of rheumatoid arthritis. Several studies involving rats suggest that supplemental vitamin E may work directly to lesson the severity of the disease.

Osteoarthritis patients treated with 400 IE per day of d-alpha-tocopherylacetate for six weeks experienced more pain relief and more improvement in mobility than controls. Those receiving doses of 600 mg per day for ten days showed significant positive effects compared to patients given placebos. Similar studies have produced like results. Antioxidants such as vitamin E, vitamin C, and pyruvate can thwart the cataractogenic effect of oxyradicals and may be effective in cataract treatment or prevention. Adults with high levels of two or more of either vitamin E, C, or carotenoids have a decreased risk of cataracts compared to those with low levels of one or more. Numerous *in vitro* and *en vivo* studies in different animals species have shown that vitamins E and C offer protective effects against light-induced cataracts as well as sugar and steroid cataracts.

Intramuscular injections of vitamin E have been shown to partially correct deficits in cystic fibrosis patients suffering from severe vitamin E deficiency and neurologic disease. Cystic fibrosis patients and patients with biliary atresia require supplementation with vitamin E to maintain a normal integrity of axons related to the gracile and possibly other sensory nuclei. Early supplementation with vitamin E may help to prevent neurologic dysfunction in cystic fibrosis patients with pancreatic insufficiency. Results of another study showed that serum concentrations of vitamin E were all but undetectable in four patients with chronic steatorrhoe, two of whom had cystic fibrosis and two chronic cirrhosis of childhood. In one patient, substantial improvement was seen following the restoration of normal vitamin E levels by parenteral therapy.

Acne patients treated with 0.2 mg of selenium and 10 mg of tocopheryl succinate twice daily for six to twelve weeks experienced positive results. Several studies indicate vitamin E supplementation may be useful in the treatment of patients suffering from neurological complications associated with abetalipoproteinemia. Studies suggest vitamin E to be an effective treatment for alcohol-related immunosuppression. Vitamin E supplementation may be useful in reversing anemia by reducing the fragility of red blood cells in regular dialysis patients. Alpha-tocopherol could be an effective means of protecting the brain against anoxic damage due to its antioxidant effects, and halting or improving neurological disorders associated with progressive ataxia. Vitamin E therapy has been shown to improve cerebellar symptoms of adult-onset celiac disease.

Children suffering from cholestasis have benefited following treatment with supplemental vitamin E at varying doses. Two months of treatment with either 150, 300, or 600 IU of vitamin E per day in women with benign breast cancer improved severe PMS symptoms. Women treated daily with 400 IU of alpha-tocopherol for three cycles also experienced significant improvements in certain affective and physical symptoms of PMS. The administration of 2 x 200 mg of vitamin E for ten weeks to high-altitude mountain climbers enhanced physical performance and cell protection. Supplementation with 900 IU of vitamin E for six weeks exhibited beneficial effects on the respiratory health of smokers. Six weeks of treatment with vitamin E improved the clinical status and normalized the proportion of OKT+4 T-lymphocytes and the ratio of OKT+4 to OKT+8 cells in the peripheral blood of children suffering from respiratory tract infections. In newborns, supplemental vitamin E has offered protection against intraventricular hemorrhage, intracranial hemorrhage, retinopathy of prematurity, and retrolental fibroplasis. Several studies indicate tardive dyskinesia patients may benefit from supplemental vitamin E, with doses averaging 1600 IU per day over a period of six to twelve weeks. Supplementation with 1200 mg daily of vitamin E for fourteen days prior to exhaustive running prevented exercise-induced DNA damage in humans resulting from oxidative stress. Animal trials have demonstrated the stress fighting activity of vitamin E as well. Studies indicate vitamin E may provide protection against the harmful effects of smoking as a result of its antioxidant activity.

Studies have linked vitamin E intake with an increased therapeutic efficiency of drugs such as AZT. Vitamin E supplementation has also been shown to result in a decrease in the progression of disease to AIDS. The incubation of human Jurkat T-cells with vitamin E acetate or alpha-tocopheryl succinate (10 microM to 1mM) exhibited a concentration dependent inhibition of NF-kappa B activation. Such findings support the possible use of vitamin E derivatives as a treatment for AIDS. Another study showed that the addition of d-alpha-tocopherol acid succinate (ATS) (doses of 5 to 15 micrograms/ml) to MT4 cells and murine hemotopoietic progenitor cells treated with AZT resulted in increased anti-HIV activity relative to the use of AZT alone. Data have shown that 1–100 mumol/l of vitamin E significantly increased the growth BFU-E and colony-forming units granulocyte monocyte from patients infected with HIV, as did 5–10 U/ml of EPO. Compared to healthy controls, tocopherol equally ameliorated the growth of BFU-E and CFU-GM from the HIV-positive subjects in the presence of AZT. A study on the effects of vitamin E in a murine AIDS model made the following observations: A fifteen-fold increase in vitamin E (160 IU/l) modulated the production of interleukin-2 (IL) in both uninfected mice and retrovirus-infected mice. Vitamin E significantly reduced the level of IL-4 secretion in the uninfected mice at four and eight weeks. Vitamin E significantly reduced IL-4 production, elevated by retrovirus infection, and significantly reduced IL-6. Vitamin E significantly increased thymic and serum vitamin E concentration previously reduced by retrovirus infection. Additional animal studies have produced similar findings.

Diabetes is another degenerative disease in which vitamin E plays an important role. Supplementation with 1 g of vitamin E per day for 35 days diminished ADP-induced platelet aggregation in type I diabetics. Doses of 900 mg per day of vitamin E for four months reduced oxidative stress and improved insulin action in noninsulin dependent diabetics. Treatment with d-alpha-tocopherol can prevent diabetes-induced abnormalities in rat retinal blood flow. In a study of middle-aged Finnish men, results showed that a low lipid standardized plasma vitamin E concentration was associated with a 3.9-fold risk of diabetes. For every decrement of 1 mumol/l of uncategorized unstandardized vitamin E concentration, there was an increment of 22 percent in diabetes risk. Low platelet vitamin E levels might play a role in the increased thromboxane synthesis demonstrated by platelets in type I diabetics. Four months' worth of vitamin E supplementation resulted in a significant improvement in glucose utilization and hepatic response to insulin in both normal subjects as well as diabetics. Daily doses of 1000 mg of vitamin E inhibited platelet activity in type I diabetics.

Treatment with 8 micrograms/kg a day of vitamin E for two weeks improved pulmonary hemodynamics, lipid metabolism, and lipid peroxidation in patients with diabetic nephroangiopathy. The use of alpha-tocopherol acetate significantly decreased lipid peroxidation activity in middle-aged patients with insulin independent diabetes. The administration of vitamin E in daily doses ranging between 600 and 1200 mg to type II diabetics stimulated pancreatic insulin-producing function and was conducive to normalization of lipid peroxidation. Supplementation with doses of 300 mg per day of alpha-tocopherol acetate normalized processes of lipid peroxidation in red cell membranes and blood plasma lipid content, reduced the blood plasma level of lipid peroxidation products and the content of total lipids in red cell membranes in diabetics. Liver function in diabetics can be positively effected by the administration of vitamin E. Decreased platelet vitamin E levels have been associated with increased aggregation, and vitamin E appears to regulate arachidonic acid metabolism in platelets. Studies have shown that platelet vitamin E levels in diabetics have a tendency to be reduced with platelet aggregation increases. Supplementation with several hundred IU of vitamin E has been shown to significantly reduce lipid peroxidation and platelet aggregation in insulin and noninsulin dependent diabetics. In nondiabetics, low doses of vitamin E (200 IU) have been seen to significantly decrease platelet adhesion and inhibit the formation of protruding pseudopods.

Research indicates vitamin E to be capable of protecting against tumor growth and carcinogenesis. Studies have also suggested vitamin E can reduce the toxicity of several anti-cancer therapies. Results of long-term follow-up studies of alpha-tocopherol serum concentrations in large trials of Finnish adults have shown a greater risk of cancer in those with low alpha-tocopherol levels compared to those with higher levels. Additional large population-based trials and case control studies have shown similar patterns across a variety of different types of cancer, including breast, colon, lung, etc. Supplementation with vitamin E has also been shown capable of limiting the course of disease as well as preventing it. One study examined the efficacy of vitamin E in the treatment of chemotherapy-induced mucositis in malignancy patients and found a total resolution of oral lesions in six of nine patients who took vitamin E. By contrast, eight of nine patients receiving a placebo showed no resolution of lesions. A review of results from eight clinical trials have shown beta-carotene and vitamin E produced regression of oral leukoplakia and that all available evidence points to a major role for antioxidant nutrients in the prevention of oral cancer. Among mammary dysplasia patients given 600 units per day of alpha-tocopherol, 88 percent responded clinically and the progesterone to estradiol ratio, abnormal in mammary dysplasia patients, increased from 30 ± 7 (S.E.) to 53 ± 11 in patients after alpha-tocopherol therapy. In a study of oral leukoplakia patients given a daily antioxidant combination including 30 mg of beta-carotene, 1000 mg of ascorbic acid, and 800 IU of alpha-tocopherol for nine months, 55.6 percent of the eighty-one patients who completed the protocol experienced partial or complete clinical resolution of their oral lesions. Results also showed that the antioxidant supplementation was most effective in those who abstained from the use of alcohol and tobacco during the study. The administration of 400 IU of alpha-tocopherol to oral leukoplakia patients resulted in a significant reduction in micronuclei frequencies in specimens from visible lesions and normal-appearing mucosa. High-risk breast cancer patients were given a combination of antioxidants that included 2500 IU of vitamin E, 32.5 IU of beta-carotene, 2,850 mg of vitamin C, 387 micrograms of selenium, 90 mg of CoQ_{10}, 1.2 g of gamma linolenic acid, 3.5 g n-3 fatty acids, and a host of secondary vitamins and minerals, experienced positive results, including partial remission in some. The topical application of 400 mg/ml of vitamin E in oil form applied to lesions for one week in patients receiving chemotherapy for oral musositis proved to be significantly effective relative to controls. The administration of alpha-tocopherol in an escalating dose schedule of 800, 1200, 1600, and 2000 IU per day for each subsequent four-week cycle until disease progression or unacceptable toxicity occurred reduced the level of major toxicities of high-dose 13-cRA in patients suffering from skin, head and neck, or lung cancer. The rate of postoperative complications in a group of gastric cancer patients taking a complex administration of vitamin C, E, and A preoperatively dropped from 30.9 percent to 1.9 percent. A study of twenty-eight liver cancer patients found that treatment with 600 mg of alpha-tocopherol, 100,000 MU of retinol, and 1.5 g of ascorbic acid for seven days prior to surgery was shown to significantly reduce the level of dialdehyde in the liver and increase the level of catalase.

Following antioxidant treatment, purulent and septic complications were 1.6 times less, as well. Animal trials also point to the promise of vitamin E as a cancer therapy; *in vitro* experiments have produced similar findings.

Much has been made of the so-called "European Paradox," which involves the paradoxically low rates of coronary heart disease in several European countries where the diet includes a relatively high intake of saturated fatty acids. Results of one large-scale, longitudinal study of coronary heart disease mortality among men in seventeen western European countries found that vitamin E intake specifically rather than the consumption of wine is most likely the best explanation. A large body of research exists supporting this idea and the use of vitamin E in the prevention and treatment of heart disease.

One study examined the effects on platelet function in low antioxidant men of supplementation with 600 mg ascorbic acid, 300 mg alpha-tocopherol, 27 mg beta-carotene, and 75 micrograms of selenium in yeast daily for five months. Results showed that relative to controls, men taking the antioxidants experienced 20 percent reductions in serum lipid peroxides, 24 percent reductions in ADP-induced platelet aggregation, 42 percent reductions in the rate of ATP release during aggregation, 51 percent reductions in serum thromboxane B_2, and 29 percent reductions in plasma beta-thromboglobulin concentration.

The consumption of one palmvitee capsule per day (containing approximately 18 mg of tocopherols, 42 mg of tocotrienols, and 240 mg of palm olein) for thirty days lowered both total serum cholesterol (ranging from 5 percent to 35.9 percent) and low density lipoprotein cholesterol (ranging from 0.9 percent to 37 percent) concentrations in human subjects. The intake of 900 mg of vitamin E per day for four months of vitamin E by elderly insulin-resistant nondiabetics has been found to be a useful therapy for coronary heart disease. Another study showed significant reductions in the indexes of oxidative stress in both smokers and nonsmokers, as well as reductions in serum platelet numbers following the intake of 280 mg per day for ten weeks of dl-alpha-tocopherol acetate. Alpha-tocopherol has specifically inhibited aorta smooth muscle cell proliferation and protein kinase C activity, findings that may be relevant to the development of atherosclerosis and related diseases.

A study of one hundred patients with transient ischemic attacks, minor strokes, or residual ischemic neurologic deficits compared the effects of aspirin plus 400 IU per day of vitamin E with aspirin alone (325 mg) for up to two years. Results showed patients in the vitamin E plus aspirin group experienced a significant reduction in the rate of ischemic events relative to patients taking just the aspirin. Significant reductions were also seen in platelet adhesiveness in patients taking the vitamin E plus aspirin. Based on these findings, the authors concluded that vitamin E plus aspirin is an effective preventive therapy for transient ischemic attacks and related cerebrovascular disorders. The combined administration of vitamin E and seventeen beta-estradiol provides protection for LDL against oxidation in postmenopausal women.

Patients receiving supplementation with vitamin E and C either immediately before or after coronary artery bypass suffered fewer ischemic electrocardiographic events and needed less dopamine perioperatively relative to controls. The ingestion of 1,000 IU per day of dl-alpha-tocopheral acetate for seven days by six nonsmoking subjects increased plasma and LDL levels of alpha-tocopherol 3.0 and 2.4 fold, respectively. The rate of oxidation showed significant decreases of 19 percent and significant elevations of LDL oxidation resistance by 41 percent.

Platelet adherence decreased an average of 75 percent after two weeks of supplementation of 200 IU of vitamin E per day in normal individuals. An 82 percent reduction occurred following two weeks of supplementation with 400 IU per day. Supplementation with 800 IU per day of alpha-tocopherol, 1 g per day of ascorbate, and 30 mg per day of carotene over a three-month period produced a twofold prolongation of the lag phased and reduced the oxidation rate by 40 percent in the twelve men studied.

Healthy volunteers administered 30 ml/day of either fish oils supplemented with 0.3 IU/g or 1.5 IU/g for three weeks experienced a 48 percent decrease in serum triglycerides and an 11 percent decrease in fibrinogen.

Male atherosclerosis patients taking 100 IU per day or more of vitamin E had less coronary artery lesion progression than those taking less than this amount, and such benefits were seen in all lesions. Intake of 60 IU per day of vitamin E has been associated with a reduced risk of coronary heart disease among middle-aged men. Similar associations have been seen in middle-aged women. Studies have shown that doses as low as 50–100 microM of vitamin E, when combined with an inhibitor of the arachidonate pathway, inhibit cyclooxygenase-independent platelet aggregation. High doses of vitamin E (200 IU/kg per day) has improved myocardial tolerance to ischemia and reperfusion by decreasing myocardial infarct size significantly. Doses of 400 IU per day of vitamin E can inhibit platelet adhesion to a variety of adhesive proteins by more than 75 percent. Supplementation with 500 IU per day of vitamin E for three months proved effective in hyperlipoproteinemia and may be considered a useful agent for combating the risk of coronary heart disease. The administration of vitamin E alone (400 IU to 1200 IU) over six weeks or in combination with aspirin had positive effects in patients with arterial thromboembolic diseases.

Other conditions where treatment with vitamin E has shown promise include disseminated granuloma anulare, endotoxemia, enteritis, epilepsy, gastric mucosal injury and gastrointestinal disease, pneumonia, male infertility, flu, keloids, Keshan disease, kidney damage, lead intoxication, leg cramps, liver damage, muscle damage, spinal injury, spondylosis, steatorrhoea, stroke, thalassaemia, thymus damage, thyroid dysfunction, tuberculosis, ulcerative colitis, ulcers, uveitis, veno-occlusive disease, vitiligo, brain injury, vision problems, retinal degeneration, glomeruslerosis, hearing loss, hepatitis, yellow nail syndrome, sickle cell anemia, UV-induced skin damage, hyperlipidemia, periodontal health, Parkinson's disease, sexual dysfunction, short bowel syndrome, burns, wound healing, hemolysis, lung damage, and neurological dysfunction. In addition to its use in fighting specific problems, vitamin E has also been shown capable of enhancing the workings of the immune system in general. Supplementation with 800 mg of vitamin E for thirty days improved immune responsiveness in older healthy adults. Repletion of vitamin E deficiency has been shown capable of dramatically improving T-cell function and improving neuropathy in patients with intestinal malabsorptive disorders. The administration of 25 mg/kg daily of d-alpha-tocopheryl-polyethylene-glycol-1000 succinate to enhance absorption of cyclosporin could be an effective means of decreasing the high cost of immunosuppression in recipients of pediatric liver transplants. Healthy older adults taking 800 mg of vitamin E for thirty days experienced an improvement in some *in vivo* and *in vitro* parameters of the immune function relative to controls. Supplementation with vitamins A, C, and E in elderly long-stay patients can improve the aspects of cell-mediated immune function. Patients given 40 mg/kg of vitamin E 3.5 hours prior to open heart surgery experienced a decreased rate of immunodepression in the postoperative period.

Vitamin K

Vitamin K is a fat-soluble vitamin both made in the body and found in nature. It consists of three related substances: phylloquinone (K1), found in foods; menaquinone (K2), produced in the intestinal bacteria; and menadione (K3), a synthetic compound of the first two. Vitamin K is found in green leafy vegetables such as alfalfa, broccoli, and spinach; in polyunsaturated oils; and in animal products like eggs, fish oils, milk, yogurt, and liver. Vitamin K is most noted for its central role in proper blood clotting. Studies have shown it also capable of inhibiting tumor growth and may be important for the prevention of osteoporosis and tooth decay. Deficiencies of vitamin K are rare; there is presently no RDA. An optimal dietary intake per day is approximately 300 mcg.

Zinc

An essential trace element in the body, zinc is involved in many biological functions including cell division and differentiation, programmed cell death, gene transcription, biomembrane functioning, and countless enzymatic activities that make it central to the aging process itself. Zinc has been shown to protect against the deteriorating vision associated with age-related macular degeneration. When taken as a supplement, zinc can improve cell-mediated immunity in the elderly. Zinc has also produced benefits in patients suffering from arthritis. In one study, 220 mg of zinc sulphate was administered thrice daily over a period of twelve weeks to patients suffering from chronic, refractory rheumatoid arthritis. Results showed significant improvements in patients taking the zinc with respect to joint swelling, morning stiffness, walking time, and subjective patient reports of own conditions.

Arthritic patients in another study received 600 mg per day of oral zinc sulphate for six months, which was followed by significant reductions in the number of swollen and tender joints, the need for nosteroidal anti-inflammatory drugs, and erythrocyte sedimentation rate relative to controls. The administration of oral zinc doses at either 50 or 75 mg per day over a twelve-week period significantly reduced serum high density lipoprotein cholesterol levels in young adult males. Oral doses of zinc sulphate of 200 mg taken three times per day significantly reduced serum cholesterol and beta-lipoproteins and significantly increased alpha-lipoproteins in stablized ischemic heart disease patients. Cancer patients have experienced enhanced immune activity after taking 250 mg per day of oral zinc gluconate over a period of three weeks. Animal studies indicate zinc can also protect against stroke and ameliorate the effects of chronic stress in mice.

Numerous studies point to the efficacy of zinc in treating skin disorders such as acne, herpes, and eczema. AIDS patients have experienced beneficial effects on the immune system from supplemental zinc therapy. Doses of 200 mg per day of zinc sulfate improved responsiveness to delayed hypersensitivity skin tests in patients suffering from alcoholic cirrhosis. Many elderly people experience symptoms of anorexia and thus fail to obtain the nutrients they need through a normal diet.

Doses of zinc ranging from 40 to 90 mg per day have had positive effects on weight gain in anorexic patients. Intake of zinc has led to improvements in patients suffering from cerebral palsy, inflammatory bowel disease, leprosy, sickle cell anemia, and Wilson's disease. When taken in the form of zinc gluconate lozenges, zinc has shown consistent beneficial effects against the common cold. Doses of 50 mg three times per week of elemental zinc over a period of six months have shown significant increases in plasma zinc, serum testosterone, sperm count, libido, and frequency of intercourse in patients undergoing hemodialysis. Supplemental zinc administered immediately after injury was associated with more rapid neurologic recovery and visceral protein concentrations in severe closed head injury patients relative to controls. Zinc has shown promise in the treatment of male infertility. Obese patients have experienced significant weight loss following eight weeks of supplementation with 600 mg per day of zinc sulfate. Zinc has been found useful in the treatment of gastric ulcers (zinc sulphate), ulcerative stomatitis (zinc sulphate), and venous leg ulcers among the elderly (topical zinc oxide). It is an important part of treating periodontal disease in elderly patients. Zinc can also reduce enlarged prostate size in men.

HERBS

Aloe

Aloe has been considered a miracle plant by cultures the world over for thousands of years. It is approximately 96 percent water, with the balance of its active contents consisting of essential oil, amino acids, vitamin, minerals, and enzymes. Aloe's primary strength as a healing agent lies in the fact of it being able to regenerate damaged tissues. Such actions have long made it a powerful therapy for wounds such as burns, cuts, and bruises. But this is just the tip of the iceberg.

A traditional remedy for diabetes in the Arabian peninsula, several peer review studies indicate aloe may indeed be an effective treatment for symptoms associated with the disease. In one, results showed the intake of half a teaspoon of aloe daily for four to fourteen weeks significantly reduced the fasting serum glucose level in all patients. Fasting plasma glucose was significantly reduced in diabetic mice by glibenclamide and aloes after three days as well. Another study found that five noninsulin dependent diabetics experienced a mean reduction in fasting blood sugar of 273 to 151 mg/dl following fourteen weeks of taking a half teaspoon 4 times daily of aloe. In a five year trial of 5000 atheromatous heart disease patients, results showed that dietary intake of Husk of Isabgol and aloe vera to the diet led to a marked reduction in total serum cholesterol, serum triglycerides, fasting, and post prandial blood sugar level in diabetic patients. Clinical profiles showed decreased frequency of anginal attacks and gradually, the drugs, like verapamil, nifedipine, beta-blockers and nitrates, were tapered. Animal experiments support such findings with respect to the potential of aloe as a valuable therapy for diabetes, and have demonstrated its anticancer properties and ability to inhibit arthritis in rats. A host of studies indicate aloe can produce strong anti-inflammatory, antibacterial, and wound healing effects. Aloe has also been used successfully as a laxative, may be effective for ulcers, and can protect against skin damage when used topically. Current research points to aloe's potential as an effective immune system booster and possible treatment against AIDS.

American Creosote Bush

One year of treatment solely with an aqueous extract of American creosote bush has been reported to have produced a dramatic tumor regression in an eighty-five-year-old male suffering from a malignant melanoma in his right cheek with a larger cervical metastasis. An extensive review article on the herb has also noted that its active constituent, NDGA, has been the subject of numerous studies on its efficacy as an antioxidant, anti-inflammatory, anti-carcinogen, anti-microbial agent, etc.; many of which have produced findings supporting its use and calling for the need for additional research into the overall health benefits of the plant in general.

Angelica

Angelica has been found to possess potent anti-tumor properties, and to protect against arrhythmia in rats during myocardial ischemia and against myocardial dysfunction and injury in rabbits. Angelica has exhibited antibacterial, anti-inflammatory, and sedative acitivity. It has proven safe and effective in the treatment of patients suffering from psoriasis. One review article has cited results from numerous studies supporting the use of Angelica sinensis as an effective treatment for a variety of conditions, including PMS, dysmenorrhea, amenorrhea, cardiac arrhythmia, high blood pressure, anemia, and acute icteric hepatitis.

Astragalus

Astragalus root is popularly used throughout the world as an immune enhancer and general body tonic. Indeed, studies have demonstrated its direct positive effects on the immune system in animal models and have pointed to its antimicrobial activity *in vitro*. In patients suffering from leucopenia, 10 ml equaled to 15 g of astragalus twice per day for eight weeks led to an 82.76 percent rate of effectiveness. Patients receiving 10 ml equaled to 5 g of astragalus over the same schedule experienced a 47.3 percent rate of effectiveness. Astragalus may benefit the digestive system, protect against liver injury, boost the immune system of lupus patients, counter alcohol-induced memory loss, improve sperm motility, and help heal burn injuries. The astragalus fraction, F3, has exhibited significant immunorestorative effects on mononuclear cells taken from cancer patients. Similar results were seen *in vivo* using a rodent model. The anti-tumor activity of LAK cells was greatly enhanced by the action of Shengmaisan with astragalus membranaceus at concentrations of 100 micrograms/ml.

In a study of nineteen congestive heart failure patients, treatment with astragalus membranceus ingredient, the astragaloside IV (XGA) produced a relief in chest distress and dispnea in fifteen patients after two weeks of treatment. Improvements were also seen with respect to left ventricular modeling, left ventricular end-diastolic volume and left ventricular end-systolic volume and heart rate.

The administration of astragalus membranaceus decreased the ratio of pre-ejection period/left ventricular ejection time, increased superoxide dismutase activity of red blood cells, and reduced the lipid peroxidation content of plasma in acute myocardial infarction patients. Astragalus membranaceus is a successful therapy for ischemic heart disease patients, proving more effective than Nifedipine and Tab. Animal studies point to the efficacy of astragalus as a heart disease therapy as well.

Bee Propolis

Apitherapy refers to the practice of using products obtained from bees such as honey, pollen, beeswax, royal jelly, and propolis for medicinal purposes. Peer review studies have shown that apitherapy is far more than just an ancient folk remedy. Several have demonstrated its antibacterial, anti-inflammatory, and antioxidant activity. Ethanol extracts of propolis can increase the rate of ossification in cases of artificially induced bone tissue loss. Bee propolis has exhibited anti-cancer effects both in animal trials and *in vitro*. It has produced cardioprotective and anti-flu effects in rats. Women suffering from acute cervicitis experienced significant positive results from 5 percent propolis dressings applied to vaginal dressings for ten days. Doses of propolis ranging in concentration strength from 10 percent to 30 percent are an effective treatment for patients suffering from giardiasis.

One study found that ocular medical propolis films applied behind the lower eyelids before bed over a period of ten to fifteen days cut recovery time in half in patients with postherpetic trophic keratitis and/or postherpetic nebula. The propolis constituent, 3-methyl-but-2-enyl caffeate, reduced the viral titer of herpes simplex virus 1 by 3 log 110 and reduced viral DNA synthesis thirty-two-fold. Rats treated with 100 mg/kg of Cuban red propolis extract experienced hepatoprotective effects against CC14-induced liver damage. Propolis also exhibited beneficial antioxidative properties in rats suffering from toxic liver damage and acute hepatic ischemia. Apitherapy has proven to be a useful treatment in patients suffering from ischemic insults, pulmonary tuberculosis, rheumatic disorders, panaritium, abscesses, phlegmons, and infectious wounds. Clinical and X-ray exams point to the efficacy of a 4 percent alcohol solution of bee glue added to root-canal fillings in severe cases of periodontitis. Another study showed that an ethanol extract of propolis stimulated the regenerative process on damaged dental pulp and led to a decrease in circulatory system disorders and degenerative processes. Animal and *in vitro* studies have produced similar findings.

Bilberry

Animal studies indicate bilberry contains effective promoters and enhancers of arteriolar rhythmic diameter that also have been shown to reduce ischaemia reperfusion injury-induced microvascular impairments.

Bilberry has exhibited significat vasoprotective and antioedema effects in animal trials as well.

Black Cohosh

Black cohosh in tincture can be useful in the treatment of depression. The herb has also been shown to have beneficial effects in women suffering from menopausal symptoms. Black cohosh can be a useful therapy during the early stages of measles, and additional studies have found it to be effective in influenza, mumps, measles complicated with pneumonia, congenital syphilis, and tonsilitis as well.

Black Walnut

Black walnut is a rich dietary source of protein, iodine, chromium, potassium, manganese, vitamin A, and vitamin C which has been used to relieve symptoms of constipation and poor digestion going all the way back to the time of ancient Greece. It is a widely recognized blood cleanser and oxygenizer, blood sugar stabilizer, and is often used topically to treat bruises, rashes, herpes, fungal infections, boils, canker sores, and gum disease. Studies have shown the consumption of 84 g per day of black walnuts can significantly lower serum cholesterol levels in healthy men. Results of animal trials point to the cardiovascular benefits and anti-cancer properties of black walnut as well.

Carrot

A carrot-only diet over a course of several days a week has been found to significantly delay death by cancer in rats. Properties from carrots have also exhibited strong antimicrobial activity *in vitro*, and can protect against liver damage in mice.

Common Plantain

Results of one study involving twenty-five chronic bronchitis patients treated with common plantain for a period of between twenty-five and thirty days found a quick effect on subjective complaints and objective benefits in as many as 80 percent of the patients with no toxic effects. Common plantain has been shown to inhibit the onset of tumors and lower blood pressure in animal trials. When administered in ointment form, common plantain has exhibited anti-inflammatory action on the skin.

Cranberry

Results from numerous studies have shown that consumption of cranberry juice is an effective treatment against bladder and urinary tract infections. Animal experiments indicate that components of cranberry can lower blood pressure as well.

Dandelion

A popular liver remedy, dandelion is an herb loaded with vitamins, minerals, protein, etc. Dandelion extracts have exhibited anti-tumor and hypoglycemic activity in animal studies. Evidence indicates that it may also be effective in treating additional conditions, including liver problems, hepatitis, gallstones, kidney trouble, and weight loss.

Echinacea

A common remedy for colds and general immune enhancer, echinacea is a plant native to America's Great Plains and long used by Native Americans. Echinacea has exhibited anti-cancer activity *in vitro* and been shown to enhance immune function, protect against skin damage, and exhibit anti-inflammatory activity in mice.

Evening Primrose Oil

Evening primrose oil administered at doses of 6 g per day in one study and 20 ml in another has been shown to produce beneficial effects in patients suffering from rheumatoid arthritis. It also holds promise for diabetics. Animal studies point to its ability to lower systolic blood pressure and total cholesterol levels and potential for treating skin conditions such as dermatitis.

Feverfew

Feverfew has exhibited evidence of anti-thrombotic potential and inhibits platelet aggregation *in vitro*. Feverfew extract has exhibited anti-candida activity *in vitro*. Daily consumption of fresh feverfew leaves can also prevent migraines.

Flaxseed Oil

Results of animal studies point to the anti-tumor activity of flaxseed with respect to colon and breast cancer. The consumption of 40 g per day of flaxseed oil over a period of twenty-three days has also been shown to have cardioprotective effects in healthy young men. Daily intake of 30 g of flaxseed has proven useful in the treatment of patients suffering from lupus.

One study found that the consumption of 50 g per day of flaxseed for four weeks increased bowel movements by 30 percent and reduced LDL cholesterol by as much as 8 percent in healthy young adults. Dietary flaxseed and flax oil have attenuated renal function decline and reduced glomerular injury with favorable effects on blood pressure, plasma lipids, and urinary prostaglandins in rats.

Garlic

A popular herb for centuries the world over, garlic is available in varying forms such as raw, oil, powder, dried, or in a host of different commercial products. Studies have shown that garlic can extend the life span and improve cognitive deterioration in mice, and has exhibited anti-aging effects on human fibroblasts *in vitro*. Garlic has also been of benefit to patients suffering from AIDS. HIV-positive patients receiving 5 g per day of aged garlic extract over a period of six weeks followed by six weeks of 10 g per day produced significant improvements in immune parameters and opportunistic infections. Garlic extracts have inhibited the growth of candida and cytomegalovirus, *in vitro*, as well as exhibited a broad spectrum of antimicrobial and antioxidant activity. Results of one case study showed that large doses of powdered garlic produced partial palliation of symptoms in a patient with severe hepatopulmonary syndrome. Garlic and onion compounds can protect against liver damage in rats.

The intravenous administration of garlic extracts exhibited anti-Cryptococcous neoformans effects in patients suffering from cryptococcal meningitis. Several animal studies have demonstrated the antidiabetic effects of garlic.

Large population-based studies have found strong inverse associations between the consumption of garlic as well as onions and the risk of cancer. Results from *in vitro* and animal studies also point to the powerful anti-cancer activity of garlic. Even more impressive than these findings is the growing body of literature suggesting that garlic may be highly beneficial for the prevention and treatment of heart disease.

One study examined the effect of raw garlic on serum cholesterol, fibrinolytic activity, and clotting time in fifty medical students. Students were given 10 g of raw garlic per day following breakfast for two months. Results showed a significant decrease in serum cholesterol and an increase in clotting time and fibrinolytic activity relative to controls. Healthy volunteers fed garlic for six months followed by two months without garlic experienced significantly lower serum cholesterol and triglyceride levels.

A group of sixty-two coronary heart disease patients with high serum cholesterol fed garlic for ten months experienced a significant decrease in serum cholesterol levels relative to controls. In another study, forty-two healthy middle-aged adults with a total serum cholesterol level of greater than or equal to 220 mg/dl received 300 mg three times a day of standardized garlic powder in tablet form. Results found that the garlic treatment significantly reduced serum total cholesterol levels. A meta-analysis of five placebo-controlled studies examined the effects of garlic on total serum cholesterol levels in subjects with cholesterol levels greater than 5.17 mmol/L (200 mg/dL) and showed that garlic was effective in reducing total cholesterol levels and is best used at doses ranging from one half to one clove per day. Hypercholesterolaemic outpatients taking 900 mg of garlic powder per day for four months demonstrated significantly lower total cholesterol, triglycerides, and blood pressure levels than controls.

Results showed a significant decrease in supine diastolic blood pressure and significant reductions in serum cholesterol and triglyceride levels in a double-blind, placebo-controlled study of mild hypertension patients who received a garlic powder preparation for twelve weeks. A popular garlic preparation containing 1.3 percent allicin at a 2400 mg dose taken by nine severe hypertension patients reduced sitting blood pressure approximately five hours after the dose, with a significant decrease in diastolic blood pressure from five to fourteen hours following the dose.

Eating one fresh clove of garlic per day for sixteen weeks reduced serum cholesterol by 20 percent and serum thromboxane by 80 percent in middle-aged men. The daily ingestion of 800 mg of powdered garlic over four weeks led to a significant inhibition of the pathologically increased ratio of circulating platelet aggregates and of spontaneous platelet aggregation in juvenile subjects with cerebrovascular risk factors. A meta-analysis of eight trials on the effects of 600–900 mg per day of dried garlic powder administered for twelve weeks on blood pressure found that it was of benefit in some patients with hypertension.

Ginkgo Biloba

Ginkgo trees have existed on earth for more than 200 million years. Their leaves have been used for medicinal purposes for centuries, particularly in China. In recent years, ginkgo biloba in the form of various extracts has been championed as one of the growing number of so called "smart drugs" that directly attack the aging process and can potentially reverse it.

Ginkgo is perhaps best known of late for its restorative effects on the brain. Results of one study showed that ginkgo biloba extract exerts a specific effect on the noradrenergic system and on beta-receptors, which suggest central effects of a drug acting on cerebral aging, connected specifically to reactivation of the noradrenergic system in the cerebral cortex.

A double-blind, placebo-controlled study found that elderly subjects with age-related memory impairment experienced significant improvement in the speed of information processing following treatment with either 320 or 600 mg of ginkgo biloba extract one hour prior to performing a dual-code test. Another showed that patients over age fifty with some level of memory impairment who received treatment with oral doses of 120 mg of ginkgo biloba per day experienced significant beneficial effects on cognitive function at both twelve and twenty-four weeks.

Ginkgo biloba extract significantly improved memory after six weeks of treatment and learning rate after twenty-four weeks in cerebral insufficiency outpatients. A study of cerebral insufficiency in patients with depressive moods noted as a leading symptom found that those treated with 160 mg per day of ginkgo biloba extract experienced a significantly greater degree of clinical improvement than controls. Ginkgo biloba extract and dihydroergotoxine treatment for six weeks led to improvements in elderly patients with cerebrovascular disease.

Healthy female subjects given ginkgo biloba extract in doses 600 mg per day experienced significant improvements in memory. Ginkgo biloba extract administered to patients suffering from senile macular degeneration showed significant improvements in lost distance visual acuity. Patients with classical symptoms of organic syndrome were tested for the therapeutic effects of ginkgo biloba extract administered in doses of 120 mg per day for eight weeks. Results showed a significant improvement after four and eight weeks of therapy. A meta-analysis involving seven double-blind, placebo-controlled clinical trials found ginkgo biloba extract (mean dose of 150 mg per day) significantly effective in reducing clinical symptoms associated with cerebrovascular insufficiency in old age. The administration of 120 mg per day of ginkgo biloba extract led to clear improvement in vigilance among geriatric patients with cerebral insufficiency. A ginkgo extract administered over a period of eighteen weeks enhanced memory processes in mice.

The scientific literature increasingly points to the positive effects ginkgo can also have on the heart. Results of one placebo-controlled study found ginkgo biloba extract significantly decreased erythrocyte aggregation and increased blood flow in the nail-fold capillaries of healthy subjects. Patients suffering from peripheral arteriopathy experienced significant improvements in the degree of pain-free walking distance, maximum walking distance, and plethylsmography recordings relative to controls following treatment with ginkgo biloba extract. The administration of ginkgo biloba extract for fourteen days led to significant improvements in hypoxic hypoxia fixation time of saccadic eye movements and complex choice reaction time in healthy male subjects.

Supplemental ginkgo biloba taken for twelve weeks at doses of 240 mg per day led to significant improvement in fibrinogen levels and hemorrheological properties in patients with a history of elevated fibrinogen levels and plasma viscosity, as well as a host of different underlying diseases. A single injection of ginkgo biloba extract at doses of either 50, 100, 150, or 200 mg had positive effects on whole blood visco-elasticity and microcirculation in patients with pathological visco-elasticity values. In a study of fifteen patients with arteriosclerotic lesions in the extracranial brain who received an infusion of 250 ml physiological NaCl and 25 ml ginkgo biloba extract, results showed significant increases in perfusion relative to controls. Ginkgo biloba extract improved contractile function following global ischemia in the isolated working heart of rats due its ability to inhibit the formation of oxygen radicals. The administration of ginkgo biloba extract over a period of three months provided protective effects on the hypoxic myocardium in rats. Ginkgo can protect against cardiac ischemia reperfusion injury in rats, and early ventricular tachycardia by coronary reperfusion in dogs.

Arthritis patients receiving a ginkgo biloba extract for sixty-five weeks experienced significantly more pain relief and walking tolerance after six months than did patients taking a placebo. Ginkgo has also produced benefits in hepatitis, tinnitus, and Parkinson's patients. Visual field damage caused by a chronic lack of blood flow in elderly patients can be reversed by treatment with ginkgo biloba extract at doses of 160 mg per day for four weeks. The administra-.

tion of ginkgo biloba leaves at doses of 120 mg per day for two months reduced plasma clastogenic activity to control levels when measured on the first day following treatment in workers exposed to high levels of radiation from the Chernobyl accident.

Such positive effects lasted for a minimum of seven months. Three months' worth of gingko biloba extract at the same dose led to improvements in some cognitive functions in elderly patients with moderate arterial insufficiency. Diabetics suffering from early diabetic retinopathy showed statistical improvement following treatment with ginkgo biloba. Diabetic rats treated with gingko biloba experienced a significantly greater amplitude in electoretinograms than controls. The treatment of women suffering from idiopathic cyclic oedema with ginkgo biloba extract led to complete correction of the biological anomaly in ten cases receiving oral and five receiving intravenous administration.

Ginkgo has promoted hair regrowth in rats. Results of a study of patients with idiopathic sudden hearing loss existing no longer than ten days who were given treatment with either ginkgo EGb 761 (Tebonin) + HAES or Naftidrofuryl (Dusodril) + HAES showed that, after one week of observation, 40 percent of the patients in both treatment groups experienced a complete remission of hearing loss. Another study showed that treatment with ginkgo biloba extract led to significant recovery in patients with acute cochlear deafness caused by ischemia, ginkgo can protect the intestinal mucosa of rats against ischemic damage through the reduction of lipid peroxidation and neutrophil infiltration. A study of ten neuropathy patients with an autonomic disregulation of skin who were intravenously administered a combination of 87.5 mg of ginkgo biloba extract standardized to 21.0 mg Flavonglycosids and 3 mg folic acid over a period of four days experienced significant improvements in nerve function following treatment. Ginkgo has proven effective in relieving symptoms associated with PMS. Both *in vitro* and *in vivo* studies showed that sesquiterpene bilobalide, extracted from ginkgo biloba leaves, might be useful for therapy of and prophylaxis against P. carinii infections in humans. Ginkgo has exhibited protective effects against spinal cord injury in rats due to its antioxidant activities.

Ginkgo has demonstrated anti-stress activity in rats and mice. Several studies have demonstrated ginkgo's antioxidant effects. The use of ginkgo biloba has shown promise in the treatment of hypoxia/ ischemia, seizure activity, and peripheral nerve damage. Ginkgo biloba extract had a significant protective effect against experimental retinal damage in rabbits. Ginkgo biloba extract had excitatory effects on the lateral vestibular nuclei neurons in guinea pigs. Vertiginous patients treated with ginkgo biloba extract over three months experienced a significant improvement in the intensity, frequency, and duration of their condition relative to controls.

The intravenous administration of ginkgo biloba extract resulted in dramatic recovery in severe cases of hypovolaemic shock related to monoclonal. Experimental models of ischemia, oedema, and hypoxia have shown that ginkgo biloba extract reduced vascular, tissular, and metabolic disturbances, along with neurological and behavioral consequences associated with them.

Ginseng

Ginseng is a potent adaptogenic herb that has been used the world over throughout history. There are several different types of ginseng, all adaptogens, including Korean, Chinese, Siberian, and American. Adaptogenic herbs primarily act as stress fighters by restoring homeostasis. A growing body of peer review literature supports such actions. One review article examining over 300 studies on ginseng published in China since 1982 found ginseng to possess a large variety of therapeutic effects on the body, including benefits to the central nervous system, cardiovascular system and endocrine secretion, immune function, stress, aging, etc. Chinese ginseng preparations have exhibited protective effects against experimentally induced stress in mice. Another study found that Vietnamese ginseng crude saponin suppressed the effects of psychological stress in mice. Ginseng therapy restored the thyroid and adrenal functions inhibited by dexamethasone treatment in rats. In a study examining the anti-aging activities of American ginseng in those over sixty, results showed that symptoms of Kidney-Yang deficiency improved and subjects experienced a decrease in functional months of age from 751.77 ± 5.215 to 743.53 ± 5.144, the effective rate being 68.57 percent. The intake of 50 mg tablets of Ginseng-Rhizome taken three times a day for two months exhibited anti-senility effects and led to the relief of age-related symptoms in a group of middle-aged and elderly subjects. In addition to these findings, the treatment had significant benefits with respect to coronary heart disease.

Ginseng has also exhibited direct anti-aging effects on rats. Korean red ginseng has exhibited positive effects on immune markers in subjects infected with HIV. Panax ginseng administered at doses of 100 mg capsules of either an aqueous or standardized extracts led to significant enhancement of cell-mediated immune functions in healthy volunteers. Animal and *in vitro* studies have pointed to the benefits of ginseng on the immune system as well.

Cancer and heart disease are two other areas where ginseng has proven useful. Results of one Korean case-control study showed an inverse association between oral intake of different types of ginseng and the risk of various cancers in humans, including lip, oral cavity, pharynx, esophageal, stomach, colon-rectal, liver, pancreatic, laryngeal, lung, and ovarian. A large-scale trial by the same authors found a significant inverse association between the consumption of ginseng and risk of gastric and lung cancer in adults over the age of forty.

An earlier study also revealed an inverse association between a history of ginseng intake and the risk of cancer. Ginseng extract and powder proved more effective than fresh sliced ginseng, the juice, or tea in reducing cancer risk. Results from animal and *in vitro* studies support such findings. As to heart disease, one study found that red ginseng was a safe and effective treatment in patients suffering from congestive heart failure and proved to be synergistic with digoxin in exhibiting even stronger improvement of hemodynamical and biological indexes.

Total ginsenoside and ginsenoside Rb have been shown to protect against myocardiac ischemic and reperfusion injuries in open heart surgery patients. Injections of ginseng principles (fraction 4) can reduce elevated plasma levels of cholesterol and triglyceride. Panax ginseng delayed experimentally induced impairment of rat heart mitochondria and muscle contraction deterioration. Ginsenosides have attenuated ischemic myocardium and protected against reperfusion injury of myocardium in dogs. Wisconsin ginseng root powder added to the diet was effective in lowering total serum cholesterol levels of chickens.

Numerous animal studies have pointed to the possible benefits of using ginseng to improve cognitive function, particularly memory and learning. The same is true for diabetes. In a study of newly diagnosed noninsulin dependent diabetics, intake of 100–200 mg per day of ginseng for eight weeks elevated mood, improved psychophysical performance, and reduced fasting glucose and body weight. The 200 mg dose improved glycated hemoglobin, serum PIIINP, and physical activity. Other conditions ginseng may benefit include stroke, sleepwalking disturbances, ulcers, kidney damage, and narcotic addiction.

In addition, Panax ginseng has been shown to be capable of enhancing the rate of blood alcohol clearance in healthy men. The consumption of two capsules containing a preparation of ginseng extract, dimethylaminoethanol bitartrate, vitamins, minerals, and trace elements per day for six weeks increased work capacity due to improved muscular oxygen utilization in healthy male sports teachers. The administration of Korean red ginseng had significant positive effects with respect to penile rigidity and girth, libido and subjective reports of satisfaction relative to controls in men suffering from erectile dysfunction.

Goldenseal

The herb goldenseal has exhibited antimicrobial activity *in vitro*, and has been shown to counter E-coli–caused diarrhea in adults. It is also a powerful immune enhancer and liver cleanser, and animal studies show its isolates to have anti-cancer and cardioprotective effects. However, you should not take this herb if you are pregnant, or for more than one week at a time.

Grape

In addition to possessing strong antioxidant potential, grape extracts have shown anti-cancer and anti-inflammatory effects in mice, reduced the risk of colon cancer in monkeys, and exhibited cardioprotective effects *in vitro*.

Green Tea

The cancer-fighting effects of green tea on animals and *in vitro* are well documented in the scientific literature. Human studies also point to its potential benefits in this regard.

In one case-control study, smoking, alcohol, and green tea were examined as potential stomach cancer risk factors in patients already diagnosed with the disease. Results showed smoking of cigarettes and the consumption of alcohol were associated with an increased risk of stomach cancer, while an inverse association was found between the consumption of green tea and stomach cancer. Another study examined the effects of green tea consumption on the risk of esophageal cancer in a group of 902 esophageal cancer patients between the ages of thirty and seventy-four. Results showed green tea consumption had a significant, dose-dependent protective effect against esophageal cancer in women and significant protective effects in male and female smokers.

A population-based, case-controlled inquiry into the effects of drinking green tea on the risk of stomach cancer in subjects under the age of eighty showed an inverse association between the two variables. Regular consumption of green tea may counteract the ill effects of mutagens and/or carcinogens produced in meat cooked under high temperature. Green tea extract inhibits gastrointestinal malignant tumors in humans.

Green tea may also be effective against heart disease. In a study of 1371 Japanese men over forty, results showed an inverse association between the daily consumption of green tea and serum cholesterol levels. Consumption of more than ten cups per day was correlated to a reduced concentration of hepatological markers in serum, aspartate aminotransferase, alanine transferase, and ferritin.

A study of 1306 Japanese males found total serum cholesterol levels to be inversely related to the consumption of green tea. Dental health is another area where green tea has shown promise. Japanese green tea's polyphenolic compounds can inhibit the attachment of Streptococcus mutans strain JC-2 to saliva-coated hydroxyapatide discs. Rats infected with S mutans JC-2 (c) and fed a cariogenic diet and/or drinking water containing green tea polyphenols have exhibited fewer carries than did controls. Chinese green tea polyphenols are effective preventive agents against dental carries. Fluoride in green tea may increase the cariostatic action in combination with other properties in the tea. Extracts of green tea has also exhibited antibacterial action against twenty-four bacterial strains isolated from root canal infections. Green tea may also help prevent stroke. Results of a four-year, follow-up study of 5910 Japanese women who neither smoked nor drank alcohol showed that the rate of stroke and cerebral hemorrhage was at least twice as high as those consuming less than five cups or green tea daily compared to those consuming five or more cups per day. In a cohort study aimed to evaluate the effect of drinking green tea on longevity involving 3380 female practitioners of chanoyu (Japanese tea ceremony) living in Tokyo, standardized mortality ratios were estimated 0.55 when all Japanese women were used as standard population and 0.57 when women living in Tokyo were used, indicating the possibility that green tea is a protective factor for several fatal diseases. Both green and black tea exhibited antioxidant effects on tissue lipid peroxidation in rats. Other conditions green tea can benefit include liver damage, pancreatitis, and diarrhea.

Hawthorn

Hawthorn leaves, berries, and blossoms have all been shown to have healing properties and have been used in China and Europe for hundreds of years. Hawthorn extract administered at a dose of 600 mg per day over a period of eight weeks has been found to significantly reduce the blood pressure and heart rate in middle-aged patients suffering from chronic heart failure. Doses of 100 mg per day of Hawthorn leaves administered to angina patients over a four-week period led to an efficacy rate of 84.8 percent. Animal studies have shown similar results with respect to the cardioprotective effects of hawthorn.

Hibiscus

Hibiscus is a common ornamental plant, the flowers of which have historically been believed to contain anti-fertility properties, particularly in women. The herb is also popularly taken for its soothing effects on the mucous membranes that line the digestive and respiratory tracts. Both animal and *in vitro* studies indicate that extracts from hibiscus possess anti-cancer and cardioprotective effects. Hibiscus has exhibited antioxidant effects *in vitro* as well.

Licorice

Low doses of the licorice extract glycyrrhizine (150 mg per day) have been shown to be effective against hyperkalemia in patients suffering from diabetes. Similar results have also been seen in studies involving diabetic rats. Licorice has exhibited antiviral effects *in vitro,* including an ability to inhibit the growth of herpes virus.

Licorice has also been used in the treatment of cirrhosis and chronic hepatitis, ulcers, and hepatitis.

Lovage

Studies have found lingusticum chuanxiong in tablet form to be a significantly effective treatment in patients suffering from angina pectoris and high blood pressure, as well as those suffering from ischemic cerebrovascular disease. When taken at doses of 3 to 9 g daily as an oral decoction, extract, or tincture, it may also be of benefit for headache, vertigo, and prolonged postpartum lochia. Lovage has also exhibited anti-inflammatory and sedative effects in rats.

Marigold

Marigold extracts have exhibited anti-cancer activity against mammary tumors in mice, and against leukemia and lung cancer *in vitro*. Flavonoids from marigold leaves have also exhibited antimicrobial activity against Gram positive and Gram negative microorganisms *in vitro*. Marigold extracts produced anti-odematous activity in mice as well.

Mistletoe

Mistletoe has been found to be beneficial against high blood pressure and is a well-documented treatment for cancer. Results of one study involving thirty-six women with breast cancer found that subcutaneous injections of the optimal immunomodulating mistletoe extract dosage (1ng/kg body weight, twice a week) for twelve weeks induced a significant increase of beta-endorphin plasma levels, a reduced decrease of defined peripheral blood lymphatic subsets after standard chemotherapy, and an evidently increased *in vitro* cytokine release by mononuclear immune cells after adequate stimulation. In another study examining the cellular aspects of the immunomodulating activity of propriety mistletoe extract in 20 mammary cancer patients, results showed that subcutaneous injections of the different dosages (0.5 and 1.0 ng ML-1/kg body weight, twice a week, for five weeks) led to statistically significant increases of defined peripheral blood lymphocyte subsets (helper T-cells, natural killer cells), which are generally believed to be involved in anti-tumor activity. The mistletoe preparation T mali has produced positive effects in oral cancer patients. Postoperative treatment of breast cancer patients with Iscador (Viscum album) significantly increased survival rate relative to controls. Subcutaneous injections of 1 mg/kg per body weight of galactoside-specific lectin from mistletoe (ML-1) twice a week for four weeks significantly increased helper T-lymphocytes and natural killer cells and enhanced the expression of interleukin (II)-2 receptors on lymphatic cells in breast cancer patients. Iscador has significantly enhanced phagocytic activity of granulocytes, natural killer cell and antibody-dependent cell-mediated cytoxicity activities in patients with breast cancer as well. Another study of breast cancer patients found that a single intravenous infusion of Iscador significantly increased natural killer cell and antibody dependent cell mediated activity within 24 hours of administration.

Advanced breast cancer patients have also shown significantly higher white blood cell counts and leukocyte levels relative to controls after chemotherapy when treated with a mistletoe preparation. Numerous *in vitro* and animal studies also point to the anticancer effects of mistletoe.

Motherwort

Motherwort extracts have been shown to suppress the incidence and growth of mammary tumors in mice. Results of one study on the effects of the herb on blood hyperviscosity in 105 patients found that intravenous doses of 10 ml in 250 mil of 5 percent glucose over a period of fifteen days produced clinical benefits with respect to reduced blood mammary viscosity and in fibrinogen volume as well as an increase in the deformability of Rbc, decreased time of Rbc electrophoresis, and enhanced anti-platelet aggregation.

Pumpkin Seed

Patients suffering from benign prostatic hyperlasia have experienced significant improvements in urinary flow and other symptoms as result of taking a combined preparation of pumpkin seeds and dwarf palm plants. Pumpkin seeds administered at doses of 80 g three times daily for one have proven highly effective against symptoms associated with acute schistosomiasis, including fever, anorexia, and liver tenderness.

Red Clover

Red clover is a purple flower found across the United States which is high in protein, phosphorus, and calcium. Daily supplementation of 100 mg of red clover has been shown to be effective in the treatment of patients suffering from metastatic renal cell cancer. Studies indicate red clover can also inhibit the growth of prostate tumors in rats, and exhibits chemopreventive activity *in vitro*. More traditional uses of red clover have been as a remedy for childhood skin problems, and also for psoriasis in adults. It is a popular herbal treatment for throat conditions such bronchitis and whooping cough, and is often used as a blood, kidney, and liver cleanser.

Rhubarb

Rhubarb isolates have been shown to inhibit the growth of human breast carcinoma cells and enhance immune response *in vitro*. Processed rhubarb can significantly inhibit pregnancy-induced hypertension in women and has exhibited cathartic effects in rats. Rhubarb has also exhibited strong antibacterial effects *in vitro*, been effective against hemorrhagic pancreatitis in rabbits, and helped alleviate suffering in patients with chronic renal failure.

Rosemary

Rosemary is a popular herb which is known for the soothing effects of its leaves and twigs when used as an oil on the nervous and digestive systems. Other common uses of the herb include treatment against headache, depression, muscle pain, flatulent dyspepsia, fatigue, gum disease, anxiety, warts, high blood pressure, and hair loss. Rosemary has exhibited anti-cancer activity in numerous animal studies and been shown to inhibit the initiation of carcinogenesis in human bronchial epithelial cells *in vitro*.

Saw Palmetto

Saw palmetto is a small, fruit-bearing palm tree native to Florida. Results from numerous studies point to the effectiveness of saw palmetto extracts in the treatment of benign prostatic hyperplasia. In one trial, 88 percent of 505 patients suffering from the disorder experienced significant improvement following three months of twice daily doses of a 160 mg extract.

St. John's Wort

While widely used in Europe for decades, St. John's wort (Hypericum perforatum) has received a lot of attention in the U.S. of late as a promising new treatment in the fight against depression, and for good reason. St. John's wort contains hypericin which inhibits monoamine oxiadase, a chemical that is associated with depression. Results from dozens of studies indicate that the herb is an effective alternative to more conventional pharmaceutical approaches that often are accompanied by serious side effects. Dosages in such studies have generally ranged between 100 to 900 mg per day.

As users of the herb have known for centuries, St. John's wort is, however, far more than simply a remedy for depression. Studies have shown it can reduce the intensity level of enzymatic and non-enzymatic processes of lipid peroxidation of rat liver microsomes *in vitro* and *in vivo*. It has demonstrated anti-herpes in vitro. Contemporary research points to the herb's promise as an effective therapy for cancer, AIDS, alcoholism, hepatitis, and isomnia. St. John's wort has been used historically against symptoms associated with PMS and as an reliable treatment for wounds and burns. It can be taken as a tincture, tea, decotion, oil, or capsule.

Stinging Nettle

Several studies point to the benefits of stinging nettle extracts in the treatment of benign prostatic hyperplasia. In one, patients who received capsules containing either 300 mg of the root combined with 25 mg of Pygeum africanum bark extract or two capsules with half this dose twice a day over a period of eight weeks experienced significant reductions in symptoms related to the condition. Similar results have been noted in other trials.

Sunflower

The intake of a linoleic acid–rich diet, applying 12 percent sunflower seed oil in rat food pellet for four weeks, has been shown to reduce the occurrence of life-threatening arrhythmias in rats. Patients suffering from scaly dermatitis have experienced benefits from the cutaneous application of sunflower seed oil on the skin for two weeks.

Turmeric/Curcumin

Turmeric is a common spice also known as Indian saffron. Results of more than a dozen studies indicate turmeric exhibits powerful anti-cancer activity in animal models. Turmeric has been shown to inhibit tumors of the skin, colon, forestomach, duodenum, and breast. *In vitro* experiments support such findings, as do those involving human subjects. In one, turmeric proved to be an effective anti-mutagen in smokers. Another showed that patients with external cancerous lesions experienced significant relief following treatment with an ethanol turmeric extract and a curcumin ointment. The administration of 500 mg per day of curcumin for seven days has been shown to significantly reduce the level of serum lipid peroxides, increase HDL cholesterol, and decrease total serum cholesterol in healthy human subjects.

Oral curcumin (turmeric) significantly reduced increased lipid peroxidation in different mouse organs including the brain, liver, lung, and kidney; and significantly reduced serum and tissue cholesterol levels in mice as well. Curcumin and quinidine has also prevented ischemia-induced changes in cat hearts; and inhibited arachidonate, adrenaline, and collagen-induced platelet aggregation in human blood. *In vitro*, curcumin has provided protection against lipid peroxidation–induced cataractogenesis in rat lenses.

Dietary curcumin administered over an eight-week period led to an enhanced metabolic status across numerous diabetic conditions in rats. Curcumin has decreased the incidence of gallstone formation in mice, reduced liver damage in rats, and exhibited anti-HIV, anti-fungal, anti-inflammatory, antioxidant effects as well.

Valerian

Valerian root has been used as a sleep aid for thousands of years and is presently the most widely used sedative in Europe. It is a perennial plant found in North America, Europe, and Asia. Valerian's active ingredient is valerenic acid and it is commonly taken either as a tea, powder, tincture or in capsule form. In addition to its sleep promoting effects, valerian is used across a large variety of conditions, including digestive disorders, anxiety, muscle spasms, high blood pressure, and fever. Peer review studies have shown extracts of valerian root can produce antidepressant effects in mice, and can have beneficial effects on sleep. Results of one study found that an aqueous extract of valerian root administered at doses of both 450 mg and 900 mg had reduced perceived sleep latency in healthy young adults.

Yohimbine

Yohimbine is best known for its effects on sexual performance, with a host of studies pointing to its therapeutic potential in this regard. One showed yohimbine to be beneficial for sexual side effects brought on by serotonin reuptake blockers in psychiatric patients. Another found that yohimbine hydrochloride administered at a maximum dose of 42 mg per day over a period of one month produced significant improvements in patients suffering from impotence. Supplemental doses of 18 mg per day over a ten-week period produced a 46 percent overall improvement rate in patients with psychogenic impotence. Psychogenic impotence patients have also experienced major improvements following treament with 15 mg per day of oral yohimbine coupled with 50 mg per day of trazodone over two eight-week periods.

In addition to enhancing sexual performance, studies show yohimbine can also protect against heart disease. The daily administration of yohimbine at a minimum dose of 8 mg significantly inhibited epinephrine-induced platelet formation in healthy subjects. Intake of 5 m of oral yohimbine produced significant increases in mean systolic and diastolic blood pressure and mean heart rate in patients with autonomic failure characterized by orthostatic hypotension. In depression patients suffering from clomipramine-induced orthostatic hypotension, 4 mg/t.i.d. of yohimbine significantly increased blood pressure. Animal studies also indicate yohimbine may hold promise for the treatment of diabetes. Yohimbine has exhibited anticonvulsant effects in rats and significant weight-loss effects in obese mice. Doses of 8 mg/kg per day of yohimbine proved effective in maintaining subjective wakefulness for eight consecutive working hours in narcolepsy patients as well.

THERAPEUTIC AMINO ACIDS

Alanine

Supplemental alanine and terbutaline have led to sustained glucose recovery from hypoglycemia in patients suffering from insulin-dependent diabetes. Alanine has also alleviated diarrhea symptoms associated with E-coli in male patients and exhibited beneficial effects on liver damage in rats.

Arginine

A therapeutic (or non-essential) amino acid, arginine is a precursor of nitric oxide. Since nitric oxide helps relax the walls of the arteries, supplemental arginine may help to promote blood flow throughout the body which can lead to a wide range of beneficial effects, including everything from stroke prevention to increased erection.

Results from a number of studies point to the efficacy of arginine in the treatment of patients suffering from a host of heart conditions. One double-blind, placebo-controlled trial found that oral intake of L-arginine at doses of 5.6 to 12.6 g per day over a period of six weeks had positive effects in heart failure patients.

Another study showed that 20 g of intravenous L-arginine significantly increased stroke volume and cardiac output while significantly reducing mean arterial blood pressure and systemic vascular resistance in congestive heart failure patients associated with coronary artery disease. The administration of 7 g of L-arginine three times per day over a period of four weeks has led to significant improvements in endothelium-dependent dilation in hypercholesterolemic young adults. Exogenous L-arginine has exhibited vasodilatory effects in patients suffering from various forms of hypertension. Treatment with 12 mg/kg of NG-methyl-L-arginine followed by 4 mg/kg every four hours reversed IL-2-induced hypotensive effects in three patients with metastatic renal cell carcinoma. Infants with persistent pulmonary hypertension have also experienced benefits following infusion with a 500 mg/kg dose of L-arginine over a period of thirty minutes. Animal studies have demonstrated the cardioprotective effects of arginine as well.

Cancer is another area where studies indicate arginine may be useful. Breast cancer patients taking 30 g per day of L-arginine for four days experienced a significant enhancement of host defenses. The anti-cancer activity of arginine has also been demonstrated in mice. Additional animal studies suggest arginine can help prevent stroke, reduce kidney collage accumulation associated with aging, and protect against stress. One study showed that supplemental arginine at levels totaling 2 percent of nutritional energy significantly enhanced the T lymphocyte response to PHA, CD4 phenotype expression, CD4/CD8 ratio, IL-2 production, and IL-2 receptor expression in burn patients relative to controls. Arginine has been shown to have beneficial effects against burns in guinea pigs. Intravenous administration of a 10 percent solution, 300 ml (30 g)/patient

L-arginine over a sixty–seventy-minute period produced significant analgesiac effects in patients suffering from different types of pain.

Arginine administration can protect against liver injury and ulcers in rats. Intragastric administration of 32.5–300 mg/kg per day of L-arginine accelerated the healing of acetic acid-induced gastric ulcers in human patients as well. In infertile men, the administration of 80 ml of 10 percent L-arginine HCL daily per os over a six-month period improved sperm motility. Supplemental arginine tidiacicate tablets containing 400 mg has also had positive effects in patients with chronic persistent hepatitis.

Aspartic Acid

Aspartic acid is a non-essential amino acid found in high levels in the brain and throughout the body. It is involved in many bodily functions, including the formation as well as disposal of ammonia and urea. Peer review studies have shown aspartic acid to exhibit cardioprotective, antitumor, and liver protective effects in animals. Additional research suggests it may also increase resistance to fatigue, be useful against depression, and could play a role in overcoming symptoms associated with opiate withdrawal. Suggested supplemental dose is no more than 1.5 g per day.

Cysteine

Cysteine has exhibited preventive effects against leukopenic complications associated with radiotherapy in cancer patients. Hypostatic leg ulceration patients treated with a topical cream containing l-cysteine, glycine, and dl-threonin three times per week over a period of twelve weeks experienced a significantly increased rate of healing relative to patients being treated with cream base alone. Cysteine has also been effective against allergic-contact dermatitis in guinea pigs.

Glutamic Acid

Glutamic acid holds promise as a treatment for three of the leading causes of death among the elderly: cancer, heart disease, and diabetes. Anti-cancer activity has been documented in animal studies, and in one trial of patients who received a 4 g swish of L-glutamine twice a day at the start of chemotherapy that lasted for twenty-eight days. The administration of glutamate coupled with high-dose glucose-insulin-potassium is an effective and safe treatment in patients with reversible cardiac failure. Glutamic acid has been shown to have cardioprotective effects in rabbits, rats, and dogs as well. Additional animal studies have documented its potential in the fight against diabetes, to improve adrenal function, and promote healing from burn injury.

Bronchial asthma patients treated with aevit and glutamic acid experienced clinical improvements. Athletes consuming drinks containing glutamine immediately and two hours after exercise experienced a lower incidence of infections seven days after exercise than controls. The administration of large doses of gamma-ethylester of glutamic acid to patients suffering from liver failure produced significantly positive effects with respect to such symptoms as tremors, confusion, restlessness, and reductions in blood ammonia levels.

Results of another study found that a protocol involving growth hormone, glutamine, and a high-carbohydrate, low-fat diet proved effective in treating surgical patients suffering from short-bowel syndrome or related problems of the GI tract. Intravenous administration of glutamic acid and glutamic acid diethylester worked to suppress certain forms of tinnitus in human patients relative to controls. Early glutamine supplementation can prevent stress ulcer problems associated with severe thermal injury in major burn patients as well.

Glycine

Hypostatic leg ulceration patients treated with a topical cream containing l-cysteine, glycine, and dl-threonin three times per week over a period of twelve weeks have experienced a significantly increased rate of healing relative to patients being treated with the cream base alone. Supplemental glycine has also been found to be useful in the treatment of schizophrenia, and in preventing stress-induced damage to the heart.

Histidine

Histidine is a lesser known amino acid that changes from an essential amino acid to a non-essential acid with age. A precursor to histamine, it can be obtained through most vegetable and animal proteins and is particularly important in blood cell production. Histidine is sometimes used against symptoms associated with rheumatoid arthritis and may be effective in the treatment of high blood pressure due to its calming effects on the nervous system. Research indicates that histidine may enhance T-cell function, which may in part explain its use against rheumatoid arthritis, and can also act as a metal chelator. Additional studies have shown the administration of histidine can exhibit protective effects on cardiac and brain function during cerebral thrombosis in rats. Suggested supplemental dose is approximately 1.5 g per day.

Ornithine

Results of one double-blind, placebo-controlled study found that 10 g per day of ornithine oxoglutarate administered for two months to ambulatory elderly patients recovering from acute illnesses led to significant improvements in appetite, body weight, quality of life, medical cost, and measures of independence. Ornithine has also exhibited anti-cancer effects in both human and animal studies as well as *in vitro*.

The oral administration of 34 mmol per day of ornithine salts of branched-chain ketoacids over a period of seven to ten days significantly improved electroencephalographic abnormalities and clinical grade of encephalopathy in patients suffering from chronic portal-systemic encephalopathy. Studies have shown that ornithine decarboxylase is a key factor in the repair process and restoration of small intestine mucosal function in rats following ischemia-reperfusion.

Ornithine alpha-ketoglutarate has also exhibited immunomodulatory effects in rats with severe burn injuries.

Tyrosine

The oral administration of 3,200 mg of tyrosine per day has proven effective in the treatment of patients suffering from dopamine-dependent depression. Doses of 100 mg/kg can significantly reduce stress symptoms associated with 4.5 hours of exposure to cold and hypoxia. Tyrosine has also been shown capable of increasing blood pressure in hypotensive rats, and protecting against ventricular arrhythmias in dogs.

ESSENTIAL AMINO ACIDS

Isoleucine

Patients suffering from amyotrophic lateral sclerosis who received daily oral administration of a mix of 12 g of L-leucine, 8 g of

L-isoleucine, and 6.4 g of L-valine experienced significant improvements in muscle strength and walking ability.

Lysine

Patients suffering from various rheumatic disorders have been shown to benefit from ketoprofen lysine administered in doses of 320 mg per day. The administration of 1,000 mg of oral l-lysine per day over a period of twelve months led to significant reductions in lesion frequency in patients suffering from recurrent herpes simplex labialis. Doses of 1,248 mg of oral l-lysine monohydrochloride per day decreased the recurrence rate of herpes simplex attacks in non-immuno-compromised hosts.

Another study showed that 1,000 mg tablets of oral l-lysine monohydrochloride taken three times per day over a period of six months decreased the recurrence rate of herpes simplex attacks. When taking an average dose of 936 mg of lysine per day administered over a six-month period, patients experienced a reduction of frequency of herpes infection from cold sores, canker sores, and genital herpes.

Migraine patients have benefitted from oral lysine acetylsalicylate combined with metroclopramide. The intravenous administration of acetylsalicylate of lysine to obstetrical and gynecological surgery patients exhibited beneficial effects with respect to postoperative pain in 77.4 percent of the patients examined.

Methionine

Supplemental methionine can prevent the induction of hepatocarcinogenesis in rats. Reports also point to its usefulness in the treatment of severe myeloneuropathy and macrocytic anemia associated with a low vitamin B_{12} serum levels, and hepatitis.

Phenylalanine

The administration of phenylalanine in doses ranging between 75 to 250 mg per day has produced beneficial results in patients suffering from depression. Doses of 250 mg three times per day over a period of fifteen days have been shown to prevent pain in cancer patients. Phenylalanine has also exhibited anti-cancer activity and prevented stress and ulcers in rats.

Tryptophan

Tryptophan has been shown to exhibit anti-cancer and cardio-protective effects in mice and rats. Patients suffering from depression have also experienced benefits after taking tryptophan, with one study showing doses of 8 g per day over a period of four weeks being effective in those moderately depressed.

Doses of 150–450 mg per day can ameloriate paranoid hallucinations and motor complications associated with L-dopa treatment in Parkinson's disease patients. Tardive dyskinesia is another condition for which supplemental L-tryptophan has produced positive effects, as is schizophrenia.

Tryptophan has also proved effective as a pain reliever and as a good remedy for problems associated with sleep.

Unfortunately, tryptophan is no longer legally sold in the United States due to problems stemming from a contaminated batch several years ago.

PART IV

HOW TO LIVE FOREVER

7

THE ULTIMATE ANTI-AGING PROGRAM

I can't repeat it often enough: The earlier you start anti-aging, the easier your job will be in the long run.

Most of the people who wind up in nursing homes are there, for the most part, because they did not *maintain* high levels of physical, mental, and emotional health throughout their lifetimes. Sadly, once they are unable to care for themselves—or be cared for in their own homes—their bodies are so weakened that they are unable to survive for long, even with managed care.

The current health status of many of the individuals living in nursing homes is directly related to their nutritional intake. Numerous studies have concluded that these individuals suffer from multiple nutritional deficiencies. From the Clinton Administration Report on the Quality of Nursing Homes: "The report concludes that the private Joint Commission on accreditation of Healthcare Organizations (JCAHO) survey process was not effective in protecting the health and safety of nursing home residents." Also, the office of the Health Care Financing Administration stated that "Five and a half years seems a long time for Clinton to discover that hundreds of people are still dying from malnutrition, dehydration, sepsis from bedsores and even physical abuse while in nursing homes."

The problems of malnutrition and dehydration are due in particular to the institutional food provided by vendors who have used RDA's that have been shown to be both insufficient and grossly inadequate for people who have compromised immune systems and multiple nutritional deficiencies.

This proposal carefully examines the scientific literature that cites the actual therapeutic dosages in relation to the category of illnesses that the majority of people in nursing homes fall into.

After reviewing thousands of scientific articles and using data from test groups of 300 individuals, most of whom are in senior-citizen age groups, we concluded that nutrition and exercise, as presented in this proposed protocol, played a key role in the health and well-being of the senior citizens.

THE REVERSING-THE-AGING-PROCESS STUDY

In January 1997 I enrolled 300 people into a "Reversing the Aging Process Study" that would last eighteen months. At the end of this period, sixty-five people had completed the study—235 people became controls. This was not a double-blind study. It was an observation of changes in their blood chemistry, weight, physical dimensions, physical appearance, memory, energy levels, sleep patterns, bowel movements, night-time urination, muscle strength, digestion, olfactory senses, visual senses, tactile senses, skin texture, and stress levels. This was a lifestyle modification study:

- 52 percent of participants had lower cholesterol and tryglyceride levels.
- 68 percent had increased DHEA levels.
- 78 percent had a significant improvement in their fat muscle ratio.
- 90 percent had an increase in bowel movements.
- 92 percent had a decreased need for sleep.
- 95 percent had increased energy levels.
- Stress levels were lowered by 97 percent.

In addition, numerical diaries had been kept by the participants reflecting subjective data. This data cited improvements that affected the participants in their overall quality of life.

We can also conclude that this protocol would benefit the vast majority of people in nursing homes and hospices. The following is not a theoretical model; it is an actual model.

Harry Biele, a ninety-year-old man who just ten years ago had chronic sinusitis, asthma, arthritis, enlarged prostate, a precancerous lower bowel, and main coronary artery blockage, is now a marathoner living life to its fullest. His cardiologist has taken away all medication like beta blockers, and his general practitioner has taken away his inhalers for asthma. He is not an exception. Harry is an example of someone who has taken positive action toward his own health. He improved his nutrition by applying a protocol similar to this one. Exercise became part of Harry's dialy ritual. He now appears to be closer to seventy than ninety.

Anyone—be he/she a senior citizen or a baby boomer—can improve his/her health. This is the scientific literature that justifies the use of recommended supplements in this protocol. Applying this protocol can play an important role in anyone's life.

THE PROTOCOL FOR LASTING YOUTH

The following is a breakdown to the protocol developed in the course of my Reversing the Aging Process Study.

Physical Exercise

The results of our study have also helped to conclude, by process of interviews, that most of the participants—and 100 percent of the controls in the study—were not exercising properly. In general, they were not doing enough exercise, nor were they exercising with enough intensity.

We have modified the recommended exercise protocol for senior citizens; however, I suggest you forget your calendar age and work at a rate suited to your *physical* and *mental* capacities.

- Build up gradually to forty-five minutes of aerobic activity per day.
- Take your pulse during the workout to make sure you are neither under- nor overexerting yourself. A heart rate monitor is very useful and can be purchased at any sports store.

  Generally, the target heart rate is determined by taking 200, subtracting your age (this is the maximal heart rate) and then multiplying the result by 50 to 60 percent. So, an eighty-one-year-old person would have a rate of 220 minus 81 times 50–60 percent, or, seventy–eighty-three beats per minute. After a few months of training, you can increase to 70 percent of the maximal heart rate.

- As well as aerobic exercise, do weight training three times per week.

It is no secret anymore. Exercise is an essential element in the overall health of people at any age. As we age our tendons shrink and our muscle mass decreases. In order to keep the body as youthful as possible, muscle mass needs to be retained, and if possible increased. Tendons need to be stretched. As we get older, we actually need more exercise and longer stretching. All forms of exercise should be preceded with a thorough stretching routine. Stretching will elongate and strengthen the tendons and get the muscles warmed up and ready for movement. Senior citizens in general will take a longer time to warm up.

Some exercises that are recommended for senior citizens are: fast walking, low-impact aerobics, weight lifting, yoga for stretching; T'ai Chi or Chi Gong for treadmill and the stair-climbing machine. All exercises that are not too impacting on the joints are beneficial.

More detailed information regarding aging is included in Part V.

The purpose of this protocol is to improve the health of the nursing home population with an intervention based on diet and behavior modification, the intake of whole foods, exercise, and vitamin, nutrient, and herbal supplementation.

To modify your dietary habits, I suggest the following:

(1) Intake of animal protein be reduced (1x week) and consumption of cold-water fish be increased (5x week).
(2) Additional protein should be derived from whole grains, legumes, and seeds. If needed, a protein powder supplement may be used.
(3) The diet should provide forty–fifty grams of fiber a day.
(4) At least one (preferably three) servings of a cruciferous vegetable should be provided daily: Brussel sprouts, broccoli, cabbage, or cauliflower.

(5) 2–4 glasses of dark green leafy vegetable juices/day. The juice should also include one-inch-length of ginger, aloe concentrate, and protein powder (optional).
(6) One-half–one gallon of water and juices ingested daily.
(7) Caffeine, soda, white sugar, and refined white flour products should be reduced to a minimum. For optimal results, they should be eliminated completely.
(8) Olive oil should be used for cooking purposes.
(9) Supplements should be taken with meals in divided doses where noted.

As far as supplements go, use the following chart as your guide. Do *not* take all of these at once. Begin with those supplements listed as group I and take each at $\frac{1}{5}$ the dosage listed here for the first three months. Then, with each subsequent month, add another group, again taking the supplements at $\frac{1}{5}$ of the suggested dosage. Over time, once you are taking all the supplements, you can gradually increase the dosages to optimal levels. You may find it easier to take a quality multiple vitamin that includes many of the vitamins listed here. If you are taking any medications, check with your physician to make sure there are no counterindicated effects.

Vitamins, Nutrients & Herbal Supplements	Suggested Dosages	Dosaged Based on Peer-Reviewed Journal Articles*
I B Complex	50 mg	10–200 mg
Folic Acid	400 mcg	2.5–35 mg
Choline	500 mg	500 mg–16,000 mg
Vitamin E	400–800 IU	30–4,800 mg
L-Methionine	500 mg	2,000–10,000 mg
Vitamin C	2,000–15,000 mg	30–17,000 mg
II Silybum Marianum	50 mg	140–600 mg
Garlic	500 mg 4xday	3,000–10,000 mg
Evening Primrose Oil	500 mg 2xday	3,000–6,000 mg
Fish oil lipids	1,000 mg	2,600–24,000 mg
III Ginkgo Biloba	60–120 mg	50–600 mg
Lecithin	5 gm	0.500 gm–16 gm
N-Acetyl Cysteine	500–1,000 mg	300 mg–42,000 mg
IV DHEA	5–25 mg	30–500 mg
DMAE	100 mg	

Vitamins, Nutrients & Herbal Supplements	Suggested Dosages	Dosaged Based on Peer-Reviewed Journal Articles*
Phosphatidyl serine	200 mg 3xday	50–800 mg
Acetyle L-Carnitine	500 mg 2xday	1,000–3,000 mg
V Co-enzyme Q-10	100–300 mg	30–390 mg
Calcium/Magnesium	800–1,400 mg	1,000–1,400 mg (Ca + +)
VI Niacin	100–500 mg	500–1,000 mg
Glutathione	500–1,000 mg	2,500–5,000 mg
VII Curcumine	250 mg	500 mg
Alpha Lipoic Acid	200 mg	100–600 mg
Melatonin	3 mg	0.3–10 mg
Pregnenolone	10 mg	70 mg (based on 70 kg male)

PRECURSORS TO GROWTH HORMONE

Take these only if you are deficient in Human Growth Hormone.

Arginine	1,000 mg	4,000–20,000 mg
Ornithine	1,000 mg	10,000–18,000 mg
Glutamine	1,000 mg	1,500–4,000 mg
TMG-Betaine	500 mg	6,000–10,000 mg
Linoleic acid (Conjugated FA)	500 mg	

HERBS FOR CLEANSING

These should be used for one month only as a part of your detoxification program.

Apple pectin	25–50 mg	8,500–20,000 mg
Bee Pollen	25–50 mg	
Burdock root	25–50 mg	
Chrysanthemum	25–50 mg	
Dandelion root	25–50 mg	
Hibiscus	25–50 mg	
Kelp	25–50 mg	
Oregon	25–50 mg	
Peppermint	25–50 mg	Enteric-coated capsules
Psyllium	25–50 mg	3,400–15,000 mg
Red clover	25–50 mg	100 mg (Coumarin)

*Therapeutic doses are based on Peer-Reviewed Journals with a focus on human trials and studies. These articles are cited within the proposal. Please refer to reference section for details.

VITAMIN AND MINERAL INDEXES

Nutrients	Recommended Adult Intake	Source of Recommended Intake	Therapeutic Intake Range based on Peer-Reviewed Journals**
Vitamin A	5,000 IU	USRDA**	
Vitamin D	400 IU	USRDA 400	
Vitamin E	400 IU	USRDA 30	30–2,800mg
Vitamin C	1,000–15,000 mg	RDA** 60mg	30–17,000mg
Thiamin (B₁)	50 mg	USRDA 1.5mg	10–200mg
Riboflavin (B₂)	50 mg	USRDA 1.7	10–400mg
Niacin (B₃) (nicotinamide)	100 mg	USRDA 20mg	500–3,000mg
Pyridoxine (B₆)	50 mg	RDA	50–200mg
Folacin	400 mg	USRDA	.02mg–35mg Folic acid
Biotin	2.0 mg	USRDA	
Pantothenic acid (B₅)	200 mg	USRDA	
Calcium	1,200 mg	RDA	1,000–1,400mg
Phosphorus	50 mg	RDA	
Magnesium	1,200 mg	USRDA	
Iron	15 mg	USRDA	
Zinc	50 mg	USRDA	
Copper	2 mg	ESAADDI**	
Iodine	300 mg	USRDA	
Selenium	200 mg	ESAADDI	

**RDA-Recommended Dietary Allowances; USRDA-United States Recommended Daily Allowances; ESAADDI-Estimated Safe and Adequate Daily Dietary Intakes. Shils, et al. 1994. *Modern Nutrition in Health and Disease,* Eighth Edition Volume 2. Lea & Febiger, p. 1582.

8

DETOXIFICATION: THE FIRST STEP TOWARD HEALING

B efore we can begin *any* program to rejuvenate and heal, we must clean up our act—literally as well as figuratively. You see, one of the primary reasons we are aging prematurely and are, across the board, so unhealthy is the accumulations of toxins in our environments and in our bodies.

Poisons enter our bodies and become stored in adipose (fat) and nerve tissue. The "little bit" of lead and other toxic metals and bacteria in the water that comes through the tap into our kitchens, where we use it in cooking, joins with the airborne pollutants—from carbon monoxide to industrial wastes—and the pesticides used to make fruits and vegetables picture perfect and larger than life, and the antibiotics and growth hormones administered to make chickens lay more eggs, cows give more milk, and livestock of every sort, from poultry and pig to sheep and steer, grow huge, to invade our bodies with amazingly unhealthy regularity. The cumulative effect of these toxins, as well as from the preservatives in packaged foods, antibiotics, and other medications, and all sorts of other substances impair immune function and reproductive capacity over time.

It's an unfortunate fact of life in the modern world: Toxic substances routinely pervade our food, water, and air.

More than 100,000 toxic chemicals are commonly found in our environment, and those are just the ones we know about. Even so-called "good chemicals"—such as antibiotic and antiviral medications, cleaning agents, cosmetics, etc.—have repeatedly been found to do tremendous damage to our bodies.

Most of our water sources are polluted. Our water systems are full of chlorine and flouride, which are known to impair thyroid function. We are swimming in a sea of toxins.

If we cannot eliminate or lessen the body's burden of these poisons, it becomes irrevelant how many vitamins, herbs, or juices we put into our systems. We constantly undo the positive effects of these nutritional forces with our intense exposures to negative forces. It would be much like having someone hug you once a week and then scream at you every other minute for the next week until the next hug. That's what it means to be in a toxic environment and then try to do something to neutralize some of the toxins. You can never get enough of the positive to overcome the negatives.

Much disease results from toxic congestion. We eat too much, drink too much, and don't get enough quality sleep. In time, the cumulative effect of these factors catch up with us. Even if you are particularly aware and concerned about your health, there are so many pollutants in our environment that, unless you detoxify, you will become sick. Surely you will never achieve your maximum physical potential.

THE CLEANUP BEGINS

Because of these toxic forces, any successful protocol must begin with a thorough cleansing: of the body, mind, and spirit; of the environments of the home, work, and community; as well as of family, friends, and all other people within these environments.

When you look at the causes of aging and disease, you must look at heavy metals. These include mercury, cadmium, and lead. Your brain, kidneys, and immune system are particularly vulnerable to these toxins, yet millions of people knowingly put more of these poisons in their bodies every day. When you look in the mouth of the average person, you see a lot of silver amalgam fillings. These fillings are leaching mercury into the body, which then goes to the brain. That can affect neurological changes. Mercury also can go to the liver and kidneys, which can affect renal function and the synthesizing of essential nutrients in the liver. It's not a matter of "Do these mercury vapors cause problems?"

Undisputedly, they do.

But in each person it can be a different type of problem. When individuals with multiple sclerosis have had their mercury fillings taken out, there have been substantial improvements in their conditions. The same has been found to be true for other medical problems. We've seen people with neurological damage, including Alzheimer's disease and other forms of dementia, improve. People who have suffered from chronic fatigue syndrome for many years have shown marked improvement after the removal of mercury amalgam fillings from their teeth.

Then, we have aluminum from antacids and cookware. Long suspected to be a contributing factor to Alzheimer's disease and senile dementia, aluminum cookware and aluminum foil continue to be used every day. And while antacid tablets are touted as great forms of calcium, little is said about the potentially toxic effect of this poisonous heavy metal on our brains.

It is estimated that one hundred million Americans are chronically ill. That means that they are on the prescription bandwagon. Common thought has it that the older you get, the more drugs you take. The average senior citizen in a nursing home could be taking upwards of fifteen *different* prescribed medications, many of which are very likely to have contra-indications to each other. That's why the third leading cause of death in the United States is iatrogenic or medically induced death from misprescribed and overprescribed medications.

This is not to suggest that we don't need medication and drugs. We do. They can be life-saving, even essential. It would be irresponsible to suggest otherwise. But it is equally irresponsible to suggest that people be given broad-spectrum antibiotics every time they come down with a cold. Colds stem from viral infection, not bacteria. Antibiotics work specifically on bacteria, not viruses. Yet the average person who consults a conventional allopathic physician with a cold will be given antibiotics. Frequent use of antibiotics lowers the immune system and promotes imbalances and pathogens throughout the intestinal tract.

Here in the West, we're given antibiotics for almost every physical ailment. And we're given way too many drugs. In fact, drugs are the first order of business when you come out of a doctor's office. I've heard doctors say that patients actually feel cheated if they don't get a prescription. They feel that they're not getting something for their money and time.

We may be accustomed to getting drugs, yet none of these drugs have made major changes in restoring our health. At best, they can stop some of the effects that are rapidly escalating, taking away some of the inflammation.

Generally speaking, most medications mask symptoms, which make them harder to diagnose. For example, you take something for pain. This medication may bring relief, but it does not stop it at its source—it simply inhibits or blocks the way the brain *perceives* the pain. Therefore, you still *have* pain; you're just not feeling it. The condition is unchanged. In fact, you may be setting yourself up for more—and more serious—injury by making it possible for you to do things, such as walk on a sprained ankle, that pain would have prohibited.

So, by being an overly medicated society, we have become a toxic society. It is estimated that over 1 million people are sick and just not aware of it.

Look at it this way: Beta blockers, channel blockers, calcium blockers—all these can interfere with phosphatidylcholine, a necessary neurotransmitter going from the brain to the penis to allow an electrical charge that helps the male to get an erection. When it is no longer present, it becomes very difficult to have an erection. That is one of the main causes of impotence. We then take Viagra, which gives us nitric oxide as a gas for smooth muscle contractibility, so that we can engorge the penis with blood, instead of using arginine and phosphatidylcholine, which would do it naturally.

With medications, we're not looking at natural approaches to these conditions, we're looking at proprietary approaches. If proprietary approaches were nontoxic, that would be great. But there are serious side effects in each of these medications. And the more drugs you take, the more side effects you have.

What is never taken into account is the fact that there is never a model in which a drug is given in a test where all other drugs that the person could be exposed to are also given in a test to see what the effects are. It's a purely mathematical theoretical model that if you take this drug and that drug you might have this reaction. In real life, it doesn't work that way—everyone's body composition is different. So again, we are toxic with medications.

Alcohol, even in small amounts, will destroy folic acid, B$_6$, and B$_{12}$. That, in turn, makes you more susceptible to homocysteine, which is a greater predictor of heart disease than cholesterol levels. We know that homocysteine leads to the pathogenesis of the aging of the heart. We are now telling people to take alcohol for their heart when there's no evidence that drinking helps. This belief was never based upon a real study. It was based upon a mathematical model that said that because a small group of individuals who drank had less heart disease or less of a specific type of heart disease, therefore they were protected by the alcohol.

In point of fact, I read the same study and saw that it was not the alcohol, but rather the grapes themselves that gave the protection. It is the proanthocyanidins, the bioflavonoids, the quercitin, and the antioxidants that protect the tissue from oxidative stress.

Oxidative stress comes from normal living, exercise, environmental pollutants, foods, alcohol, smoking, low-level radiation, and electromagnetic pulses. This oxidative stress proliferates free radicals and is the number-one cause of aging and disease. It, therefore, predisposes you to having an unhealthy body.

Although it may seem that way, ill health doesn't happen overnight, and that's the problem. The body has an amazing capacity to rejuvenate itself. You're experiencing a constant, twenty-four-hour-a-day barrage of free radicals hitting your cells. And if the inside of the artery is getting multiple hits, you're creating an oxidative stress that leads to tiny lesions.

These lesions are then healed, and part of the healing process involves the formation of scabs. When this process occurs internally, such things as cholesterol, fats, and different types of lipids collect onto the scabbed areas, adhering and building plaque or scaling. This is frequently the initiation of the plaque, but instead of being reasonable and looking deeper at the problem, we look at what was in the plaque. Then we say that cholesterol is a primary ingredient in the plaque, i.e., cholesterol is the cause of atherosclerosis, a thinning of the passageway in the artery through major occlusion. In truth, it is the lesion in the arterial wall and the original cause of that lesion that cause the problem.

Homocysteine can precipitate all that, and cholesterol is only one of the factors. In fact, free radicals are the primary cause.

Alcohol consumption causes free radicals. So, the very thing the so-called experts are saying will help us will not. What the researchers fail to mention is that the incidence of cancer in those people in one area of France who said they were protected from heart disease was actually higher. It's much like telling a woman to take Tamoxifin to prevent breast cancer, when it's associated with a higher incidence of endometrial cancer. That's not a good trade-off, but that's the reality. So, we have to look at oxidative stress as our primary cause of disease, our number-one cause of premature aging. We have to do this every day.

As I've already said, few people have a problem eating fifty french fries or three scoops of ice cream, but ask them to take three vitamins, and you would think they had been asked to tear out their hearts. "I've got to take all these? I won't have any time to live."

People will be ultraconservative about what they do for their health, but extremely liberal—have no boundaries—in what they do that promotes disease and aging. It's insane. It should be just the opposite, but that's not how we live. We're accustomed to having all the things that are bad for us—the fried foods, red meats, caffeine, carbonated drinks, highly processed foods—in our diets. We don't want to change. In fact, we use any excuse not to change, as if it's too much effort to save our own lives.

But it's not too much effort to do things that are harmful. I had to build into the protocol something that helps address that question; hence, behavior modification is the backbone of this program. Through the early study groups, I found that, if you just gave a diet to people, they wouldn't stick with it. If you just give antioxidents, they'll take them once in the morning and forget to take them the rest of the day. If you just give juices, when you're enriching the body with chlorophyl and enzymes, maybe they'll juice occasionally, but they'll do anything to try to get out of it. "I don't have a juicer. I don't have organic products." Always an excuse.

So, I'm showing you what to do, and how effective it has been for the thousands of people who have participated in the studies that generated this protocol.

WHAT TO CUT DOWN ON

The first step we must do is to become extremely aware of every-thing around us. The vast assault on our systems is overwhelming and is getting worse every day, so it behooves us to develop a height-ened sensitivity to the environment.

Increase your awareness of not only your health but the health of the planet. Some of the primary causes of aging that surround us—solvents (such as those in our cleaning products), formalde-hyde (a chief preservative in cigarettes), the pesticides and herbi-cides, the chemical additives and the bacteria in our foods all play a huge role in our overall well-being.

There are endotoxins and yeasts and parasites in the most un-likely places. When you drink tap water, you are allowing a stew of poison into your body—from the lead and other heavy metals leached from pipes and water mains to bacteria and decay from or-ganic matter in the water.

Anything that is toxic that goes into the body creates a body threshold. In other words, there is a limit as to how much your body can accept of a toxic substance before something finally gives way. How many parasites can you take in? Parasites can live forever in your gut. Millions can be teeming inside your intestines without your being aware of them. Parasites don't pass through the body. They latch on, eating into the mucosal lining of the stomach and intestinal tract, and they set up house there. Everything that's alive creates waste products. The waste matter produced by parasites, like giardia lamblia, can get into the bloodstream, go to the brain, and cause what we call brain fatigue. I believe that the reason that many people are so fatigued today is because they're so toxic. Their bodies have become overwhelmed by these toxic products.

In addition, there are a lot of bacteria in the atmosphere. People are very cavalier. They'll pick up a piece of fruit, wipe it on their pants, and take a bite of it. When you just wipe any fruit or vegeta-ble, all you do is smear any contaminants on the surface even more uniformly. You never clean anything by wiping it; you have to disin-fect it, wash it in a natural solvent that will remove bacteria, pesti-cides, and other contaminants.

Even organic produce should be cleaned, perhaps even more

than nonorganic foods, because organic fruits and vegetables are grown in fertilizer made from manure. Hence, coliform bacteria are present. When the rain hits the fertilized ground, these bacteria bounce up onto the produce. Someone harvests it and puts it in a box. That person has bacteria on his hands. Dozens of hands—each with their own bacterial "gloves"—could touch that produce before you eat it.

So, you may think it's "safe" because a food is organic and neglect to wash it. This is not good. Everything you eat should be washed, even sprouts. Everything you drink should be washed before it is juiced—zero exceptions.

While there are several commercially manufactured vegetable washing liquids, you don't have to hound your health-food store or supermarket for them. This recipe, made from things you already have in your home, can be used to remove bacteria and other toxic matter from fruits and vegetables.

SIMPLE SOLVENT

1 gallon filtered water
¼ cup hydrogen peroxide
¼ cup apple cider vinegar

Combine ingredients in a sink or basin. Soak fruits or vegetables in this solution for four to five minutes to dissolve material adhering to the plant surface. Agitate vigorously to lift the particles off the surface. Discard this solvent solution, then rinse vegetables in filtered water.

WATCH—AND WASH—YOUR HANDS

We think we're being diligent, but we're not. We handle doorknobs and money and hangers in subways. And we shake people's hands. Just spend an hour in traffic watching how many orifices people can stick a finger into on their way to work. Then realize that they're going to be touching doorknobs that you will be touching; handling money that you're going to handle; shaking hands with you. And you're going to use the telephone or ATM they touched—that stuff doesn't just go away. Bacteria can live for long periods of times outside the human body, as can viruses and parasites.

When I give a lecture to hundreds of people in an auditorium, I tell them this story: If I put a petri dish on every seat in the auditorium and, after spraying a nonpathogenic bacteria into my mouth, talk at a normal conversational velocity while standing in front of the room, by tomorrow every single petri dish would be contaminated. What you cannot see is that every time we talk, we each create a high velocity spray of saliva, with thousands upon thousands of water molecules coming out of our mouths. These microbe-contaminated molecules can waft around in the air for hours. You come into the space and inhale them. They go into your eyes, nostrils, and mouth, thus getting into your system.

If you are strong, if your immune system has been very diligent and you have fed it the right nutrients, you can trap them and destroy them before they make you ill.

But what if you're the average person who's sick to begin with? You don't have a diligent immune system. Now you come into an area where a lot of people are talking. Think of all the different microbes floating around in the air. Think of being in an airplane where they don't have recycled air. The same air circulates through the plane's cabin, and you're breathing it the entire time you're on board. What if there is a passenger who has tuberculosis? It has been shown that TB can be dispersed in an airplane. But, remember, anything else that can be breathed can be dispersed as well. Once it's dispersed, it wafts around in the air. Now you've got that in your system. The problem is that we don't take any of this into account. We think it's not important. After all, real men don't get sick. Well, real men die every day. Bacteria are a real factor to be reckoned with.

You don't have to be obsessive-compulsive to have clean hands. Wash them often, or use a disinfectant hand rub throughout the day. Simply put some in your palms and rub it around to cover your entire hands and fingers. It's not as much trouble as one would think.

Whenever you go into a bathroom—even at home—touch everything, from doors to toilet handle to taps, with a paper towel. If this seems too bothersome, just think about the other people who have used this facility. Someone walks over to the tap after having just used the toilet. They turn on the tap, wash their hands, and turn off the tap. Well, who was the person before them who turned the tap on and off? When you turned on the tap, you contaminated it, too. Turning it off doesn't decontaminate it just because you washed your hands.

It escapes me why we use so little common sense in this area. If you doubt me, take a culture off any of the faucets in any bathroom in America. Instead, use a paper towel to turn the faucet on and off, and open the door with it to further minimize your exposure to bacteria and other contaminants.

We cannot be paranoid because we must co-exist, but we can take precautions. I'm just asking for a healthy caution to minimize the cummulative contamination of the body, because, ultimately, bacteria will bring you down. Bacteria are pleomorphic, changeable. Bacteria from your gut can migrate to your lungs, your brain, and your liver. Parasites can migrate into the blood system, and they can be there for a very long time, doing harm, before you realize they are there. All the while, your body is creating local, focal infections.

These infections tax the immune system so that all the nutrients you consume go to repair where the body is damaged. In effect, they are used to extinguish these local brushfires throughout your body.

If you live like the average person with a deficient diet—full of excess fats, animal proteins, sugars, bacteria, viruses, parasites—have mercury fillings, and are exposed to pollutants from the air and water, then you have a whole body filled with these contaminants that are more than the body's immune system can handle. Then you start to show it externally where before it only showed up internally. A gene that is predisposed to balding, thinning, or graying is going to do exactly that because there's nothing there in abundance to change the gene. It has exceeded the genetic threshold.

Our processed diet is filled with food additives and preservatives. Never eat anything that won't go bad. That should tell you something. What do you think those chemicals are doing to your system? There is no evolutionary mechanism to deal with food preservatives and additives, emulsifiers, plasticizers, foaming and antifoaming agents, and texturizers. We have nothing it can be used for in our bodies—it is purely and simply a toxin. A small amount of a toxin doesn't mean that it isn't a toxin. And when it joins up with the little bits of toxin from other sources, the result can be staggering.

There's something called a pigmy rattlesnake. It's a tiny snake with a tiny bite, but it has tons of toxins in its venom. It won't necessarily kill you, as a larger rattlesnake could, but get bitten a few times and you will die. So, every time you have that piece of processed white bread that you didn't think anything of, it's no big deal. But you are building up toxins. It's cumulative, because what the body can't use it tries to store and protect you from. Unfortunately, the body has only so much storage room.

One of the areas in which the body stores toxins is fat. Hence, the fatter you are, the more toxic you will be. I don't care about your weight per se, because being overweight in itself is not a primary indicator of aging, but since toxins are stored in fat, every moment that you're burning fat for fuel or dieting, you're actually flooding your body with herbicides, pesticides, and growth-stimulating hormones stored in your fat tissue. It's like you have become a toxic dump site.

As a rule, the leaner you are, the healthier you are. Ideally, woman should be about 12 to 17 percent body fat; men, 9 to 14 percent body fat. If everyone had that kind of lean: fat ratio, we'd be an enormously healthy nation.

OTHER FACTORS ASSAULTING OUR IMMUNE SYSTEMS

If pesticides and pollutants were the only culprits wrecking your immune system, that would be bad enough. However, no matter how much you detox your life, it will do you no good unless you also take positive and aggressive measures to eliminate the huge influx of stress in your life.

Stress is equal in its capacity to harm you as seriously as any environmental pollutant with which we normally come into contact. It creates a cascade of powerful hormones, including cortisol, epinephrine, and adrenaline. These are important factors necessary to a fight-or-flight response; however, they can be harmful if not abated.

The body cannot distinguish between merely having a bad day or being argumentative, thinking negative thoughts, and having negative emotions from an authentic, fight-or-flight situation, when you are in danger. Your body cannot differentiate between the actual and the imagined in this regard, so it will respond as if it was being threatened. If you start a whole push of these hormones, you can be in this state all day.

To put it another way, as long as you are under any anxiety, depression, fear, or anger, your body is in the death mode. You are promoting hormones that can destroy you. Think of how negative, or angry, the average person often is. Any negative emotion creates negative hormones. And it's instantaneous. That's why our thoughts are a very powerful part of the healing—or age-reversal—process.

Our thoughts are never neutral. Thoughts have power because you can only feel what your thoughts create. You can only be happy if you think happy thoughts; sad if you think sad thoughts; angry if you think angry thoughts. Remember, the thought always precedes the emotion, but the process can be so fast that you don't have time to stop and think about it.

It is an automatic, defensive, reactionary energy that comes right out like an emotional minefield ready to detonate. Someone steps on it and then *boom*—it explodes. Then you look around for justification. It was their fault; they made me angry; I'm upset. But that's not what it's all about.

So, if you want to age, to kill yourself, if you want to get cancer, arthritis, diabetes, heart disease, go ahead: Keep being negative. You're gambling on disease, and you'll get it. You will always win and get your disease if you're under continuous stress. It's not a matter of *if* you'll get sick, it's a matter of *when*.

Under these conditions, under which most of us operate every waking moment of every day, you will absolutely, unequivocally, definitely, get sick. It's when, and to what degree, it will manifest that is the question.

WHAT TO ACCENTUATE

Let's start with something positive—let's start with what you can do about it. Start by becoming aware that nothing should go into your body that doesn't heal or nourish it. Those are the only two reasons you should be eating or drinking anything: for nourishment and healing. Often we eat because we're sad or anxious or because of a social event. While that's not an excuse for eating foods that are not nourishing, that's exactly what we do, and then make excuses for it.

So, instead of excuses, let's make decisions.

First, we want to change the quality of our protein. We want protein from nonanimal sources. Animal sources are putrefying and disease-promoting. Get your protein from nonflesh sources—grains, nuts, seeds, and legumes.

Protein—especially from animal sources—at every meal is a myth. We routinely eat far too much protein. Unless we are very active or have a disease, we should consume about 60 to 70 grams of protein—from *any* source—per day. The average person eats closer to 120 grams.

The human body is not able to store protein, so it converts protein into fat. This process dehydrates the body and overtaxes the kidneys and the liver, making this an expensive and toxic way to get the fat the body needs for proper metabolism.

We should be eating things such as millet, buckwheat, brown rice, spelt, rye, quinoa, raw vegetables and fruits of all types, tempeh, tofu, nuts, tubers—yams, potatoes, sweet potatoes, and cruciferous vegetables like broccoli, cabbage, and cauliflower. And the only oil we should use in cooking is macadamia oil, because it's the only one that is heat stable. Canola oil, from new information published recently, is not stable. As a result, it is potentially dangerous to your health. Use canola oil only in salad dressings, not in cooking. Virgin olive oil and flax seed oil should be used in salads or at the very end of cooking, when the heat is down.

In addition, you should have at least four glasses of mixed vegetable juice per day and two glasses of fresh fruit juice per day, all organic. There are a lot of different vegetables and fruits to choose from.

The heart of this anti-aging program is cleansing with juices. I found that when I was taking all the right foods and supplements and exercising, my health still didn't improve. When I started juicing, I noticed a difference. And when I concentrated the juices with extra chlorophyll, that made the biggest difference . . . especially in my hair, which I found to be an indicator of my health and youth.

Once when I was out on a tour in the Midwest and knew I

wouldn't be able to get the healthy, organic foods I usually eat, I took several gallons of a vegetable powder that I had made at my ranch in Texas.

I had taken all my fall harvest of vegetables and juiced them. I knew this guy who had a little apparatus that could dry this powerful liquid into a powder in a vacuum chamber. So that's what I did.

While I was on the road, I drank vegetable juice laced with this powder throughout the day. Generally, it was carrot mixed with other fruits or vegetables. I kept throwing a scoop of this powder into some water. That's all I had for about twenty-five days.

This somewhat unorthodox diet gave me enormous energy, and I felt really great. I was lecturing and doing media work nonstop day after day, traveling from city to city. Instead of being fatigued and worn out, I was always raring to go. In fact, the day I returned home, I ran a 50k national championship in Central Park.

Over the next twelve weeks, I ran—and completed—five marathons. That's the kind of energy I had. I kept on taking this powder in water several times a day, every day. Over the next fifty-seven weeks, I ran fifty-seven races and won every one. I was at the top of my health.

About four weeks after this, while sitting at my desk and rubbing my forehead, I felt little bristles. Looking in the mirror, I noticed new hair growth. Little dark brown stubs were all over my head. This startled (and pleased!) me, and I started looking through my hair. I realized that the gray, which I'd had since I was a teenager, was no longer completely gray. The root, the tiny little base near the scalp, was brown. I analyzed my situation and realized that the only thing that I had changed was that I was adding the juice with the chlorophyll to my diet.

That's when I realized that the key to detoxification was to flood the body with chlorophyll. Eating vegetables wasn't enough, because every time you eat a vegetable, only a relatively small amount of that chlorophyll gets into the body. Most of it is indigestible fiber that goes in the stomach and the intestines. Only the organic water that's inside gets to come out and get into the blood. When you juice that, you get the full amount, and when you increase its potency it by adding extra chlorophyll powder, you really concentrate the nutrients. ·

I did an analysis, and I was eating the equivalent of one hundred pounds of vegetables a day, but in juice and powder form. Then I started looking at different phytochemicals that prevent cancer, that repair DNA, that help fight bacteria and viruses and fungi. I saw that every single vegetable is loaded with anywhere from 75 to 200 phytochemicals. I pored through the literature and found out which phytochemicals do what.

Then I realized that if these phytochemicals can repair DNA, they can not only clean the body but also help to stall aging. I started loading up on the phytochemicals from the vegetables and fruits that were specific for DNA repair. As a result, wrinkles that I acquired from sun exposure were gone. My skin became smooth, and my nails were very pink and growing very fast.

Then I started measuring my hair. It had slowed down its growth, from about three inches per month to about a quarter inch per month. However, within eight months I had a whole new head of hair. Mind you, I did everything else the same. I exercised, did stress management, had air and water purifiers in my apartment, had hardwood floors and natural cotton sheets. All that I've been doing for years. The only thing that had changed was the addition of that powder. So when people ask me how I am able to work twenty-two hours a day, I tell them it's because I'm "nontoxed."

That's the most crucial part.

If you're emotionally toxic, you're going to be tired. You're going to require more sleep, more rest just to live. And if you're physically toxic, too, you're going to be even more tired. If you're emotionally and physically toxic, you have a real body burden, and an emotional burden that you have to unload first. When you get that all cleaned up so you're not worrying about your previous obsessions, you have cleared the way for exuberance and glowing health. It's like an albatross that's been lifted from around your neck—you can really feel the lightness of your life, and always remember, health is light. You can breathe, you can move, you can glow. And the juices are what does it.

About ten years ago, a lot of Americans began buying juice extractors, but they didn't use them. The pattern was, they'd use them once and then thought it was way too much work. They'd put their juicers away, after promising themselves that they'd just buy a gallon of juice once a week and that'd do the trick. However, they soon found themselves right back in their old patterns, and nothing substantive had changed. It's like we get on these little health jags and then go off of them. If you stick with the juicing, that's just the beginning. But if you don't juice, nothing else will help, because it won't be as effective. In fact, you won't have begun the process of cleansing. You'll get the bacteria and parasites out of your body because the phytochemicals—especially from the mustard family—are also antiparasitic. And once they go in, they start repairing the DNA.

Say you drank at one point, and your liver is damaged. Juicing will definitely help to repair that. I've worked with a lot of recovering alcoholics and helped them repair their damaged livers. Regular, organic juicing and antioxidants throughout the day is the real epicenter of the program. It's a natural process of purification all the time.

Just being around happy people makes you feel good, and being around negative people brings you down. One makes you feel drained and tired, while the other makes you feel good and energized. It's the same with food. You have a cup of coffee, and you get a temporary boost before you crash. In contrast, you have juice, and it glides right up and keeps you up.

You have to realize that the average American has tons of toxins in his intestines. They are loaded with pounds and pounds of debris that shouldn't be there in the first place—it's putrefying. And if you think it's bad when that quarter pound or half pound of waste comes out of you, imagine how bad it is when it's still in you. That's what's cleaned out with the juicing. You clean your intestines more than you ever thought possible.

Added to the juice, we should take aloe vera. Aloe vera is the single most healing of all the herbs. It's anti-cancer, anti-parasistic, and it repairs DNA. It protects us from viruses and bacteria. Every time I take juice, I take aloe, and it makes a big difference.

You should drink at least a gallon of purified water a day. Most of us drink only at mealtime and when we're noticibly thirsty. Wrong. You can develop a habit of *not* drinking water and walk around being 66 or 67 percent water, instead of 72 percent, which is what your body needs.

When you don't have the water in you, you won't have the energy you need. The very first thing I do to get people's energy up is to increase the amount of water in their diet. Immediately, their energy goes up.

When someone has dementia, the first thing I do is give them lots of cold water all day, every day. About three weeks later, I start to see their dementia dissipate because they have rehydrated their brains. Unfortunately, your brain actually shrinks as you dehydrate. By drinking lots of pure water, you get better neuron activity and better cellular chemistry, and you're able to detoxify the cells with water.

A reminder: I am recommending that you drink water *in addition to* the fruit and vegetable juices suggested as part of this protocol.

You then need to increase the nutrients, like B complex, vitamin B_{12}, and vitamin C. The amount of vitamin C needed will be different for each person. If you go out in the sun, you need more vitamin C because the sun causes free radical damage. When you've been in a stressful situation, you need more vitamin C, which is very important, as is alhpalipeic acid.

Evening primrose oil nourishes joints and the immune system. Garlic is a great detoxifier, especially when taken at bedtime. About 2,000 mg is needed, and will work overnight to lower blood pressure, lower cholesterol, and cleanse parasites as well as harmful candida and bacteria out of the intestines. Ginkgo biloba feeds the brain by increasing circulation to the brain and scalp.

Then you have acetyl carnitine, and phosphytidyl serine for the brain; DHEA, our master hormone, and glutathione, which protects cells, especially the eyes and the brain cells. There are really only two antioxidants in the brain—melatonin and glutathione. Both are crucial to help the brain stay fit.

Other important nutrients include calcium/magnesium from citrate; curcumin, which is from tumeric; green tea; potassium; cycopene, from vegetables; bee propolis, which is a natural antibiotic; acidophilus; astragalus; boron for your bones; bromalane for digestion; genostine to protect against cancer; quercitin for bruising, capillary strength, lowering cholesterol, helping your heart, and declogging your arteries; DMAE at 100 mg; NAC; and cleansing herbs, like apple pectin, burdock root, dandelion root, hibiscus, gotu kola, chrysanthemum, peppermint, licorice, Oregon grape root, red clover, and fo-ti.

One thing you have to do is to completely avoid all refined sugars, except for raw honey. In addition, do not eat foods containing yeast, MSG, dairy, caffeine, or chocolate. Stay away from wheat, meat, chicken, fried foods, food additives, preservatives, coloring agents, artificial sweeteners, and artificial flavors.

Magnetic therapy can also be used to help. I've seen four thousand Gauss magnets placed at the base of the head to not only stimulate hair growth, but to help balance mood swings as well. More melatonin is produced because the magnets pulsate into the pineal gland, allowing the brain to produce more melatonin. The melatonin helps fight cancer and depression and protects the brain. That's just some of what it does. Leave the magnet in place for about an hour and it will do the job.

In addition, exercise aerobically for at least forty-five minutes to one hour each day, six days a week, to increase circulation and remove toxins from your musculoskeletal system. Try power walking, stair-climbing, jumping rope, jogging, or heavy biking—meaning in heavy, not light, gear—anything, as long as it's fun. Weight training will further tone your body and cleanse your system.

The last major component in detoxifying the body, mind, and spirit is behavior modification. It doesn't do a whole lot of good to get healthy if you don't know who you are, or if you continue in the same toxic, or negative, behavior patterns. You need to understand how to honor your life and feel good about it.

This is not the same as working hard at feeling good. You shouldn't have to work hard to feel good; that should come as a natural process of honoring who you are. And if you have to work on honoring who you are, then what you're honoring is not who you really are, because the process shouldn't be forced.

So, we work on that and we have a whole protocol for behavior modification, a protocol for stress management, a protocol for exercise, and a protocol for eating.

DEALING WITH THOSE WHO TRY TO SUBVERT YOU

Just as we must flesh the poisons from our physical bodies, it is also essential that we purge the toxic people, places, and things from our lives if we are to be.

Think of people in relationships. Like the woman in one of my health support groups was in an abusive relationship. Her identity, her very being, was tied up in this grueling, toxic relationship. In fact, she confessed to the group, this was only the most recent in a long line of toxic men into her life for the past ten years. That prevents her from getting on with her life.

Think of how many times *you* have made an excuse for someone else's toxic, negative behavior. No doubt you felt you were redeeming yourself through suffering by acting as caregiver, knowing that the other person would then create a co-dependent relationship with you. A toxic co-dependency never becomes positive. You're only going to get hurt. And the other person's not going to change if you're going to be responsible for them. If you're going to cook their food and give them a free home and free clothing, then why should *they* change?

You must *choose* to make the break. In short, you must choose to detox your life and eliminate the poisonous relationships in your life.

Granted, there are *some* people—parents and siblings, for openers—who cannot be completely removed from your life. It's up to you, however, to limit your contact with these people, both in frequency and duration. It's not as difficult as you might imagine, once you put your mind to it.

DETOXING YOUR HOME

As you've no doubt gathered, detoxification involves far more than ridding your body of as many poisons as possible and eliminating the toxic relationships in your life. Twentieth-century environmental toxins are an unavoidable reality, especially for those who live in densely populated urban areas.

No one will consciously drink water from a polluted river. Nor will they willingly expose themselves to asbestos or lead-based paint or chemical fumes without taking hazardous-materials precautions. The obvious pollutants are easily avoided. It is, however, the chronic, day-in, day-out exposure to small toxins that do us in.

In the process of protecting ourselves from the insidious presence of dangerous materials around us, we must be rigorous in monitoring the toxins that surround us in less obvious ways.

The "sick building"—or "sick house"—is a relatively recent concept. Building materials and methods used in construction have changed considerably since World War II. Energy-efficient homes and office buildings built during the energy crisis of the seventies have heavy insulation and minimum ventilation to the outside. Air is recycled through heating and air conditioning systems that are rarely infused with fresh air, meaning we are breathing the same germ-filled air day after day after day.

Ironically, if that heating and air conditioning system goes on the blink, there is no way to open windows and let in fresh air. Back in the early seventies, a friend of mine worked on the thirty-fifth floor of a brand-new office tower in midtown Manhattan. In late April, temperatures rose into the high seventies, making indoor temperatures close to unbearable. The heating and air conditioning system of the building had not yet been converted to summer mode, so it could not be used for cooling. My friend's employer threatened to throw his desk chair through the wall of glass that provided his office with a glorious view of Central Park if the building's engineer didn't rectify the problem. Not surprisingly, a week later the building owner sent around a memo offering to install "portholes" in the exterior walls to allow "independent ventilation."

Materials used in construction, as well as the furnishings—carpeting, fabrics, furniture—are often more convenient, cheaper, lighter, man-made components unheard of in pre-war buildings. Particle board, which is so useful in modern construction and furniture, is a silent time bomb, giving off invisible, odorless—but no less dangerous—vapors many years after it is installed.

Formaldehyde is a major culprit in the modern home or office building. Particle board; new synthetic carpets, draperies, and upholstery fabrics; insulation; many interior paints and even permanent-press fabrics can give off this invisible gas. In its gas form, formaldehyde—the very same compound that preserved those earthworks and other specimens you dissected in high school biology—is invisible and, unless in high concentrations, odorless. Its vapors can cause burning eyes, headaches, and even more serious symptoms such as asthma and depression.

Combustion heating appliances, using natural gas, oil, coal, kerosene, and even wood, create by-products that are potentially toxic. While expensive, electrical heat and air conditioning are safest.

While moving or completely rebuilding your home or changing your place of employment may not be possible, you can still take steps to detoxify your surroundings.

- Remove all gasoline, pesticides, fungicides, herbicides and fertilizers, paints and thinners . . . everything that would vaporize and seep into your house . . . from your attached garage or basement.
- Seal off any ducts or vents between your garage and house.
- When working in your garden or lawn, remove your shoes before coming indoors.
- If you're working with chemicals, immediately wash your work clothes so that the contaminents are not carried into your home.
- Seal off exterior walls and do everything possible to minimize moisture in your basement. This dampness is enough to support a healthy growth of mold that can permeate your home. A forced-air heating system can carry spores throughout your home.
- Be aware of fermented foods, including mushrooms, that can cross-react with air-borne mold spores that can trigger allergic reactions.
- Take care that your kitchen is thoroughly vented to prevent build-up of gas burn-off from stoves and pilot lights.
- Make sure your microwave oven is not leaking; a defective microwave creates unhealthy conditions within eight feet.
- Make sure there are no freon leaks from your fridge.
- Discard all aluminum-based cookware.
- Do not use aluminum foil in cooking; it can oxidize microscopic amounts of the metal into your food. Foil *is* safe to use when storing cooked foods.
- Do not use Teflon or other nonstick cookware; it can easily get into your food and body.
- Discard all ammonia-based cleansers. It's very toxic.
- Invest in a negative ionizer to eliminate airborne toxins— mold spores, dust, cigarette smoke, hydrocarbons, pet hair and dander, positive ions—in your home.
- Use distilled water in your humidifier; otherwise mineral deposits from the water will end up on your carpet, floor, and furniture.

- Use plants—especially leafy green, nonflowering varieties that don't produce pollen—to improve air quality in your home. They're natural air purifiers!
- Use full-spectrum lightbulbs in your home to provide the same quality of light as natural sunlight. This nurtures and improves the condition of the hypothalamus in the brain.
- Have your home heating system inspected and repaired if necessary, to make certain there are no leaks of fuel and fumes.
- Clean up the clutter in your life—the garage, the kitchen, your closets and dressers, your car, your office. Dust mites thrive in a paper- and clutter-filled environment. So do disease-carrying insects like cockroaches and rodents.

Terry C., who lives on Long Island, one of the participants in the studies that gave rise to this protocol, confided that detoxifying all aspects of her life was not without obstacles. "The next obstacle [after dealing with caring for her elderly mother and expanding the ways that she cared for her own body] was to not let people run my life and make me do what I don't care to do. I know it sounds simple, but I just say no. It's just as simple as that, and it makes a world of difference. In the past, negative comments by others would always lower what I thought of myself (feeling that I was not good enough or worthy enough). By examining the conditioned beliefs about myself and now knowing that the comments come from their fears and not mine, the arrows of emotional hurt do not hit their target. This has contributed to my staying more on an even course of being happy during the day.

"The clutter obstacle is a tough one. I keep picking at it and, bit by bit, things have changed. I threw out all the carpeting—I am allergic to dust, mites, and mold—and I now have bare wood floors. The basement is almost empty and the garage is next. While typing this, I am sitting next to bags of blankets I am giving to a personal aide to the mother of a friend who is poor. I am treating this cleanup like a marathon, and I know that I cannot stop until all of this useless stuff is gone."

Terry continues: "How do I see myself now? I see myself as a person who wants to continue to help other people but without having me, as a person, become suffocated by it. I want helping others to be a part of my life, not all of it. I want to experience as much as I can and enjoy the excitement of the world, to learn new things, and to be healthy and continue to grow."

PART V

YOU'RE AS YOUNG AS YOU MOVE

9

THE BENEFITS OF EXERCISE

You may eat the most nutritious foods, swear off cigarettes and alcohol, and think only positive thoughts, but if you don't exercise, I guarantee that you will never reach the state of optimum health you seek.

Exercise does not promise you eternal youth, but if your body is not moving, you are not alive. Quality of life is an important issue to many people as they get older. What we enjoyed in our youth no longer interests us—staying up all night listening to loud rock music is just not exciting anymore. But unless we make a conscious effort to choose and improve the quality of our experiences, we have a tendency to fall into predictable ruts that dull our senses and put our brains on automatic pilot.

We become complacent, and bored . . . and a bored person is boring, especially to ourselves. One way out of this predicament is to increase our body awareness and viability. The only way to do this is to exercise.

HOW EXERCISE HELPS YOU RIGHT NOW

Fitness is a lifelong commitment. The physical benefits of getting fit and staying that way are numerous. Exercise firms muscles, strengthens the heart and lungs, improves blood circulation, builds strength and endurance, burns off excess calories, strengthens

bones, limbers up the joints, improves digestion, and relieves constipation. If you are starting on a program to lose weight, all this may
not be as important as being able to deflate that spare tire. It's easy
to think of exercise as merely a way to control one's flab.

While that is important, it doesn't get to the essence of why you
want to change your life through exercise. Make no mistake about
it: Regular exercise will dramatically alter you in ways you might
not imagine when you do those first few push-ups or run that first
mile.

In the beginning, simply making a commitment and sticking to
it is an incredible accomplishment for many people. The act of, say,
jogging three times a week, is an intense adjustment to make. Making that promise to yourself to jog, then getting up and actually
doing it and keeping your promise, is a wonderful thing. If exercise
did nothing else, it would confirm your sense of self-worth by this
alone. But this viewing of exercise as a strictly mechanical act is at
the heart of why most exercise programs fail after a few months.

In setting up my program, I found that when people saw exercise as a strictly physical phenomonen with no mental or spiritual
component, they were unwilling to continue their exercise program
after their initial reasons for doing it in the first place had been met.
If you've doing aerobics to lose weight, and then you lose the
weight, that's great. However, unless you are willing and able to
change your whole paradigm of how you view yourself and your
universe, it is unlikely that you will keep up any exercise program
for more than a few months.

HOW EXERCISE HELPS YOU OVER THE LONG HAUL: THE MENTAL AND PHYSICAL BENEFITS

Even if you have not been able to do an exercise program before,
you know the benefits of making a commitment and sticking to it.
In doing so, you feel good about yourself, you feel empowered, and
you feel that you have control over your life to a degree that you
may not have had before. These things are admirable goals, and
certainly can be accomplished through the practice of regular exercise.

Physically, regular exercise will increase your body's immune system, so you will be ill less often. Over time your sleeping habits will improve. You will feel more rested with less sleep, because the rest you get will be deeper. You will have more energy and be less susceptibile to injury. In addition, you will have a lower risk of some degenerative diseases such as heart disease, colon cancer, and breast cancer. Stronger bones—a particular need for women to fend off osteoporosis—will occur. And your heart and lungs will be much more efficient. Stress will be more effectively managed, and you will have much less anxiety.

All this is wonderful, and if exercise just did these things alone, it would be worth it. However, the main benefits as I see them are to your spirit and self-image.

How many of us are living the lives we really want to live? Doing what we really want to do, with our whole heart, our whole mind? The discipline of exercise gives us internal rewards that go far beyond the ability to run a mile in five minutes.

In our exercise programs, we learn to differentiate between what others expect of us and what we expect of ourselves. When we run or swim or skate merely to look good to others, we are only skimming the surface of how truly transforming our programs can be for our spiritual growth. When we do the same things for ourselves, because we learn about who we are and what our place is in the universe, we reap rewards far beyond breaking records or winning trophies. We connect with our deepest selves, tuning in to both the positive and the negative aspects of who we truly are. As you do your exercises, ask yourself: Who am I doing this for? And why? I think you will find that a host of false images will first come to mind. Maybe you're doing an activity to lose weight, to gain muscles, or to increase your aerobic capacity. Great. That in itself is admirable. But what if you changed your perspective of why you exercise? It has been said that a novice sets goals to attain goals, but a master sets goals to illuminate his way along the path of life. In exercise, it truly is the journey, not the destination, that counts. When we dig deeper into ourselves, we come to realize that all life is connected, and that we simply do not have to be anything other than who we are. That in itself is a source of illumination. How many things do you find yourself doing to please others' false expectations of you? I think if you were to add them all up, you'd have a pretty long list.

With a truly intergrated exercise program, you set goals to experience levels of achievement, to be sure. But the real achievements are always of the spirit. When you love what you're doing, there is no separation between who you are and who you say you are. A good exercise program that feeds your spirit as well as your muscles will give you that, and more. Consider what Krishnamurti said: "Real life is doing something you love to do with your whole being." When you do that, there will be no contradiction between what you are doing and what you want to be doing.

AEROBICS, ANAEROBICS, AND OTHER "ICS": WHAT'S THE DIFFERENCE?

Simply put, aerobic exercise increases your heart rate. This in turn increases your blood circulation, which brings more oxygen to your muscles. Exercises that involve steady, rhythmic motions of your major muscle groups and burn oxygen for more than a brief spurt are considered aerobic because they force your heart and lungs to work at anywhere from 60 to 85 percent of their capacity. Running is a good example of an aerobic exercise.

An anaerobic exercise isolates the movement of muscles but doesn't add any extra oxygen to the blood. Isometrics or weight lifting are good examples of anaerobic exercises. They were designed to increase muscle size and strength, but not to necessarily to help oxygenate your blood.

10

WARMING UP AND COOLING DOWN

EASE INTO YOUR WORKOUT

No matter what your chosen sport, no exercise program should begin without a warm-up. Just a few minutes of light activity gets your muscles loosened and, most important, warmed up so that you may exercise more vigourously without fear of injury. By doing this, your body does warm up in the truest sense of the word—increased activity starts the blood flowing to the muscles and your body begins to feel both more alive and more relaxed.

Most sports authorities agree: a good warm-up, one that lasts at least ten minutes, does help prevent injuries. One way to do this is to do something that will make you sweat, but not tire you out—after all, this is just the warm-up, not the whole program! You can take a brisk walk, ride a stationary bike, do push-ups, or sit-ups—anything that will make you break a light sweat. Then, follow this with stretches and, after that, ten minutes of any easy performance of the activity in question.

As you get into better and better shape, it is tempting to think that you no longer need to do any warm-up activities. After all, you've been working out a while now and feel confident about yourself. While confidence is vital as a mental construct for success, it will not replace the actual activity of warming up. When you do your beginning warm-up exercises, the muscles are saturated with blood, and this increases their elasticity. In this way, the muscles, tendons, and ligaments can take a more intense level of strain without injury.

In addition, quite a few important changes occur during the warm-up process. As you warm up the muscles and flex the joints, the strength and speed of muscle contractions improve, which allows them to perform to their full range of motion. In addition, you also conserve energy, and therefore can exercise longer because it takes less energy to produce the necessary movements. Your blood becomes thinner and flows more easily. This means that it can get nutrients to the muscles more quickly, and therefore the removal of waste products such as lactic acid that may cause cramping are also removed more quickly.

Here are some stretches to get you started. Take your time, and relax. It is important to do these preliminary exercises slowly. Remember, your muscles are going to be tighter warming up than they will be in the cool-down phase of the program. Stretching should take five to ten minutes.

1. To stretch your arms: hold one arm straight out from your side, keeping it level with your shoulder. Make a circle by lifting your arm straight up, then lowering it to your side. Then hold your arm out again. Swing it across your chest as far as you can, but not to the point of being uncomfortable. Hold your arm straight out in front of you, bending your elbow in a right angle with the palm toward the floor. Without moving your upper arm, move your forearm straight up in the air and then straight down again. Do this three times in a row; then do it on the other side.

2. To stretch your back: Stand with your legs apart about two feet. Raise your arms straight above your head, keeping them even. Gently and slowly lean your head back approximately four inches, or to your comfort level. Reach for the sky, stretching your shoulder muscles as much as possible. Hold for at least five seconds, longer, if possible. Keep your breathing slow and steadily while doing this. Relax, lower your arms, then repeat the process two to five times.

3. To stretch your legs: Stand up straight and balance yourself with your hand against a wall or a chair. Bend one knee, grasp the ankle, and gently pull the leg up and back. Hold for five seconds or longer. Release and relax. Repeat on the other side.

It is important to breathe normally during these warm-ups. Never hold your breath when you stretch. Do these exercises slowly, gently, and gradually. Never bounce—a strong, fluid motion is your goal. Stretch fully, but always well within your comfort level. You may stretch to the point where you can feel some resistance, but not pain. If you feel any pain or discomfort, stop immediately.

THE LOW-DOWN ON COOL-DOWNS

Most experts agree that a cool-down is even more important than a warm-up. Even though you may think you don't need it, but you do, and here's why:

A five-minute cool-down:

1. Allows the heart rate to slow down gradually. It is very dangerous to suddenly stop after vigorous exercise like jogging. Deaths involving joggers are rare, but when it happens, you usually find that the runner didn't do a lengthy cool-down and then went into cardiac arrest.
2. It significantly reduces the build-up of lactic acid, which causes cramps, sore muscles, and pain. Even if you feel okay at the time, your body still has not gotten rid of all the waste products produced by exercising, such as lactic acid. That's why you frequently feel so sore the day after vigorous exercise—the lactic acid is still in your muscles.
3. It prevents blood from pooling in the legs. Again, joggers come to mind. After a hard run, you have so much blood pooling in your legs, combined with great amounts of adrenaline coursing through your body. This affects the heart, sometimes fatally. The easiest solution is to simply keep moving for about five to ten minutes. Nothing strenuous; just walk around for a bit. That will do the trick.

11

THE POWER OF AEROBICS

In constructing an exercise program, you must ascertain the optimum heart-rate levels you want to reach during the exercise period. I recommend that aerobic exercises be performed three to five days per week.

During a fifteen- to sixty-minute exercise period, a healthy person's heart rate (the number of beats per minute) should equal 60 to 90 percent of his or her maximum rate. This rate depends on his or her age. To determine this maximum rate, simply subtract your age from the number 220. The result is the most number of times that your heart should ever beat per minute. Highly conditioned athletes may add another 10 percent. For the purposes of aerobic workouts, however, you must establish a 60 to 90 percent "target range" of this maximum rate—and then stay within that range. Anything less than 60 percent will not tax the heart enough to produce results; anything in excess of 90 percent could prove too strenuous.

A healthy forty-year-old, for example, would calculate his or her maximum rate and target range as follows:

Maximum rate:
$220 - 40 = 180$

Low target:
$$60 \text{ percent of } 180 = 180 \times 60$$
$$= 100$$
$$= 108$$

High target:
75 (MAX) percent of 180 = 180 × 90
$$= 100$$
$$= 162$$

YA GOTTA HAVE HEART

During the course of exercising, use your pulse count to determine whether your heart rate is within the target range. Your wrist or temple will provide the most accurate pulse reading. Do not use the carotid artery in your neck because the rate may slow down when you press on this artery. If your pulse rate is a bit high during the exercise period, either do the exercises more slowly or use less vigorous motions to lessen your energy output; if your pulse is too low, exercise a little harder to increase it.

By exercising regularly, you will decrease your resting rate because the heart begins to operate more efficiently, pumping more blood with fewer strokes. The average resting pulse rate for men is 80; for women, 72. For those in good condition, the resting rate is often much lower. As your conditioning improves and your resting rate lowers, you will have to exercise harder to reach your target range.

After you stop exercising, the amount of time it takes your heart to return to its resting rate provides a good indication of fitness. Take your pulse as soon as you stop and every few minutes after that. Then judge your recovery rate according to these guidelines: six to eight minutes indicates good condition; eight to ten minutes indicates fair condition; more than ten minutes indicates poor condition. Eventually, it should take less time to recover, providing you with measurable evidence of fitness improvements.

The cardiovascular benefits of aerobic work are greatest during the first twenty to thirty minutes of exercise. Beyond that, you still benefit, but to a lesser degree. Therefore, the best approach is to maintain a regular schedule that gets your heart rate into the target area for thirty minutes at least three times a week. Realize that skipping a few days of running won't disrupt the program, but skipping a couple of weeks will.

You get a great deal of energy by exercising the first thing in the morning. To determine how energetically you should exercise on any given morning, take your pulse before you get out of bed and compare it to your average awakening rate. (This can be determined by taking your pulse immediately upon awakening each morning for a week and then dividing the total by seven.) Go easy if the rate is two to three beats faster per minute that day; avoid aerobic exercise totally if the rate is five to six beats faster. When the rate exceeds the norm by that amount, it means the body is already stressed.

BREEZING THROUGH BREATHING

Aerobic exercise promotes a series of events in the body that deliver large amounts of oxygen to the muscles. This process begins with the respiratory system, which delivers oxygen to the blood as you move. The blood then carries oxygen and fuel to millions of body cells. As your muscles burn this oxygen and release energy, they alternately tense and relax.

For the muscles to receive this oxygen, the respiratory and circulatory systems must be able to deliver it to the blood. This process then works in reverse to eliminate such waste gases as carbon dioxide. First the gases move from the muscles to the blood, and then to the lungs, where they are released from the body. When you do aerobic exercises on a regular basis, this process operates more efficiently, which in turn helps your heart operate at its maximum performance.

One of the first things to do in this process is to visualize. That may not sound important, but many professional athletes have attributed their winning performances to this. As you breathe, imagine your lungs filling slowly with light. Inhale to the maximum and then release the air while seeing all your stress and cares leave you with each exhalation.

JUMPING RIGHT IN—TEN FUN AEROBIC CHOICES

Not every aerobic workout has to be in a mirror-filled gym with a hyperactive instructor who looks like an animated Barbie doll or an intense dancing athlete. Here are ten forms of exercise that provide aerobic benefits with little need for equipment or, in some cases, special skills. Best of all, they're fun, which makes it more likely that you'll do them. After all, *thinking* about going for a long run, or *planning* to go for a bicycle ride, does not tone muscles, get your blood flowing, and provide the benefits of the run or the ride.

WALKING

One of the main benefits of walking is its mobility. Other than a good pair of shoes, you need no equipment, and it can be done anywhere you are. This is particularly good for those whose jobs include a great deal of travel and are concerned about disrupting their exercise routine.

A gentle form of cardiovascular exercise, people of all ages and all levels of conditioning can do it. It does take some time to get the greatest cardiovascular results. It would take ninety minutes of walking to achieve the same aerobic benefits offered by a thirty-minute run. However, the stress on your joints is much lower, and the chances of injury are minimized.

It is important to realize that exercise places marked demands on the body's metabolism. The heart rate increases as you begin. This in turn increases the circulation of blood, oxygen, and nutrients to all of the body tissues. As your muscles contract and relax, you utilize minerals, such as magnesium, calcium, and potassium.

The longer you exercise, the greater amount of oxygen is delivered to the tissues, and the more you depend on oxygen for energy production. This explains why, if you've been exercising regularly and you miss a few days, you'll feel tired. Your body has gotten used to operating at peak efficiency and is depleted from the lack of oxygen it has been used to.

Before you start, be sure to take your pulse. When you walk, use a rhythmic gait that takes the foot from heel to toe and allows your arms to swing naturally. Don't shove your hands down into your pockets or press your elbows close to your sides. Let them swing freely. It is important not to carry anything that will unbalance your body or add extra weight.

Walk twenty to thirty minutes on three to five days a week for the first couple of weeks. Every two or three weeks after that, increase the time by 10 percent until you have reached ninety minutes. Each time you walk gradually build up to your target heart rate and then hold your pace. Check your pulse every ten minutes or so. Be sure to slow down if you feel tired, or even stop and rest; then slowly build back up to your normal pace.

Of course, the best place to walk is in the country. Nature is the most effective tranquilizer going. However, if you can't do that, go to your local park and walk. Always choose grass or even bare dirt over concrete. If the weather is bad, you can walk in the hallways of your apartment building or inside your house.

RUNNING

The benefits of running are tremendous. Runners seldom have problems keeping their weight down, as it is a highly effective form of aerobic exercise. In addition, the heart's health is vastly increased by the influx of oxygen-rich blood due to increased circulation. Your immune system is improved, and your musculoskeletal system is strengthened.

Running helps flush toxins from the system, and the benefits to the body from that cannot be overstated. Also, running is incredible for reducing stress, which many feel is at the basis of all illness. Best of all, running requires little investment in equipment, with the exception of good running shoes, which are most important.

BIKING

Biking is another versatile exercise. You can bike outdoors during good weather, and you can also use an indoor exercise bicycle during inclement weather. This form of exercise strengthens the anterior muscles in the front of the legs, thereby helping to prevent injuries to the rear leg muscles and the knees. Bicycling also puts less stress on the joints and muscles, which makes it perfect for those recovering from arthritis.

To get the best cardiovascular results from this aerobic activity, you must develop a steady pace that puts your heart rate into the middle of your target range. The cardiovascular conditioning that you want will take a much longer time to achieve if the pace is too slow. An overly fast, sprinting pace will lessen the training effect.

So, moderation is the key. Don't ride so hard that you continuously exceed 80 percent of your maximum rate.

Instead, use what is called "interval training" to achieve optimum results. Interval training improves speed and stamina, which improves your aerobic conditioning. Here's how you do it: First, sprint for thirty seconds and then ride more slowly at your normal rate for thirty seconds. Repeat the sequence three to five times in a row.

Before starting a bicycling program, get a good quality pair of bicycling shoes. They will protect your feet from the force of pedaling. If you cannot do that, the second best choice is to wear good running or walking shoes. Either way, use foot clips to keep your feet on the pedals.

It is very important, especially for women, to get a bike that is the correct height. Make sure it's constructed solidly and feels right to you. Get a seat that's comfortable and durable. When buying your bicycle, realize that at the correct seat height, your knee will be slightly bent when the pedal hits its lowest point. Pant clips or rubber bands will keep your pants from getting caught in the chain. If you ride outdoors after dark, be sure to wear light-colored or reflective clothing, and use a red light on your bike.

There is very little difference in riding a stationary bike. You can alleviate the strain on your lower back and improve your body alignment by straightening up the handlebars from the racing-style position. The attitude you bring to this is the same as with an outdoor bicycle—if you are reading a book while you are riding, you're not working hard enough. If you can't carry on a conversation while riding, you're working too hard. Generally speaking, getting a more advanced bike—one with a computerized counter and screen—will keep your attention and lessen the chances of boredom.

DANCING

Dancing is by far the most social way to get your aerobic training. It lifts your spirits, increases your vitality, and you get to move with your feelings, so it becomes an expressive exercise as well as an aerobic one. You can work at your own pace, and there are many different kinds of dancing you can do. You can stretch, isolate, and work individual muscles groups, and it can be as aerobic as the mood and the music inspires you.

SWIMMING

Swimming is a gentle yet incredibly effective way to exercise. Because of the water's buoyancy, your body's "real" weight is minimized, thus making it easier to move. This is why so many sports doctors are recommending swimming for those are recovering from injuries. By exercising in the water, you can increase your flexibility while building incredibly powerful arm, shoulder, and rear leg muscles.

Nonswimmers can start out by simply walking in the water. After taking your pulse, simply walk slowly from one side of the pool to the other in water that's about waist deep. Build up the intensity and duration slowly until you have reached your target heart rate and can sustain it for twenty to sixty minutes.

When you feel stronger, you can vary this by deep-water "running." This consists of wearing a special life vest and running as one would on land. The effects are the same as with regular running, but the stress on your body is much less. Start slowly. At first, you may only be able to sustain the motion for one or two minutes. However, as you keep on, you will find it much easier to reach your target goal, which is sustaining the running for twenty to sixty minutes. Any style of running is fine, with speed and range of motion as the variables.

If you know how to swim, you can develop a program that resembles the running routine—twenty to thirty minutes of aerobic work done three to five days per week. Start with an easy stroke, such as the sidestroke or free-style stroke, and gradually work up to your target heart rate. If necessary, vary your swimming technique to get to the twenty-minute mark.

Just as with any other exercise program, skip a day or two a week to allow muscles to recover from the stress of swimming. You can also use interval training with swimming to increase your speed and cardiovascular endurance. Sprint for up to thirty seconds and then return to your normal pace for thirty seconds. Repeat the sequence three to five times consecutively. It is important to stretch your leg muscles after you swim.

Swimming is versatile and less injury-inducing than many other aerobic activities. Be sure to wear a bathing cap or ear plugs to protect your ears. Good-quality goggles add immeasurably to your swimming comfort.

ROWING

Rowing is good for the heart because it increases the aerobic activity. It is considered one of the ultimate aerobic exercises, and increases coordination as well. When you row, you are fully stretching and contracting your muscles, which improves your muscle tone, especially in the upper body. While you need special equipment (i.e., a boat), in the winter you can work on the rowing machines in your health club, and thus still reap the benefits of the sport.

CROSS-COUNTRY SKIING

In addition to being out in nature, this exercise provides even more benefits than any other exercise, according to some experts. It requires you to use the muscles in your upper and lower body to their utmost capacity, which in turn increases the aerobic effect. You can ski outdoors during the season or use indoor cross-country skiing machines year-round.

JUMPING ROPE

This aerobic exercise is perfect for those whose goal includes losing weight. Jumping rope will burn more calories per minute than many other aerobic exercises. It may look easy, but, in fact, it is a tough cardiovascular workout. You must begin very slowly and build up your tolerance over a long period of time. If you work out too strenuously at the beginning, you could seriously injure your lower back and legs.

At first, just jump for two to four minutes. If you are heavier or really have not exercised in quite a while, do even less. Begin by walking or running in place, picking up speed until your feet are coming off the ground at a fast pace. Be careful to jump on a surface that "gives," such as a wooden floor or carpet. Try not to pound into the floor heavily; be as light-footed as possible. Then, jump on both feet at the same time for ten to thirty seconds, with or without a rope.

Rest by walking or jogging in place for a few minutes until you can breathe easily again. Repeat the process until you have jumped for no more than four minutes. The total workout time is twenty minutes for beginners.

As with other forms of aerobic training, do not overstress the body by jumping every day. Every two or three weeks, boost your jumping time by 10 percent. Eventually, you will be jumping for twenty to thirty minutes per workout, using interval training if desired. It is important to do this gradually, as it will allow your bones and muscles to adapt to the stress. Doing too much too quickly could damage your lower back and calves and even lead to stress fractures of the leg and foot bones.

One of the main advantages to jumping rope is its mobility. You don't need a lot of space or special equipment. You can do it almost anywhere—the yard, the basement of your home, or inside the house if your ceilings are high enough. This is especially good for people who travel frequently. A jump rope takes up very little room in your luggage, and you can do it wherever you are.

SKATING

Whether on sidewalks or ice, skating is a marvelous way to get low-impact aerobic activity. Figure skating does much the same things for your body as dancing, and is just as social. Racing is much like running, with its increased aerobic activity. It helps your coordination and is a low-impact way to get your heart rate up. While you need special equipment and a specific place to ice skate, you can also purchase rollerblades and keep up your training when you are away from the rink.

GETTING INTO INTERVAL TRAINING

This is a great combination of aerobic and anaerobic exercising, which improves both speed and endurance. The sequence is as follows: During your aerobic workout, get as close as possible to your maximum heart rate for thirty to sixty seconds and then ease up for thirty seconds at about 70 percent of the maximum rate. Remember that if your heart rate drops below 60 percent during the "resting period," the aerobic effects will be lost. Repeat the sequence three to five more times.

These general principles can be applied to any type of aerobic activity, including running, walking, bicycling, and swimming. Once you become accustomed to this, you can vary the pace by increasing the number of sequences, increasing the intensity of the sprinting, or even increasing the length of the sprinting period. The length of the "rest period" can be reduced as well.

12

KEEP MOVING! THERE'S EVEN MORE

Neither the need nor the ability to exercise and remain fit ceases once we reach a certain age. Here's what some of the older athletes who follow this powerful protocol to remain young and vital do well past what the calendar says is youth.

Sid, age fifty-nine "Even though I had been an athlete in high school, running track, from the ages of seventeen to thirty-nine I did nothing physical but work. In the eleventh grade, I failed wood shop and math and wasn't eligible to run track anymore. So a month later, I quit school and joined the Air Force. I ended up weighing 156 after four years. I had no clue about nutrition. I ate everything and anything, and I especially loved extra-sweet drinks.

"Before I met Gary, my motivation to change my diet was purely visual—I just wanted to look better. I really didn't care about my health. Gary was my first step to evolution. The first thing I did was stop drinking coffee with creamer, drinking alcohol, smoking cigarettes, and taking drugs. I started eating only chicken and fish, then gradually weaned myself off them. All the time I was evolving, I kept in mind what Gary had said about positive thinking. 'Whatever you say, you become.'

"I started feeling so good about myself and my health was consistently improving, so I quit eating dairy products altogether—even cheese. In the middle of all this, I was always reading and thinking. I realized that they were all connected, that you couldn't be a vegetarian and in peace and harmony with the earth, and then go home and curse out your wife. It's all the same thing; it's all connected. This is a way of life that must be practiced every day, in all phases of my life.

"I am a highly competitive runner, and am ranked first in the U.S. in the half-mile indoor race. I have more than eighteen national titles; last year I ranked fourth in the world in the South Africa 800. I have been U.S. champ in both the 800-mile and the 1500-mile races. I run six days a week, five to six days when in training. When racing, I may run three to four days a week. I am running at the bottom of the fifty to fifty-nine age group. I finished fifth in my age group in the Trump Fifth Avenue run.

"I'm really looking forward to turning sixty. Running is the only sport where athletes want to get older, because it puts you a new age level. I just got my bachelor's degree in social work at age fifty-nine. I never would have had the stamina to do this without my diet and exercise routine.

"I eat one big meal a day, usually around midday. I have fruit and juice in the morning, and at night I have fresh organic juices, such as carrot, celery, fresh ginger, apple, and garlic. This is the most incredible power drink I have ever had.

"At fifty-two, I ran a 4.43 mile, and was one of three men to break the record. I have worked hard, gone to school, and taken care of my wife during her long illness. If I were to give advice to anyone wanting to change their life, I would say that we must honor the earth and all its components."

Joan R., age seventy-two　"Heart disease is endemic on both sides of my family, but it took my mother's heart attack to get me to change my eating habits. At that time, I became a vegetarian. However, I did no exercise whatsoever until 1975, when I joined a health club.

"Then I took a one-day course in racewalking, and entered my first race the next day. Much to my delight, I won! That exhilarating experience totally changed my life. I began training in earnest, and to date have won over forty racewalking competitions.

"I think the most powerful thing I've learned from Gary is the importance of attitude. In fact, that is what governs one's emotional and physical state. I think it would be impossible to maintain your health without a clear, focused, and positive attitude.

"This thinking is what has gotten me through my life. I have survived the death of four of my children, who were diagnosed as neurologically damaged. I have survived living with an alcoholic, abusive husband. I have survived and overcome my childhood, which was one of constant stress, as my sister is a violent schizophrenic.

"Through positive and focused thinking, I have made a good life for myself, and have joy and peace in my life. I have been a musician and conductor and have owned an art gallery. My love of life was definitely enhanced by Gary's program. In that, I took from his what was most applicable, such as dietary and exercise suggestions, and added it to my already rich storehouse of knowledge."

Dolly, sixty-eight, and Ed, seventy-six   Dolly and Ed have, as they say, always been in "pretty good shape," although Dolly, a teacher for home health aides in private health care, says, "I always had three or four colds a year."

Ed, who is a retired insurance broker and real estate investor, has been a runner for twenty-five years, logging five to six miles a day. Dolly joined him on the course two years later—"to keep warm," she laughs, recalling how cold she'd get sitting in the car grading papers while her husband trained during the winter months.

Ed says that in 1990 he was diagnosed with a carotid artery with more than 90 percent blockage. When he refused a surgical procedure to treat the condition, his cardiologist—and his son-in-law and daughter, who are both physicians—tried to intimidate him by saying that he was a "walking time bomb."

"We listened to Gary on the radio and were impressed," Ed explains. "At the time we ate a conventional diet of processed food, meat, dairy . . . but no simple sugars and no coffee."

"The hardest thing for us," Dolly adds, "was making the commitment to becoming vegetarian—organic vegetarian. Changing wasn't hard; making the decision to change was." Today, the only animal food they eat is an occasional piece of cold-water fish, such as salmon.

The couple went to Gary's lectures and then joined the Reversing the Aging Process Study Group. "We have actualized everything he had lectured about. We bought his books, videos, and supplements, and we juiced every day," Dolly interjects. "We really followed the protocol 100 percent."

"The juicing—raw juicing—is really important. We drink juices morning, noon, and twice at night," Ed adds. The couple also brings their own vegetables to family functions because they have not yet "convinced them that *organic* really is important."

In addition to their rigorous adherence to the diet recommended by the protocol, the couple maintains a strong physical training schedule. Ed runs about five miles every other day, and on the days he doesn't run, he walks everywhere—to the bank, the library. Dolly gets up at five A.M. every day, runs every other day.

They usually race on the weekends. "One mile, 5-K, five miles, 10-K, even half marathons," Ed notes. "I'm leading in my age group—seventy-plus—in long distance running in the Metropolitan Athletic Congress Grand Prix." This is a series of twenty races around the Metropolitan New York-New Jersey-Connecticut area.

Dolly's leading in her group of women between the ages of sixty and sixty-nine. "Every year Dolly is nominated by the New York Roadrunners Club for her age group," Ed boasts.

Dolly had four silver amalgams [fillings] in her teeth, which meant that her body was toxic with mercury. After having them removed, she took extensive steps to detoxify the mercury from her cells by having intensive intravenous vitamin C and ozone treatments at Gary Null's healing center.

Dolly also credits the positive thinking techniques Gary Null advocates with making their progress possible. "The biggest tip I'd give anyone wanting to reverse aging is to think positive," she states.

PART VI

EATING TO LIVE

13

WHAT'S FOOD GOT TO DO WITH IT?

What's food got to do with health and wellness? Can it slow or even reverse aging? Will the quality of your life be that much improved simply by changing what you eat? If you partake of a traditional Western diet—the answer is no. If you look to the centuries-old tradition of the Chinese—the answer is a resounding yes.

We may think the concept of "holistic eating" is new, but the Chinese idea of considering everyday food as medicine goes back nearly five thousand years. It was first started by the Emperor Shen Nong, who introduced agriculture to the Chinese people in the three thousandth century B.C. According to legend, Shen Nong was intrigued by the vast numbers and varieties of plants around him and began to experiment with them in search of food sources for his people. He and his disciples tested millions of these plants—tasting them, cooking them, and making teas and meals from them.

In the process of their dedicated study, they observed that many of these plants not only tasted good and satisfied hunger, but they also enabled people to stay vigorous and strong. Some induced sleep, while others kept people awake; still others removed pain or helped people recover quickly from even the most serious illnesses. They found that some plants and herbs would make the skin soft and beautiful, while others enhanced youth.

Despite the thousands of years this philosophy of food-based medicine—and the millions of Chinese who have practiced it through the ages—traditional Chinese medicine and accompanying practices such as acupuncture, *Chi Gong*, and other exercise techniques that incorporate breathing and movement as well as concentrated thought, are not considered "scientifically proven" by Western medical practitioners. Consequently, many Americans are denied this knowledge, or are at least discouraged from practicing these principles.

In recent years, many people have become discouraged with their health and their health-care practitioners. They have been reading about foods and alternate diets, and have been actively revamping their nutritional programs. In the forefront of this are the so-called "baby boomers," who are not willing to surrender their active lives for ones of immobility and senility. Searching for newer ways of living fully, they are investigating alternative practices of health care. One result of this awareness is the preponderance of organic food stores and vitamin shops. Thankfully, organic, wholesome foods are being stocked by ordinary supermarkets in every community.

GOOD FOOD KEEPS US GOING!

Staying youthful is synonymous with staying healthy. And staying healthy is controlled, to a large degree, by daily habits of eating. If your eating habits have become just a habit, with little thought put into them, you will find that your diet will not only be calorically imbalanced, but nutritionally imbalanced. This, in turn, will make sure that you are not on an even keel either. Intention makes design, as the philosopher said, so it would be good for both your body and spirit to take some time out to consider what you are putting into your body, and why. Are you eating from boredom? Are you eating because it's noon and time to eat, rather than listening to your body tell you when it is hungry? Are you eating to fill an inner emptiness that food will never fill? All these things and more can change if you alter your thought patterns. Going from mindless noshing to deliberate, consecrated eating takes some effort but is worth it.

One thing you can do is to make each meal a ritual of sacred nourishment. Standing in front of the fridge mindlessly shoveling down tofu is as useless as eating half a cow. Remember, thought always precedes action. Especially if you live alone, you may be tempted to eat on the run, and not take time to properly prepare a meal, or to judiciously and consciously observe what you are doing.

Take each meal as an opportunity to treat yourself to the highest good you can. By sitting at a table, set with your best plates and silverware, and ritualizing the meal, you have the power to consciously be there, at one with your self, your food, and your spirit. In that way, you will automatically take more care in preparing good, nourishing meals that satisfy all your senses. The smell of freshly cooked onions sizzling in the pan, the aroma of freshly steamed vegetables, the spark of raw garlic—all these things speak to us as sensual, living beings. Contrast that with standing at the sink chewing on a raw carrot before running out the door! The quality of life starts at the nourishment level. Keep this in mind in incorporating any new dietary concept, and the rewards will be much greater.

Another thing to consider while restructuring your eating program is to keep a diary. Nothing elaborate; just a few notes to yourself on what you ate, what you felt as you ate it, and how your body reacted after eating it. In this way, you may catch any food allergies and/or adverse reactions to your eating patterns, as well as noting what foods in particular gave you a lot of energy.

In this diary, you can also keep notes on the nuts and bolts of your eating program. Dr. Hans Kugler, president and founder of the International Academy of Alternative Medicine and author of *Tripping the Clock: A Practical Guide to Anti-Aging and Rejuvenation*, offers these dietary guidelines that you can incorporate into your notes:

Know your daily caloric maintenance level Be aware of the amount of calories you need to maintain your ideal weight. Then you can easily make adjustments for weight gain or weight loss, as needed.

Vary the amount of food you eat according to the time of day Eat like a king at breakfast, a prince at lunch, and a pauper at dinner.

Reduce overall fat and sugar intake Experts say that total fat intake should be no more than 30 percent of your weekly total calories. Eliminate refined carbohydrates from your diet and substitute complex carbohydrates that have lots of fiber, such as oats, barley, bran, beans, soy products, apples, cranberries, currants, and gooseberries.

Eat a variety of carbohydrates, vegetables, and whole grains These foods are the building blocks of good health. Include such foods as fruits, vegetables, whole-grain breads, cereals, whole-grain pastas, starchy vegetables, and beans.

Have lean or nonfat protein at every meal Though important, we now know that more is not better. We do not need vast amounts of protein as we once thought. Rather, we should distribute small amounts of protein throughout the day. This will keep our energy levels high and eliminate that "sinking feeling" that sometimes occurs in the late afternoon.

Include organically grown foods in your diet Chemically laden foods are a burden to the body. Even small amounts of toxins accumulate and eventually wear it down. Be kind to your body by keeping your diet as pure as possible. Organic produce is now more commercially viable, so that even in the smallest towns there will be at least one health food store. Patronize it!

DIETARY DOWNFALLS

Forty years ago, roughly a third of every grocer's inventory was natural, fresh produce. Today, it's a different story altogether. Fresh fruits and vegetables barely fill an aisle in most modern supermarkets, and even that is likely to be altered. Fruits and vegetables are routinely grown with artificial fertilizers, sprayed with pesticides, and treated with hormones and chemicals to control ripening and facilitate mechanical harvesting. They are dyed, sprayed with chemicals to prevent ripening during shipping and to induce ripening once delivered, or they are coated with waxes to give them a glossy appearance.

Once known as "the staff of life," most modern bread is virtually without nutritive value. Wheat and other whole grains provide a rich source of nutrients—complex carbohydrates, protein, oils, and roughage, as well as an excellent balance of vitamins and minerals. Grinding wheat with stone rollers blends these ingredients together, providing a product so nutritionally rich that it is quick to spoil. It is also susceptible to attack by vermin and fungi if not used immediately. As bakers endeavored to make a product that could be trucked over long distances and stored for weeks, not days, processing was increased and preservatives added, and white flour—and a product rendered incapable of sustaining life—was born.

White flour begins with steel rather than stone rollers, flattening and separating nutrient-rich bran and germ from a chalklike dust. While bran and germ are routinely sold as animal feeds, the remaining powders are further bleached with chlorine gases, and processed to make a spoilage-resistant flour. This product is then "enriched" with synthetic versions of some of the vitamins removed through earlier processing. Not coincidentally, vitamins considered necessary for this enrichment are those most easily synthesized—barley malt, ferrous sulfate, niacin, thaimin mononitrite, riboflavin, corn syrup, partially hydrogenated vegetable shortening, yeast, salt, calcium sulfate, sodium stearoyl lactylate, mono- and diglycerides, whey, dicalcium phosphate, calcium propionate, and potassium bromate.

One of the most common additives in processed foods is sugar. As a result the average American eats 160 pounds of sugar yearly. After processing, many foods are so lacking in taste that there would be no taste at all without the addition of large quantities of sugar and salt. Both are preservatives and both are inexpensive. Both are also addictive. Many processed foods—even those you don't expect to contain sugar and salt—contain large amounts of one or the other, if not both. Just read the labels. You may be in for a surprise!

You may picture farms being like those we see on television or that we remember from our childhood, but those farms exist only in the collective imagination. In reality, instead of fertile fields alive with lush crops and chirping chickens and oinking pigs roaming around a farmyard, we have huge agribusiness complexes that have nothing to do with what we may fondly recall as farming.

Instead of bucolic fields with contentedly grazing herds of cattle, commercially grown livestock are kept in conditions that cannot by any stretch of the imagination be considered humane. Kept in cages where they cannot move, chickens are raised by the thousands in huge buildings where they will go from birth to death and never see the sky. A conveyor belt brings them food and water and carries away their waste. A chicken may spend its entire short lifetime without ever even walking a step, and certainly without touching the ground. Some modern breeds grow so fast, their legs cannot support their weight.

Today, a steer is born, taken from its mother, and put on a diet of powdered milk, synthetic vitamins, minerals, and antibiotics. Drugs in its food reduce its activities, thus saving on feed. Next it is actually allowed to eat pasture grass, though this is supplemented with processed feed, premixed with antibiotics and growth-promoting drugs. At six months, this animal weighs five hundred pounds and is ready for the feed lot. Here it is doused with pesticides and placed in a pen that is lit around the clock to alter natural sleep patterns and encourage continuous feeding. Commonly feed consists of rendered dead animals including diseased dogs, cats, cows, pigs, chickens and sheep, along with ground up corn husks, urea, carbohydrates and sewer sludge. After four months in the feed lot, the steer weighs twelve hundred pounds.

Plant crops are similarly manipulated. Hybrid varieties of common fruits and vegetables are grown in nutrient-depleted soil and treated with poisonous chemicals, which are known and proven to be carcinogenic. These chemicals are absorbed into the plants and cannot ever be washed away, as they are in the cellular structure of the stems and leaves. No amount of rinsing or cooking can destroy these chemicals, and they are passed along to us as we eat the foods. It is small wonder that so many of us are sick. Modern agribusiness is a huge conglomerate, with annual sales well over $200 billion per year. Every single year well over $500 million worth of poisonous chemicals are added to our foods, and this is a conservative estimate. The industry of agribusiness fosters a way of eating and living that disconnects us from the natural processes of life. That is why it behooves us to think before we buy our foods, and realize that all life is interconnected. The toxins that are in the ground today will be in your bone marrow tomorrow.

Fortunately, we have ways to combat this. One of these is the practice of vegetarianism. And not simply vegetarianism, but *organic* vegetarianism.

VIRTUES OF VEGETARIANISM

Is it possible to eat without filling our bodies with the poisons perpetrated by commercial farming? Yes, it is. A natural food diet, which is filled with nutritious fresh fruits and vegetables, whole grains, legumes, seeds, and nuts, and avoids unnatural additives is a major step in the right direction. Cutting down on your meat intake or, ideally, cutting it out altogether, is even closer to optimum healthy eating.

There is irrefutable scientific evidence that proves the adequacy—indeed, the superiority—of a vegetarian diet. Medical literature is filled with testimonials and fact-laden studies that show that the common degenerative diseases we think of as inevitable are linked with a diet that is high in meat, sugar, fat, and chemical residues. Being a vegetarian offers many dietary benefits, not the least of which is a supple, youthful body and a sharp, clear mind.

Eating healthy foods rejuvenates the life force by supplying the body with multiple anti-aging nutrients. They also help to resist the onset of disease—most cancer is diet-related—and may even reverse chronic conditions. Dolores Riccio, author of *Superfoods for Life*, says the best foods are those given to us in nature, such as:

Fruits and Vegetables Most fruits and vegetables contain valuable nutrients for anti-aging. Especially noteworthy are the cruciferous vegetables—broccoli, Brussels sprouts, cabbage, kale, radishes, and watercress—for their anti-cancer properties. Melatonin, for immunity-boosting and better sleep, is found in bananas, corn, and tomatoes. Chromium helps regulate insulin and can be found in apples, broccoli, grapes, raisins, mushrooms, and potatoes. Magnesium defends against asthma and heart disease, and is also a memory booster. Good fruit and vegetable sources include avocados, bananas, and dark green vegetables. Vitamin E's helper, selenium, is found in onions, shallots, mushrooms, and garlic. These foods help the heart and keep the skin elastic.

Intense color and flavor indicate health-giving properties. Dark green and orange vegetables, for example, are high in carotene, which protects against cancer. And bitter greens help the liver. Citrus fruits, such as oranges, lemons, and grapefruits, help rid the body of free radicals, keep the skin looking young, and accelerate healing.

Grains and Legumes These fiber-rich foods keep our digestive tracts healthy. They are high in B vitamins, which work to support the brain, and rich sources of vitamin E, making them good for the heart and skin. In addition, whole grain fibers, such as brown rice, contain zinc, for nourishment of the male reproductive system and repair of the body.

Oils   Contrary to common trends, we all need some fat in our diets. A teaspoon a day of monounsaturated fats is essential for keeping the brain and heart functioning properly, for protecting our appearance, for raising HDL (good) cholesterol and lowering LDL (bad) cholesterol, and for keeping our hair and skin from becoming dry. Good sources of monounsaturated fats are olive oil and canola oil.

Avoid saturated fats—those found in potato chips, meats, cheeses, coconut and palm oil.

Polyunsaturated fats, like those found in flaxseed oil and fish, are precursors for omega-3's, such as DHA and EPA, which prevent clotting of blood and stickiness of platelets. Research shows that these fats can get into the blood vessels and stabilize plaque. People who eat one fish meal a week have a 50 percent reduction of sudden deaths compared with people who don't. Healthy sources of fish are deep-water migratory fish, like salmon, halibut, and cod.

The Benefits of Soy   Soybeans and soybean products are staples of Japanese diets, and for good reason. Scientific research has identified healing agents in soybeans, called glycosides. Glycosides contain substances that protect the cell from oxidation from the low density lipoproteins found in "bad" cholesterol. Rather than relying on hamburgers, pork, dairy, chicken, and pork for protein—these foods are high in saturated fats that damage tissues—we should use high-protein soy products often. Soy products have also been found to figure prominently in the diets of women who do not get breast cancer.

IS THE FOUNTAIN OF YOUTH REALLY A WATER FOUNTAIN?

For years we have been told that we need to drink at least eight-ounce glasses of water every day in order to remain healthy. Somehow, however, the word "water" has been overshadowed by other liquids—coffee, tea, sodas, milk, even juices. As far as I am concerned, coffee, tea, sodas, and anything else that contains caffeine are toxic and should *never* be consumed. Milk and other dairy products should also be avoided—especially by adults—because they are high in fat. They are also extremely mucous-forming and have a high potential for allergic reactions. As we age, we do not have the enzymes necessary to break down the milk sugars. Therefore we may experience gas, bloating, nausea, diarrhea, and, often, gall bladder distress.

It is imperative that we have a consistently clean supply of water for drinking, cooking, and bathing. Without this, we are allowing ourselves to consume inordinate amounts of pollutants. One of the best ways to ensure removal of toxins in our home water supplies is to buy good water filters—not only for the kitchen sink but for the tub and shower as well—because most of the nation's water supply is contaminated by agricultural run-off, manufacturing waste, fluoride, chlorine and other chemicals and chemical by-products.

All of these materials affect people adversely without their ever suspecting it. When your water supply is contaminated and you drink it, the toxic chemicals in the water go right into your bone marrow, fat, and internal organs, where they increase the chemical overload that is tearing down your system. Every tissue in your body is affected by these toxins. No wonder so many people are getting sick.

One of the problems with this kind of pollution is that the symptoms of this kind of poisoning may masquerade as something else, not readily traceable to polluted food and, especially, polluted water. Many food allergies are traced directly to the multitude of poisons in what we eat and drink.

Water has to be pure, free from fluoride, chlorine, and chemicals, which is why I recommend distilled water. To achieve optimum health, I recommend that you drink a half gallon to one full gallon per day. Caffeine, soda, and white sugar should be reduced to a minimum; for optimal results, they should be eliminated entirely.

14

MEAL PLANNING MADE EASY

While I don't insist that participants in the programs I conduct become vegetarian, I do recommend that they consider the possibility, and at least restrict their animal protein to cold-water fish. It is possible to eat without partaking of the poisoned fruits of technology by adopting a natural-food diet. This path relies on unrefined grains, legumes, seeds, nuts, and fresh fruits and vegetables, steering clear of unnatural additives, including sugar and salt. A balanced diet that cuts down or eliminates meat is even closer to an unadulterated, healthful ideal!

The degree to which you become vegetarian is determined by the specific way you eat.

Pollovegetarians eat no red meats but do eat chicken in conjunction with plant sources.

Pescovegetarians include fish in their plant-based diet. In Asia, hundreds of millions of people follow this type of diet, living on staples of rice and fish.

Lacto-ovo-vegetarians consume milk and milk products and eggs in their fruit- and vegetable-based diet. This is basically a nonflesh diet.

Lacto-vegetarians eat milk and milk products in addition to fruit and vegetable foods.

Vegans, the strictest of all vegetarians, thrive solely on plant foods—vegetables, fruits, nuts, seeds, grains, and legumes. This regimen excludes *all* animal foods—including honey and gelatin.

Time after time, we are warned against the nutritional deficiencies of "ill-planned vegetarian diets." This is not a danger, provided sufficient care is taken in planning a nutritionally balanced diet.

In truth, *any* ill-planned food plan should be avoided, no matter what foods are eaten. Care must be taken in planning and preparing all meals—vegetarian and nonvegetarian alike.

No one food is indispensable or magical. Animal flesh, for instance, is nearly void of carbohydrates, has little or no fiber, and is a poor source of calcium and vitamin C. It is high in saturated fats and cholesterol. Meat eaters get their complex carbohydrates, dietary fiber, and other nutrients from exactly the same sources as vegetarians—fruits, vegetables, grains, seeds, and nuts. By omitting meat from your diet, you sacrifice all the harmful ingredients it has, while still being able to acquire the protein necessary for health and youth from plant sources.

A nonflesh diet—or one like my Reversing the Aging Process Protocol, which limits animal protein intake to once a week and consumption of cold-water fish to small servings three times a week—will, in the long run, lower your risk of developing many diseases and raise your chances of maintaining good health. Everyone, regardless of age, can probably benefit from such a diet.

EVE HAD THE RIGHT IDEA: THE FANTASTIC FRUITS

Fruit should be the main source of sweetness in your diet. Instead of robbing your body of its vital, essential nutrients as white sugar does, whole, fresh fruit is filled with vitamin C. Linus Pauling did ground-breaking work in the field of vitamin research, and his studies and others confirm the necessity of adding large quantities of vitamin C to your diet. This can be taken in supplements, to be sure, but remember that fruit is chock-full of it.

Few things beat the taste of an organically grown apple fresh from the tree, or the first new strawberries of the season. Most of us just eat fruit because it tastes good, but it is important to remember that fruits do much more for your body than just keep you regular. It has been found that vitamin C may keep your heart healthy, help prevent atherosclerosis, and cut your cholesterol levels. And there's growing evidence that it reduces triglycerides, which are the blood fats now considered to be as important as high cholesterol in the development of heart disease. All fruits have some effect on this; however, scientists have found that the pectin-rich fruits, such as apples, grapefruit, and oranges, are particularly good at reducing your blood cholesterol levels.

As always, fresh fruit is the best, and organic fresh fruit is the best of all. Certain fruits, such as strawberries, blackberries, and blueberries, should not be consumed unless they are certified organic, as the chemicals used in producing them are especially toxic.

When buying fruits, select those that look fresh and feel firm. Don't buy produce that's soft or bruised, and don't buy more than you can reasonably use in a few days. Remember, it's a fresh product, not one filled with chemicals, and thus will spoil in a few days. Refrigerate the fruits you buy as quickly as possible. When choosing citrus fruits and pineapples, pick ones that feel heavy for their size. Wash all fruits carefully in a washing solution of water, hydrogen peroxide and cider vinegar. Just because it's organic doesn't mean it doesn't need washing. When preparing, pat the produce dry after washing to prolong freshness. Don't cut fruits until just prior to eating them; exposure to the air destroys vitamin C.

You should eat at least three servings of fruit every day. Whole fruits are low in calories, have lots of fiber, are filling, and thus satisfying.

GRAINS: THINK WHOLE FOR HEALTH

Major sources of fiber and complex carbohydrates, real whole grains—not those pasty white flours and rice most often seen on American tables—are also rich in vitamins and minerals, which we need to prevent heart disease and cancer. This superiority makes them essential to our nutritional pharmacy.

Whole grains of any variety are more nutritionally complete than white or partially processed grains, such as couscous and cracked wheat berries, which are, in turn, better for us than the more processed flours, breads, and noodles. Needless to say, whole grain products are always preferable to "refined" foods such as white breads and pastas.

A GLOSSARY OF GRAINS

Amaranth   Ancient Aztecs believed that Amaranth gave them supernatural strength, and in addition to eating vast quantities of the grain—which they called "The Golden Grain"—they used it in religious ceremonies. Cortez, who led the Spanish conquistadors in their quest to destroy the Aztec civilization, not only killed the Aztec emperor Montezuma but also ordered his troops to burn all amaranth fields *and*, as if that wasn't enough, ordered them to cut off the hands of anyone with even a single seed in his possession.

The name amaranth comes from a Greek word for "immortal"—most appropriate since, in the mid-1980s, a handful of seeds found in a thousand-year-old Aztec ruin were planted and sprouted roots on a farm in Pennsylvania. A pseudo-cereal grain that comes from a broad-leafed plant rather than a grass, Amaranth is a tiny grain—only slightly larger than a poppy seed—but it's power-packed with nutrients. Amaranth outstrips all other common grains as a source of protein—16 percent as opposed to 10 or 12—and as it is extremely rich in lysine, the amino acid that controls protein absorption, and methionine, an amino acid missing from most beans, it is more complete than most other vegetable proteins.

Jane Brody, in her *Good Food Book*, says that the quality of amaranth protein is so good that it exceeds cow's milk in its ability to sustain life, containing as much as 30 percent protein. Amaranth can be either popped dry in an ungreased skillet, one tablespoon at a time, or cooked in liquid and used for pilaf, in soups, or as hot cereal. For this method, use 2½ cups water to 1 cup amaranth. Bring to a boil, cover, and reduce heat. Cook over medium-low temperature for twenty to twenty-five minutes, stirring occasionally.

Barley   Another historical grain, barley has been around since the Stone Age. Archaeologists have found traces of cakes made of wheat and barley baked in the sun. A wholesome, low-gluten grain, barley has been grown on all continents, by almost every culture, for eons.

Three layers of skin protect each barley kernel: two inedible husks that cover the embryo or germ and a delicate, protein-rich core called the aleurone. In the center is the starchy endosperm. In processing barley for human consumption, these outer layers are almost always removed, leaving a product called "pearled" barley. Most of the nutritional value of barley is lost in this process since valuable protein, fiber, and B vitamins are in the aleurone. Therefore, the most nutritionally valuable form of barley is simply hulled, leaving most of the aleurone layer intact.

Despite the low vitamin count in pearled barley, a substance known to inhibit cholesterol production in the blood has been found in the nonfibrous portion of the grain. To cook, use 3 cups water to 1 cup pearl barley. Cook for thirty-five to forty-five minutes. To cut cooking time, presoak grain at least five hours and cook for fifteen minutes. Hulled barley must be soaked overnight and requires one hour cooking time. Cook covered; add liquid as required. Hulled kernels can be sprouted for salads.

Bran   This isn't a *kind* of grain. Bran is the fibrous seed coating of any cereal grain—wheat, oats, barley, etc.—that is separated from flour or grain by sifting or bolting. It is made of primarily noncaloric dietary fiber, notably vitamins B, B_6, niacin, pantothenic acid, riboflavin, and thiamine. Processed and unprocessed bran, used in cooking, is known to relieve constipation and prevent diverticular diseases of the intestines, as well as regulate serum cholesterol and lower blood sugar levels for diabetics.

Buckwheat   Not a grain at all, buckwheat is a distant cousin of the rhubarb. However, it is the buckwheat's three-cornered seed rather than its stem that is of value. The shell, when dried and split, reveals a pale kernel or *groat*. When roasted, buckwheat groats are known as **kasha**. Buckwheat has more than 90 percent of the protein value of milk solids, and more than 80 percent of eggs. A pound of buckwheat provides protein equivalent to a half-pound of beef.

Another plus: buckwheat also contains high amounts of all eight amino acids—lysine, leucine, isoleucine, methionine, tryptophan, threonine, phenylalanine, and valine—which the body does not produce on its own. In short, buckwheat is closer to being a complete protein than any other plant source, including soy beans. Whole buckwheat is hulled groats and stone ground "cream of buckwheat." Buckwheat groats and kasha are available whole and ground (coarse, medium, and fine). Cooking times vary with the type of buckwheat you're using.

Corn   Corn is a Native American grain that, transported to Europe by Columbus, is one of the few complex carbohydrates with the potential to feed the entire world. It is this nation's top agricultural commodity, grown on one of every four acres of cropland, in every state, as well as throughout the world. (Only wheat occupies more acreage.)

The sweet corn that stars on our summer and fall tables is a relative newcomer, not developed until the 1700s. Our forefathers ate very little fresh corn. Most of it was dried and ground into meal or flour to be used in bread and cake. While a cup of cornmeal is high in complex carbohydrates and contains .44 milligrams of thiamine, .26 milligrams of riboflavin, and 3.52 milligrams of niacin, as well as significant amounts of magnesium and potassium, it is not considered a "whole food" because it lacks two essential amino acids, lysine and tryptophan.

When buying cornmeal, look for stone-ground meal. However, because of its high oil content, cornmeal has a relatively brief shelf life. Store it in the refrigerator in airtight containers for up to three months, or twice that long in the freezer. There is a downside to this. While cool temperatures prevent the meal from turning rancid and inhibit insect infestation, vitamins are lost.

In addition to cornmeal, corn is found as **hominy** (hulled corn kernels), as well as **grits**, hulled corn that has been ground into a meal. To cook, gradually add 1 cup of grits to 4 cups boiling water. Stir until boiling; lower heat to a simmer, cover, and cook for twenty-three to thirty minutes, stirring occasionally. In case you didn't know, **polenta** is the Italian version of grits.

Millet   While most of us think of millet as birdseed, that hasn't always been so. Millet has been traced to the Neolithic Age. Look for this tiny sandlike grain in natural- or health-food stores, where it is, as a rule, sold in bulk. (The kind you find in the pet shop is, for the most part, unhulled and, consequently, inedible by humans.)

Millet is comparable to other cereal grains, with more protein than rice, sorghum, corn, and oats. A good source of B vitamins, phosphorous, manganese, iron, and copper, it is very low in gluten, making it especially attractive to anyone with a gluten intolerance.

To cook, toast 1 cup hulled millet groats in a heavy skillet for five minutes. Slowly add 1 cup toasted millet to 2 cups boiling water for twenty to thirty minutes.

Oats/oatmeal Whole-grain oats are rich with seven B vitamins, Vitamin E, and nine minerals, including iron and calcium. They are reasonably high in protein, in a form that is higher in quality than the protein in wheat. Most importantly, oats are high in soluble fiber, which helps to lower serum cholesterol levels. Unlike most grains, only the inedible hull is removed by the milling process, with the bran and germ left intact on the edible kernel. Whether you're cooking steel-cut oats (also known as Scotch or Irish oats) or rolled oats (the more traditional American oatmeal), you'll use 2 cups water to 1 cup oats for about 2 ½ cups cooked hot cereal. When adding oats to breads and cookies, soak in water or juice first to soften.

Quinoa A mini-grain that, uncooked, looks like golden caviar, quinoa was first cultivated in the Andes by the Incas. Like amaranth, it is packed with lysine and other amino acids, making it a complete protein. A cup of the cooked grain has the calcium content of a quart of milk. It is also a rich source of iron, phosphorus, various B vitamins, and Vitamin E.

Toast quinoa, a little at a time, in a dry skillet before cooking to enrich its flavor. Rinse 1 cup quinoa under cold running water; drain, and add to 2 cups water or vegetable stock. Heat to boiling, stir, cover, and reduce heat. Cook until liquid is absorbed, ten to fifteen minutes. Yields 3 cups. Cooked quinoa is transparent.

Rice Rooted in history, rice has been cultivated on almost every continent, and while it is not the most nutritious grain in the world, it is probably the most often consumed. Statistically, rice supplies 55 percent of man's daily food requirements, and one pound of rice has four times the food energy of the same amount of potatoes.

There are more than seventy varieties of rice grown around the world, yet most Americans eat two kinds, long-grain and medium-grain white. Brown rice also can be either long or medium grain. Remember: All rice begins as brown rice. It becomes white when it is stripped of its husk, bran, and germ . . . and, consequently, most of its nutrients. What's left is almost pure starch.

The milling process for rice is extremely wasteful, as only 55 percent of the original weight remains. The hulls must be removed for rice to be edible; however, the bran and germ, left intact in brown rice, contain thiamine, the B vitamins, and iron. Cover and simmer 1 cup brown rice (we'll ignore the white kind) in 2 cups water for thirty to forty-five minutes over medium heat. Yield is approximately 3 cups.

Rye Most Americans have only eaten rye in breads—rye breads, pumpernickel, and other dark loaves. While whole rye contains more protein, minerals, and B vitamins than whole wheat, whole rye flour and food products are difficult to find, even in health-food stores! Most often, rye flour is combined with wheat flour in baking.

Compared to processed rye, whole grain rye is power-packed with twice the protein, three times the phosphorous and calcium, four times the riboflavin, five times the iron and thiamine, six times the niacin, and seven times the potassium.

Whole rye berries or rye groats can be cooked in liquid and served as a porridge or side dish or sprouted for use in salads, soups, and on sandwiches. Cracked berries can be ground and cooked into a hot cereal somewhat like grits or ground into a meal to be used in combination with other flours. Rye flakes can be cooked into a hot breakfast cereal much like oatmeal.

The nutritional content of rye flours can be spotted by the color. Light and medium flour has been sifted to remove much of the nutritious bran. Dark rye flour is unbolted (not sifted) and is more nutritious.

Triticale A relative newcomer to the grain field, triticale is a rye-wheat hybrid first reported in 1876 to the Edinburgh Botanical Society. Like wheat, it is a high-yielding grain with superior baking qualities, and it has the hardiness and protein quality of rye. Triticale is 16 percent protein, higher than either of its genetic parents, and has twice as much lysine as wheat.

Triticale berries can be soaked and cooked, like wheat berries, while cracked berries can be added to bread dough for crunchiness and increased nutrition. Flakes can be cooked into a porridge or hot cereal; triticale flour can be used in baking.

A word of caution: Triticale flour, at first thought to be low in gluten like rye, does contain gluten; however, it's very delicate and must be handled with care. Knead for only a few minutes. Soak triticale groats overnight and boil 1 cup grain in 3 to 3½ cups water for forty to fifty minutes.

Wheat   Unfortunately, too many people have become allergic to wheat because they have consumed too much refined wheat flour in breads, cakes, pastas, and packaged, processed foods.

There are more than 300 different varieties of wheat, belonging to fourteen basic species. Ninety-five percent of the crop grown and consumed in the United States is *Triticum aestivum*, or common wheat. Agronomists break wheat down into two strains—"winter wheat" or "spring wheat"—depending upon the time of year the seed is planted.

Wheat also comes in two botanical categories, "hard" and "soft," indicating the volume of gluten in the grain's cellular structure. *Hard common wheat* has approximately 12 percent protein content. Kernels are tough to mill, while *soft common wheat*, which is from 6 to 10 percent protein, is starchier and significantly easier to process. The high gluten content of hard wheats such as *hard durum wheat* or *semolina*, with its ability to absorb liquid, is considered ideal for bread baking. On the other hand, soft wheat, which is relatively low in gluten, is regarded as best for pastries.

Bulgur   is wheat—specifically, wheat *berries*—that has been cracked by parboiling and then dried. It is an "old" food—traces of sun-dried wheat grains were found in ancient ruins in many areas, including Etruscan urns and Hun saddlebags. Used in such Middle Eastern dishes as tabbouleh, bulgur comes when wheat is steamed, then dried before being crushed into the desired grind. A quarter pound of bulgur contains as many nutrients as a whole loaf of whole-wheat bread: 11.2 grams protein; 75.7 grams carbohydrates, 338 milligrams of phosphorus, and 229 milligrams of potassium, as well as ample doses of niacin, riboflavin, thaimine, calcium, and iron. The amount of water you'll need to prepare 1 cup bulgur depends on how you plan to prepare it. Easiest is to place 1 cup bulgur into a heat-safe bowl and then pour 3 to 4 cups of boiling, lightly salted water over the bulgur. Let stand forty minutes, then pour into a colander lined with cheesecloth. Place in the sink and let drain. Then gather cheesecloth around bulgur and squeeze out all moisture. The bulgur needs no further cooking. Simply combine with spices.

Couscous could, quite realistically, be called "wheat grits." In reality, it is finely cracked wheat (or, in come cases, millet) that has been steamed, dried, and refined. The best way to cook couscous is to steam 1 cup of the grain over simmering hot water for 20 minutes; then put it in a bowl and add ½ to ¾ cup cold water. Break up lumps with a fork and return to the steamer and continue steaming for twenty to forty minutes longer, depending upon the recipe you're using. Fluff with a fork before serving.

Wild Rice   This gourmet grain is not really rice. It is the seed of an aquatic grass, native to North America, where it grows wild around the northern Great Lakes, mostly in Minnesota, where, under Federal law, it is harvested by Native Americans.

After the seeds are harvested, they are cured over smoke fires. Then, according to tradition, but probably not pragmatic today, the cured seeds are spread on the ground, where the young men of the tribe dance on the cooling seeds to loosen the hulls. Finally the rice is sifted through blankets to winnow out the chaff, leaving the burnt brownish-black kernels to be graded for packaging—giant (long-grain), fancy or medium grain, and select or short grain. The rarity of the grass and the complicated harvesting and cleaning process make wild rice the "caviar of grains"! While a hearty hybrid has been developed and is now in limited production, this is an obvious attempt to cut costs since authentic wild rice is inordinately high. While it can be harvested by mechanical threshers and processed by mechanical parchers and winnowers, this tame version is not much less costly and is substantially less pungent and tasty. Nutritionally

Pointers

- Store grains, including rice and cereals, in airtight containers in the refrigerator, especially in summer.
- Exposure to light will destroy the riboflavin in grains, so use either opaque or dark glass containers.
- When buying loose grains, buy from a store that sells *a lot* of grain. And don't buy more than you need.

speaking, wild rice is a quality high-carbohydrate grain—about 73 mg per cup—that is high in phosphorus, magnesium, potassium, and zinc, not to mention thaimine, riboflavin, and niacin, plus all of the B vitamins. A cup of cooked wild rice contains a mere 130 calories.

TO COOK: Use 3 cups water to 1 cup wild rice to yield approximately 3½ cups cooked rice. A short-grained variety can be cooked in as little as 35 minutes; long grains can take as long as an hour.

LET THERE BE LEGUMES

Legumes, which includes anything that grows in a pod, have been an important part of the human diet around the world for at least four thousand years.

Immature legumes, such as green peas and garden peas, are most familiar to American tables; however, the nutritive power of these foods increases considerably when they are allowed to mature and dry on the vine. Dry beans and peas have a higher protein value per dollar than any other food source, making them the least expensive way possible to meet your body's protein needs—cheaper by far than cheese, eggs, and poultry. Bean protein has also been shown to reduce the body's serum cholesterol level, the exact opposite effect of animal protein sources.

While some B vitamins, which are water-soluble, are lost in cooking, a single serving of cooked dry beans can supply as much as 40 percent of the body's recommended daily requirements for thiamin and B_6. Iron is also high on the nutritional list. For example, a one-cup serving of lentils provides 42 percent of the RDA for iron for an adult male, and 23 percent for an adult female. Serve with foods rich in vitamin C—tomatoes, broccoli, green or red peppers, citrus fruits—to increase the body's ability to absorb iron from legumes.

With the exception of soybeans, legumes are also naturally low in fat. Unless you add animal fat in the cooking process, what fat there is is polyunsaturated, providing protection against cardiovascular disease. Additionally, legumes are low in sodium, which raises blood pressure, and high in potassium, which acts to lower blood pressure.

Beans and peas are powerful complex carbohydrates, full of dietary fiber, starches, and complex sugars. They supply the body with more roughage than almost anything except cereal bran.

Legumes are also amazing insulin regulators. Because beans and peas produce such slow rises in blood sugar, the body needs to release very little insulin to control glucose. Beans, along with other foods high in pectins and gums, actually cause the creation of more insulin-receptor sites on cells, giving insulin more places to enter the individual cells rather than circulating in the system.

The only negative side to the consumption of legumes is that they have the potential to cause flatulence—that's gas, indigestion, bloat, etc. This is caused by complex sugars that are not broken down by the digestive enzymes and begin to ferment when they come in contact with bacteria in the large intestine. This problem can be curbed in the cooking process; besides, the gas will subside as your body becomes accustomed to regular consumption of these astounding foods.

A GLOSSARY OF LEGUMES

Aduki Beans/Adzuki Beans From Japan, these small, shiny, dark red beans provide a high quality protein that is easily digested. Because of this, it is considered a healing food, served to the sick and elderly. In addition to being used as beans in soups and entrees, adukis is also processed into a slightly sweet-tasting paste that is used in everything from soups to desserts. Dry beans are readily available in healthfood stores. One cup of adukis almost triple in volume when cooked in 3 cups of water.

Black Beans Small, shiny black ovals, these rich-flavored beans are also known as turtle beans. A staple in the cuisines of their native South and Central America as well as Cuba, they are also grown in the Southeastern United States. Use in soups, either whole or pureed, and with rice and spices for protein-rich entrees. Dry beans are available in most grocery stores and Spanish markets. Cook 1½ cups of beans in 4 cups of water for 2 cups of cooked beans.

Black-eyed Peas Also called cowpeas, these quick-cooking beans are small, oval, and creamy white with either a black or dark yellow spot. (The yellow ones are, naturally, called Yellow-Eyed

Peas.) A hearty hallmark of Southern Soul Food, black eyed peas are mixed with rice and onions . . . and assorted traditional spices . . . for hoppin' John, that traditional New Year's dish that generates good luck in the year ahead. Widely available, dried, frozen, and even canned, 1 cup of dry black-eyed peas doubles in volume when cooked in 3 cups of water.

Broad Beans   Depending on their color and origin, this category of large legumes is known as fava beans, English or Windsor beans, even horse beans. They range in color from a rich, dark brown to waxy white and can be purchased fresh, dried or canned. Cooking time and resulting volume for dry beans depends upon the individual bean.

Chickpeas   Called by many names—*Garbanzos* (Spanish); *Ceci* (Italian)—chickpeas are round, tan, and very hard. Widely used in Mediterranean and Middle Eastern cuisines, chickpeas roll into soups, stews, salads, and sandwiches. Mixed with tahini (crushed sesame seeds) and spices, mashed chickpeas become hummus; parboiled and ground, they can be fried or grilled to become falafel. Most often sold precooked in cans, dry chickpeas are readily available. Cook 3 cups peas in 4 cups water for 4 cups of cooked beans.

Flageolets   These luxury legumes come from France, where they are a main ingredient of that cold-weather classic cassoulet and alongside the most delicate entrees. Either white or green, these small kidney-shaped beans are available dried, flash frozen, and canned. Cooked in 3 cups of water, 1 cup of dry flageolets yields approximately 2 cups cooked beans.

Kidney Beans   Probably the most popularly used legume in this country, these large beans are named for their kidney shape and deep red color. Best known in chili—with and without meat—they also find their way into soups, salads, and casseroles. Available dry or canned, 1½ cups of dry kidney beans cooked in 3 cups of water yields two cups cooked beans.

Lentils   Small, flat red or brown seeds that look like tiny buttons, lentils can be found in almost all of the world's cuisines. Easily digested and quick to cook since they need no soaking, lentils form a protein-rich base for soups and purees, hot or cold salads, casseroles, or simply combined with rice and vegetables for a satisfying meal. One cup of dry lentils cooked in 3 cups of water yields 2½ cups cooked beans.

Lima Beans   Small fresh beans are often called Fordhooks or, down South, butterbeans, with the lima label going most often to the dry version. However, small or large, fresh or dry, these flavorful beans add variety to your menu. Mixed with whole kernel corn, fresh limas emerge as succotash, while dried beans add body to soups, stews, and casseroles. Large limas have a stronger taste than their smaller counterparts, and some cooks say they should be skinned before using them in soups or purees. Two cups dried limas cooked in 2½ cups water yields approximately 2 cups cooked beans.

Peas   Look in your market for a variety of fresh peas. Whether they are whole garden or shell peas or the two delicious edible pod varieties—the flat snow peas and plumper sugar snap peas—they definitely belong on your table. Delicate in flavor and sweeter tasting when fresh or fresh frozen, peas—both green and yellow—are also sold dried. Exceptionally well endowed with soluble fiber—about 2.7 grams per half cup—whole peas can be added to a healthy diet to help lower cholesterol, control blood sugar, and even lower blood pressure. One cup of whole dry peas cooked in 3 cups of water doubles in volume.

Pinto Beans, Pink Beans, and Red Beans   Pintos are brownish pink spotted with brown while pink beans are solid brown-rose. Red beans, on the other hand, are solid brownish red. All three varieties look like miniature kidney beans and are similar in taste. Therefore all can be used interchangeably in recipes. Cooked in 3 cups of water, 2 cups of dry pintos, pinks, or reds will yield an equal portion of cooked beans.

Soybeans   Quite possibly the most important, not to mention versatile, food on this planet, soybeans and the wide spectrum of products made from soy have been found to promote health in numerous ways: lowering blood cholesterol and unclogging arteries; preventing and/or dissolving gallstones; reducing triglycerides; regulating blood sugar; regulating the bowels and relieving constipation; decreasing cancer risk, and even replacing estrogen levels in postmenopausal women. Eating soy foods of any type six times a

How To Cook Legumes

Like grains, dried beans and peas expand greatly when cooked. One cup dried beans—approximately ½ pound—renders between 2½ and 3½ cups cooked beans. Pick through your dried beans and remove any pebbles and debris, as well as any shriveled beans that may have found their way through the packaging process. Then wash in cold water and drain.

- *Soak your dried legumes.* All dry beans and peas, except split peas, lentils, and black-eyed peas, should be soaked before cooking.

    This next step is not *essential* if you have sufficient cooking time; however, it generally produces a better product because it leaches out some of the indigestible sugars and serves to improve the flavor and texture as well as the appearance of the beans.

- *Traditional soaking method:* In a large pot, cover dry beans or peas with 6 cups cold water per pound of beans. Cover loosely with a lid or plastic wrap. Let soak at room temperature for six to eight hours or overnight. Drain, rinse, and cook. (If soaking for longer than overnight, refrigerate beans.)

- *Quick soak method:* Cover washed beans in 6 to 8 cups *hot* water per pound of dry beans. Heat water to rolling boil, stir, and cook beans for two minutes. Cover pot and turn off heat. Let beans stand for an hour. Drain thoroughly, rinse, and cook.

- *Basic cooking:* Put soaked beans into a large pot or Dutch oven. Add 6 cups fresh water per pound of beans. Add seasoning spices (but not salt—it'll keep beans from softening) and vegetables at this point. Also add 1 teaspoon cooking oil to prevent foaming. Bring liquid to a boil; cover loosely to vent top and allow steam to escape; reduce heat and simmer beans between and two or more hours until beans are tender. (Cooking time depends upon size and dryness of the beans, hardness of the water, and the altitude.) You can add a pinch of baking soda to the cooking water to speed up hard water cooking time. Another hint: Avoid adding acidic ingredients such as vinegar, tomatoes, or lemon juice to the cooking water until the beans are almost cooked as the acid deters softening.

> • *Special cooking methods*: Beans and peas can be cooked in the *pressure cooker*, following manufacturer's instructions. Cooking time will be from ten to forty minutes. You can also use a *slow cooker*, in which case beans will take ten to twelve hours at low heat; five to six at high heat. Follow manufacturer's instructions.

week has been proved to reduce abnormally high blood cholesterol by as much as 20 percent. Because the beans themselves require a very long cooking time, soybeans are most often consumed as a processed food—flour, tofu, miso paste, milk, and even fermented as soy sauce. If you want to cook dry soybeans to use in soups or stews, 2 cups beans, cooked in 2 cups water, yields approximately 1½ cups cooked soybeans.

Split Peas   Very small and flat on one side, split peas require no soaking and cook very quickly. (Don't use your pressure cooker or you'll have a mess on your hands!) Most often, green split peas are used as the basis of a hearty soup or puree enriched with potatoes, carrots, onions, and leeks . . . plus assorted herbs and spices. Yellow split peas are the *pease* in British Pease Porridge and Indian dal. Both varieties have a soft, grainy texture marked with a distinct, rich flavor. One cup dried split peas, cooked in 3 cups water, yields 2¼ cups cooked split peas.

White Beans   You can find several varieties of white beans in any grocery store: Great Northern, cannellini, navy or Yankee beans, marrow beans and pea beans or pigeon peas. Smaller navy or pea beans are favored in traditional Boston baked bean dishes, while Great Northern are easily substituted for flageolets in cassoulets and casseroles. Cannellini, which are also called white kidney beans, are popular in Italian foods. The yield varies with the size of the individual beans, averaging 2 cups cooked beans per 1½ cups dry beans cooked in 3 cups water.

THE POWER OF PROTEINS

We Americans eat vast quantities of animal proteins, far more than could ever be considered healthy. We have been brainwashed into thinking that not only do we get adequate nuitrition from this, but that meat and fish are the only good, not to mention complete, sources of protein available. This is patently untrue!

Grains, legumes, nuts, seeds, and green leafy vegetables are absolutely packed with protein. It would be almost impossible to eat a two thousand-calorie vegetable-based diet that includes all six categories of vegetarian foods without ingesting fifty grams of complete protein. We have been told that we need forty to fifty grams of protein per meal, when in fact our bodies require a mere forty to fifty grams of protein per day.

Protein provides the body with the building blocks that make muscles, blood, hormones, and new tissue. While it is a vital and necessary component of one's diet, the most recent research shows that most Americans consume as much as five times more protein than is necessary to meet their actual metabolic needs. Research has shown that too much protein is not healthy, and has been actively connected to tissue-breakdown diseases such as arthritis.

The protein found in animal muscle tissue is far more concentrated than the plant protein found in whole grains, dark green vegetables, and legumes. When you eat a meal heavily laden with animal proteins, it overloads the body. Concentrated protein has been proven not only to leach calcium from the bones, which leads

Potent Vegetable Sources of Protein

Whole Grains:
   millet, corn, barley, brown rice, quinoa, amaranth, triticale, etc.

Legumes:
   lentils, chickpeas, alfalfa sprouts, aduki beans, lima beans, soy and soy-based products, etc.

Dark Green Vegetables:
   kale, collards, broccoli, spinach, etc.

Nuts and Seeds:
   almonds, cashews, walnuts, pecans, pistachios, macadamias, and nut butters made from them.

to osteoporosis, but it also damages the kidneys by clogging the filters. This has been known to lead to kidney failure.

In contrast, a balanced vegetarian diet supplies the body's protein needs without dealing a damaging blow to the system. The false idea promulgated by the meat industry that plant protein is incomplete and lacking some vital amino acids is a complete myth. Nature simply cannot make a soybean, potato, or grain of wheat without using all the same amino acids (the "building blocks" of protein) required by the metabolism of humans.

Vegetable proteins, eaten throughout the day in a well-balanced vegetarian diet, are each "complete" in their own way and will be metabolized quite completely, finding their way to the liver and other tissues where they will be used as needed.

Another selling point for a vegetarian diet: combining protein-rich vegetable dishes increases protein absorption by approximately 30 percent.

FATS FOR FITNESS

In the average American diet, we receive nearly half—that's 45 percent—of our total calories from fat. This has taken its toll in making Americans some of the least nourished and most overweight people in the world. While we should not avoid fat completely, numerous studies have confirmed that a high percentage of fat intake is a huge contributing factor in all kinds of diseases, from breast cancer to heart disease.

That said, it is important to differentiate between the kinds of fats, and what they each will do to the body. Omega-3 fatty acids, which are found in some fish, have been shown to be good for the heart. The essential fatty acids in sesame seeds, sunflower seeds, safflower seeds, and soybeans are vital for the maintenance of health, growth, hormone production, and other important functions.

While it is important to have a variety of fats in the diet in small amounts, it is not necessary to add tablespoons of fat in the form of oil when grains, legumes, fish, seeds, and nuts are plentiful in your diet.

All fats are not created equal. There are two kinds—saturated and unsaturated. Saturated fats are found in animal food sources such as meat and dairy products. Unsaturated fats are mainly found in grains, legumes, seeds, nuts, and the oils derived from them, including corn oil, safflower oil, sunflower oil, and soy oil. These fats are far better for you because they provide certain essential fatty acids. These fatty acids help control high blood pressure and regulate the ability of substances to enter and leave cells.

Your daily consumption of calories from fat probably should be limited to 15 percent of your total calories, and these should be from your regular consumption of grain, legumes, nuts, and seeds.

15

WEIGHTY MATTERS

Not surprisingly, most of the people who enter *any* health-oriented program have weight issues.

Many of the participants in the study groups leading up to the development of this protocol were much like Monique J., who told me:

> I had reached a point where I refused to buy any more clothing until I lost weight. The clothes that I used to wear did not look good on me any longer, and on two occasions, I had to buy clothing two sizes bigger just to have something to wear.
>
> In addition, climbing staircases and sometimes walking fast had become a painful, stressful experience, particularly during the winter, when I had to wear a heavy coat and boots. Although I had taken part in many exercise classes and did some exercise on occasion at home, I felt that I could and should be doing better. I felt that I was stuck and needed to do something to give me a push, some kind of discipline in my life. I never seemed to find enough time to attend to all the tasks that I assigned myself for the week, in particular household tasks.
>
> There were times when I wanted to accomplish some tasks, but I did not have the energy to do so.
>
> In the course of the protocol, I have lost fifteen pounds, almost without effort, just by eliminating meat and dairy products, wheat, chicken, turkey, and by drinking the green juice daily and eating

only organic food. The nutritional supplements have also been helpful.

The exercise program has also helped. I could have done even better, if it was not for some interruptions in the exercise and time spent outside of New York on two occasions when I could not apply the protocol.

The heaviness that I used to experience before the program when climbing stairs or trying to walk fast has greatly diminished.

A participant in the study group composed of people with significant weight issues, Carol J. also had a lot to say about weight. In addition to obesity, Carol was also plagued by arthritis in her legs, knees, and neck that had her in almost constant pain.

I was significantly overweight at 215 pounds and five-feet, five and a half inches tall. It embarrassed me to be that heavy. I felt as though I was saying to the world that I had problems I could not or would not deal with—and that was correct. I felt lonely most of the time.

I was surprised to find that, after only a month of sticking rigidly to the dietary part of the program, all the aches and pains were gone. I didn't need pain killers after that first month.

Feeling better physically helped me feel better emotionally. The immediate success gave me the motivation to stick with the program. I started losing weight and have slowly but steadily lost in the past year. I had never been able to lose more than thirty pounds and never kept it off for more than a year. At this point, I have lost fifty-five pounds and I am still losing, rather than regaining, as I would have in the past.

Before you begin *any* weight management program, you need to know, first of all, what your ideal weight is . . . and how to reach that weight.

EXACTLY HOW MUCH SHOULD YOU WEIGH?

Forget about those insurance-industry height and weight charts. There's a simple formula that is used to calculate the most desirable weight for your body.

For women, allow one hundred pounds for the first five feet of height and add five pounds for each additional inch. For men, start with 106 pounds for the initial five feet and add *six* pounds per additional inch. For example, a woman who is five feet, six inches tall should weigh 130 pounds; for a six-foot man, the ideal weight is 178 pounds.

Once you know what your best weight is, it's quite simple to compute the number of calories—actually, kilocalories—your body will need to maintain this ideal weight.

If you weigh more than your ideal, you are obviously consuming more calories than are necessary to maintain this weight. To stop doing this, create a baseline that equals ten calories per pound of ideal body weight. Then add three calories per pound for a sedentary person; five calories per pound for one who is moderately active, and ten calories per pound for one who regularly exercises at a strenuous level.

I hate to break the news to you: unless you are an Olympic athlete or, possibly, the mother of three preschoolers, you are probably only moderately active at best. Most adults—and, sadly, most young people, too—are sedentary, if truth be told.

Using this formula, our five-foot, six-inch woman, whose ideal weight is 130 pounds, would need approximately 1690 calories per day to maintain that weight level. If she weighs *more* than 130, she is no doubt consuming more than 1690 calories per day to stay that way. Our six-foot man whose perfect weight is 178 pounds is a competitive runner who trains intensely throughout the year and runs in approximately thirty-five races per year. He would need 3560 calories per day to maintain that body weight while training; 2670 calories per day when not training.

By determining your ideal weight and the calories you need to maintain that weight, you will be able to divide your nutritional needs in the proper proportions for optimal health.

CHOOSE TO LOSE—BUT DON'T DIET

Diet is crucial. Eat less. Eliminate saturated fats and excess protein, which creates toxicity in our body, in our liver, while making us feel sluggish. These fats and protein create both edema or water retention *and* dehydration. I also recommend going vegetarian and organic.

Because body weight obeys the fundamental laws of thermodynamics—calories taken in vs. calories burned—weight loss occurs when the body burns more calories than it consumes. Therefore, a 155-pound woman whose ideal body weight is 130 pounds should effectively lose weight on a 1690-calorie food plan plus moderate exercise.

As I've already explained, carbohydrates—especially the complex carbohydrates found in whole grains, fruits, and vegetables, for example, rather than the simple carbohydrates found in white breads, pastas, cakes and cookies, ice creams, candies, and soft drinks—and proteins—especially from vegetable sources—are preferable to fats. You can have a *huge* bowl of rice and sautéed vegetables and feel totally satiated for far fewer calories than are in a fast-food cheeseburger with extra mayo and a side of fries.

I recommend eating six *small* meals per day rather than the traditional three squares. In this way, you will maintain a balance in your blood sugar and the level of nutrients in your body.

Eat for health and strength, concentrating on the nutritional value of your foods in the amounts you have determined will maintain your ideal body weight, and weight loss will follow.

Part VII

INSIDE MOVES

16

MENTAL GYMNASTICS

Staying young is an inside job.

This is not to say that age is only a state of mind. Still, despite the physical aspects, such as diet and exercise, self-empowerment and behavior modification have proven to be essential to the success of this program.

Most of us eagerly begin something new—such as my Reversing the Aging Process protocol—with great enthusiasm and every intention to succeed. However, as time goes on we begin to lose our focus; the energy, the joy that called us forth dissipates. We return to the plodding, lifeless pace that had governed us *before* we began this project.

The self-impowerment/behavior modification component of the Reversing the Aging Process protocol has proven extremely important. Before it was added, there were dropouts/incompletions in virtually every study group

Before we can truly make a major change in our lives, we must modify our outlook and gain deeper understanding of our Selves. We must first learn to have a sense of Self and also a love of our Self. To identify this, I recommend starting with the Self-Impowerment questions, and moving from there.

Once we have questioned our value systems, then and only then can we affect change. The protocol then becomes easy to follow and adopt as a way of life.

When we look at how the body ages, we cannot overlook the

tremendous impact our thoughts, beliefs, and values have on the acceleration as well as the slowing down of the overall aging process. While fueling the body with nutrients and supplements is vital, as is exercise and daily introspection and reflection, there is a growing body of evidence that points to the amazing affect our thoughts have on our biochemistry and our immune system. Chronic negative emotions such as anger, guilt, resentment, frustration, worry, sadness, and depression elevate the adrenal gland's production of catecholamines and cortisol, which, in consistently high levels, suppress our immune system and accelerate the aging of our organs.

Look at how our belief systems and thoughts, emotions, behaviors, and relationships affect and determine our levels of happiness and, in turn, our overall health. These questions enable you to examine your beliefs.

Set aside a period of quality time for yourself to carefully consider each question and how it affects your life. Address only one or two questions each day . . . taking care that you answer each consciously and completely. In this way, you will be sure to identify your strengths and weaknesses and the areas in your life that bear attention.

SLOW YOUR MIND TO THE SPEED OF LIFE
LIVING IN CONSCIOUS ATTENTION

1. Are our goals more important than our lives?

2. To create a new reality—step back and look—*at the facts*—what are they?

   How do they affect me or others?
   How should I feel about them?
   Do they match or challenge my preconceived view?
   What will happen if I accept them as is?
   Why and how can I rearrange and then reinterpret the data to correspond to my
      previous input?
   Do the facts invalidate my beliefs?
   Can I tolerate being wrong? What will change?

3. Wisdom is not a reaction but an awareness of the truth of the present moment.

4. What inspires your curiosity?

5. What comes from a mind that is:

    a. Overly critical and judgmental?
    b. Always analyzing?
    c. Distressed?
    d. Serious?
    e. Always trying to control everyone and everything?

6. What comes from a mind that (is):

    a. Uncontaminated by toxic thoughts?
    b. Innocent?
    c. Curious?
    d. Positive?
    e. Passionate?
    f. Accepting?
    g. Gentle?
    h. Lets everything go?
    i. Loves suprises?
    j. Is up to adventure?
    k. Can feel comfort in the moment?

7. Can you experience anything without first thinking about it?

8. Where is the center of your experience?

9. When are our experiences effortless?

10. Clear your mind and bliss will follow.

11. What makes you feel comfort and discomfort?

12. With any conflict, we use appropriate verses inappropriate tools?

13. Do we approach problems when we feel good or bad?

14. How do high or low moods alter our approach to problems?

15. What happens when you face a problem from a troubled state of mind?

16. In a happy, relaxed state of mind—how much time do you focus in:

    a. The past?
    b. The present?
    c. The future?

17. Do you overprepare for the past catching up or the future closing in?

18. How do we make a hidden problem or fear or insecurity visible? We become conscious.

19. To what do we listen with full attention?

20. If the superficial issues scare us, then we panic at the prospect of a far deeper and closer attention.

21. What would we see if we just observed and took no sides?

22. If we keep ourselves so constantly busy, then we limit what we feel.

23. What in your life is impermanent?

24. How do you deal with finite things?

25. When we suffer from being honest and true, we suffer in innocence.

26. When we suffer from being wrong, we do so in shame and guilt.

27. If you don't face the problem, you can't create a solution.

28. All good things are earned in part by being patient.

29. Silence, stillness, surrender to the moment is not the same as doing nothing.

30. We are impatient for answers.

31. When any problem cannot be fully addressed by knowledge and intellectual effort, then faith is the next step.

32. Do we feel more alive and confident: emotionally, physically, spiritually, awake? asleep?

33. What pleasures do we allow—why—how often?

34. What pleasure do we deny ourselves—why?

35. Do we only allow pleasure when we feel we've earned it?

36. What if we applied the same work ethic to the principles of pleasure?

37. Do you allow unstructured time, play, fun, pleasure—how often?

38. If you have succeeded at surviving one crisis after the next, what does this tell you?

39. Where do we feel safe, comfortable—sanctity for quiet moments, free from responsibility?

40. How do you deal with really finding the right door, but are you using the wrong key?

41. The problem (Reaction)   The solution (Transformation)

42. What boundaries have we accepted from others as if they were our own?

43. Positive EFFORTS =   Negative EFFORTS =

44. Do you find happiness in what you do or negativity in what you don't have?

45. List your peak experiences. How do you achieve them?

46. Are you motivated by anticipated need or joy?

47. Do we try to perform tasks and obligations for acceptance or because these things give us pleasure and feel right?

48. Some self-detrimental behaviors are the only pleasures an individual allows one-self.

49. What pleasures do we oppose?

50. Do we experience life or merely perform life?

51. Material gains generally equal social and personal and professional validation.

52. If you could self-actualize your natural needs, what would be different?

53. Do you try to *prove* your faith, love, friendship, rather than feel it?

54. To show a life well lived, must we suffer?

55. Because you have suffered, this should not allow you to feel a moral superiority.

56. How do we make good people feel bad?

57. Do we control through reward/punishment or unconditional encouragement?

58. To what are we enthusiastic?

59. How can we turn low-grade pain into high-level pleasure?

60. Is your life a:

    a. Drama?
    b. Comedy?
    c. Adventure?
    d. Horror?
    e. Satire?
    f. Tragedy?
    g. Musical?

61. Pleasure expands.   Pain constricts.

62. Every step forward is challenged. How do we respond?

63. How do we become more responsible to the world around us?

64. Why do we have pets?

65. Learning is a challenge but necessary to our growth.

66. Freedom requires being vulnerable.

67. Do we have pleasure—fear?

68. Our "health efforts" could contribute to our stress.

69. Our beliefs predetermine our future actions.

70. Facts remain—Beliefs change.

71. Our highly repetitive life and beliefs convince us something is right.

72. What happens when, like the Buddha, we become wakeful and detached?

73. What are we attached to?

74. When, where, why do you feel empty?

75. Why don't we make easy decisions?

76. Do you humor and share or fear and hide your uniqueness?

77. Do you feel that your happiness and completeness depends on others?

78. Why can't we make up our minds?

79. Society rewards personal relationships and not autonomy?

80. Are you self-directed or do you seek others' approval?

81. We only appreciate challenges if the effort is difficult and requires sacrifice.

TRANSFORMING YOUR CRISIS

1. How do we live and experience an integral life?

2. What or who creates or influences our beliefs?

3. How do your thoughts, experiences, decisions, feelings, and needs affect your beliefs?

4. With every honest effort to change there is a corresponding urge to resist.

5. Are we born gifted or do we develop these special qualities? If so, at what costs and rewards?

6. Are we willing to begin a new chapter in our lives? Write it out. If we are not willing to begin a new chapter, what in our previous chapter draws us back?

7. Experiement with your life. Do so both in and out of the context of social acceptability.

8. In order to grow we must surrender. What have we refused or not refused to surrender?

9. Lasting growth requires commitment to consistent quality effort; within this growth there are peaks, plateaus and valleys.

10. When you look at what you want to transform, is it in the context of the part or whole of your life?

11. How adaptable are you?

   a. Feelings.
   b. Perceptions

12. What is the purpose of self-control—social control—family control—religious control—educational control—medical-health-scientific-historic-geo-political control?

13. Do we expect to be taught—healed—helped in a specific manner? What if it doesn't happen?

14. What occurs when we are rigid and inflexible?

15. How do you handle a difficult situation?

   a. Complain
   b. Blame others
   c. Seek help from others
   d. Take control and seek solutions

16. How do you view people with opposite qualities from yourself?

17. If you were to carefully examine the people in your life who you've given control and power to, what qualities would they possess?

18. Do these people share common bonds?

19. Look at every problem that caused you grief. What were the lessons of cause and effect? Did you observe any early signs that something or someone was not going well? What was your response?

20. List the little and big lessons, and how they were learned. Preventative or after the fact?

21. How often do you become defensive? What does this do to your options?

22. Do you try your best—when—why—why not?

23. How often do you offer honest opinions?

24. If something doesn't make sense, how do you deal with it?

25. How often do you say exactly what you

    a. Feel?
    b. Believe?
    c. Expect?
    d. Need?

26. Which daily habits do you use that create harmony or conflict?

27. Which resolutions do you keep—why not and why?

28. What positive words do you offer to yourself and others?

29. How can you make your life simpler?

30. When and why do you challenge authority?

31. Describe what no longer works for you.

32. What do you want to learn? Why?

33. Describe all the little things that give you joy.

34. What do you like or not like about your work?

35. Which dreams have you tried to make happen?

36. Describe what anyone else does that bothers you? What have you done about it?

37. Which responsibilities would you rather not have?

38. Which of your expectations of others are not being met? How does this affect you?

39. Stop before you commit yourself to a reaction. What other choices do you have?

40. Which pressures or stresses do you allow that you shouldn't?

41. What would you do with more free time?

42. Do you work too little/ too much? To what effect?

43. Would you feel better if you worked for yourself?

44. How many things do you leave undone? Why? Do you begin something else and not finish that as well?

45. What do you do with a problem?

    a. Talk it to death
    b. Deny its importance
    c. Give it over to someone else
    d. Look for positive solutions

46. Would your changing be accepted, tolerated, or rejected by others?

47. Do you trust in the wrong people and purposes?

48. Who else would you prefer to be? Why?

49. What can you afford or not afford? How does this affect your life—health—happiness?

50. What sacrifices have you made because of the choices you've made?

    a. Gains
    b. Losses

51. Whose opinions do you value the most? Why?

WHO ARE YOU REALLY?

1. What determines our choices?

    a. Certainty
    b. Doubt

2. With certainty there is no doubt.

3. We learn so well, we don't have doubts, and we don't reflect on what we do.

4. No doubts. No choices.

5. An absolute belief—unshakable; does not mean it is correct. Nor is the phenomenon stable.

6. How does each Life Energy accept or not accept their lives?

    a. Emotional—boredom—jealousy—fear—frustration—apathy.
    b. Body—depression—overweight—no energy—sickly—indigestion—insomnia—constipated.
    c. Acting out—no risks—procrastination—passive—blaming—never sure—denial.

7. Which energy has talent?

8. What do others have that you do not?

9. Only when you know who you really are will you then know how to live.

10. Dreams can only come true when our vision is focused and clear.

11. Who or what clouded or blocked your vision?

    a. Parents
    b. Teachers
    c. Friends
    d. Society

12. Who saw no value in it?

    a. Parents
    b. Teachers
    c. Friends
    d. Society

13. Crises will frequently allow us an opportunity to bring suppressed qualities into this moment.

14. Change the name of your crisis and alter its significance.

15. How does each life energy end and begin things?

BREAK THE RULES
BE A REBEL FOR A CHANGE!

1. Prepare a detailed survey of where you are versus where you need to be.

    a. View of self
    b. View of life
    c. Your age—emotional / biological / spiritual / physical
    d. Your career
    e. Your friends
    f. Your family
    g. Your sex life
    h. Your assertiveness
    i. Your anger / anxiety / depression / boredom / joy / passion
    j. Your health
    k. Your creative self
    l. Your security
    m. Your compulsions / addictions
    n. Your education
    o. Your responsibilities / social / worldly / personal / work / friends
    p. Your spiritual self
    q. Your hobbies
    r. Your connection to the past

    s. Your fantasies

    t. Your *stuff*

    u. Your adventurer/explorer self

    v. Your communication

    w. Your quality time

2. Which is more significant:

    a. Success in work

    b. Success in society

    c. Living in peace and balance with life

3. Should you diminish the moment for what you yearn for?

4. By changing your words you change your actions

    a. I can't

    b. I don't know

    c. I'm no expert

    d. I'm stupid

    e. I'm not creative

    f. I'm unlucky

    g. I'm unloved

    h. I'm not sure

    i. I'm no hero

5. Which is real:

    a. The thought

    b. The feeling

    c. The emotion

6. To what do we consciously and unconsciously submit?

7. When we listen nonjudgmentally we hear everything.

8. Everything we attract we mirror consciously or unconsciously, we just don't always like the consequences.

9. If you have experienced love and still need love, what then are you seeking?

10. Success gives you . . . Failure gives you . . . Where will each take you?

11. How many right choices did you make today?

12. How do we affirm ourselves?

    a. Quietly

    b. Meekly

    c. Apologetically

    d. Affirmatively

    e. Demandingly

13. How well do you do everything? What determines the quality of your efforts?

14. We frequently don't make changes or take appropriate risks because we don't know how we are supposed to accomplish the task.

15. Don't ask *how*—rather, affirm *when* you will engage in a transformational process.

16. Break the rules—Do It Differently.

17. What purpose have you created for your life and legacy?

18. When are you ready to learn?

19. What keeps us within the circle of the known?

    a. Celebrity

    b. Nutrition

    c. Power

    d. Science

    e. Success

    f. Medicine

    g. School

    h. Religion

    i. Politics

    j. Business

    k. History

20. What determines how and what you think about?

21. Which is more relevant, the circumstances or your view of them?

22. What you are seeking is what you should think of.

23. Do we support Social Psychosis? Are we fervent? rigid?

    a. Cold War

    b. War and crime

    c. Sexual liberation

24. Who or what manufactures your thoughts?

25. How much do you need to achieve harmony?

26. A frequent dual exists—Intelligence vs. Action

27. We hide or run from what? It doesn't matter.

28. What is more important, the event or our response to it?

29. What happens when you don't want anything from anybody?

30. Do we give exclusively in order to receive exclusively?

31. Affirm "yes" and stand by it—don't hesitate or equivocate.

32. Do we honor our individual capacity for experience?

33. Don't overly glamorize someone or something that cannot live up to your ideas or fantasies.

34. Our lives are illuminating and dark. Which do you create—indirectly or directly?

35. Negative energy vibrates the darker side.

36. Positive energy vibrates health and healing and happiness.

37. What are you willing to connect with? Why?

17

MAKING CONSCIOUS CHOICES

Imagine that you're driving two hundred miles in a sparsely populated midwestern state, such as Kansas. The land is flat. The scenery, though pretty, is monotonous—mostly cornfields. There aren't many other drivers on the long, level highway, and those you encounter are courteous. After a while you feel you know what to expect; you sense the road is going to continue along in the same way that it has. So you become a very comfortable, complacent driver. You put on cruise control. You become a little less alert. And as long as you don't fall asleep, this is probably okay.

Now imagine that you're driving two hundred miles in a northeastern state, such as New Jersey. Road conditions are going to be changing much more rapidly and dramatically here. You'll be involved in some heavy traffic in the metropolitan New York and Philadelphia areas. You'll be traveling on congested highways with confusing intersections, and you'll have to contend with some crazy drivers, the kind who insult you for no reason and cut you off without notice. Since New Jersey is a compact state with diverse geography, you'll also be going through suburban and rural areas, and you'll see a variety of views, including industrial blight, shopping malls, lushly landscaped suburbia, and bucolic countryside. Some of the road will be flat, but you'll also hit ups and downs. In short, in this region, you're always going to be somewhat unsure about what or who is coming up next. You'll have to be alert every minute, taking in the changing scene, anticipating what's up ahead.

Here's my point: We should all be going through life as if we're driving through New Jersey. But many of us are acting as if we're on the road in Kansas. We've put on cruise control. We think we know what's up ahead. The problem is, to echo Dorothy in *The Wizard of Oz,* we're not in Kansas anymore.

Like it or not, you have to admit—life today is getting more and more like a trip through New Jersey. It's filled with the good, the bad, and the ugly, with the beautiful, the bewildering, and some rude surprises; the only constant is that the road's changing all the time.

Unfortunately, this constant change may be hard to come to grips with. It's only natural to assume that our world will continue to look and function as it has. After all, when we're toddlers first finding out about the world, we learn from past experience. If we learn on Monday that pots on the stove are too hot to touch, on Tuesday we assume that they'll still be too hot to touch. Mommy never likes us to run into the street, and she always likes us to say "please" and "thank you." Those early, basic things we learn about the world don't change, which is good, because that's how we're able to grow up in one piece.

Whole societies used to be as unchanging as the personal world of toddlers. Agrarian cultures existed for hundreds of years doing things exactly the same way century after century. But as history went on, and especially in the past three hundred years, the pace of cultural change picked up. Now, as Alvin Toffler describes in his book *Future Shock,* that pace is continually accelerating. (By the way, this book makes interesting reading, not only because it describes accelerating change, but because it illustrates it: Published in 1970, it's filled with details about technology and social trends that are now totally passé. This brilliant book embodies its own point about the rush of the future by being, in certain respects, as dated as a dinosaur!)

WHERE WE ARE NOW?

Today our world is changing so fast, it seems almost impossible to keep up. As I write this, in mid-1998, a movie is being made called *You've Got Mail.* It's a romantic comedy in which E-mail plays a central role in uniting the protagonists. The interesting thing is that the director, Nora Ephron, is quoted in the newspaper as saying that the movie has to come out "in the next five minutes," because E-mail will soon become a dated technology, to be replaced by a new communications mode with a video component. It seems as if our social and cultural environment is evolving so quickly that a year is like a decade used to be.

Let's take all this down to the personal level. If we make the mistake of assuming that the world's unchanging, what happens? Well, first of all, we may find ourselves unemployed. This has happened to millions of people. They didn't bother to learn the new skills, mostly computer-related, that are needed by workers today. Or they were living with the job world paradigms of the past. For instance, they still had that old idea about company loyalty, and assumed that if a company hired you and you did a good job, they'd keep you on for life. That one went out years ago, but these people didn't notice. Or right now, many people are still assuming that the place consumers buy things is a store. That assumption was a reasonable one yesterday, but it's not going to be tomorrow, because the so-called "e-economy," with people buying things on-line, is taking hold. Jobwise, if a person's not on his or her toes and ready to move with the changes, he's likely to find himself unemployed. Then the person winds up sitting at home, blaming the system, and wondering what happened.

What happened was that that individual made the mistake of assuming that the world was going to continue in the same way, and it didn't. We can make that mistake in the relationship area as well. People change. What if your spouse grows in certain ways that you don't acknowledge? Your marriage will founder. You can't assume that your relationship is going to stay the same as it was on your wedding day. And yet if you're a baby boomer who was brought up with the set of romantic notions prevalent in the fifties, you may be assuming exactly that.

Think about it, baby boomers. Remember fairy tales? This generation—at least the older part of it—was the last to which fairy tales were told without a sense of cynicism or irony. They were still an accepted form of children's entertainment, and society was not making fun of them yet. Consider what happens in fairy tales. People have trials and tribulations, but they always end up together, living happily ever after. And you can probably think back to what "happily ever after" meant to you as a child. It meant that the relationships of Cinderella and Prince Charming, Sleeping Beauty and her prince, Jack and the Beanstalk and his mother, and the three little pigs, were going to continue along unchanging and blissful for many, many, many years. These people were going to get real old and probably die before they had a bad day together! Needless to say, if you're unconsciously using this template for your relationships, you're making a big mistake.

On the deepest level, you can make the mistake of not acknowledging the changes in your own self. We age, and we may not want to see that. But look, aging isn't all bad. When I talk about reversing the aging process, I'm talking about undoing unnecessary damage we've inflicted on our cells and organ systems, because I believe that suffering from premature degenerative disease *is* bad. But aging as a concept has its good aspects. You can be evolving spiritually and emotionally. You can even be improving physically; I know people who are in better shape in their seventies than they were decades earlier, because they worked at improving their fitness.

You have to work with change, as opposed to ignoring it. Did you ever see a middle-aged person who's got the exact same hair style, hair color, clothes, eyeglass frames, and makeup she had when she was eighteen? Did you ever meet a mature baby boomer who acts as if it's still the 1960s and we're in the "summer of love"? There's something ridiculous about these people. It's as if they haven't bothered to open their eyes in years.

People whose eyes *are* open are always asking questions: Where am I right now? What's happening out there in the world? What's ahead, and how do I want to fit into it? Or not fit into it? What exactly is my plan—and why? Here are some more related questions and ideas.

Some things in life are permanent. Many aren't. Do you acknowledge this?

We like to think that permanency is a big part of our lives. We want constancy, stability; we want our jobs, love relationships, and friendships to last forever.

The trouble is, most things in life are not permanent. Change is the norm. So if we try to hold on to something, we usually only create stress. There are people and things in our lives that we must recognize from the beginning are only temporary. Other things can be maintained on a more permanent basis. Let's look at some important parts of life.

Relationships There is no such thing as a permanent relationship. Although some people stay with us throughout our lives, we should not feel that they must. As long as we can enjoy pleasure and beauty in a relationship, we should maintain it, but once that is no longer happening, it may be time to let it go.

The fact that someone's been in your life for a while does not mean you can take them for granted, and this applies to friendships as well as to more intimate relationships. Each year on January 1, I make a list of my friends. I'll look at each name and ask, "Am I really a friend? Do I honor the relationship? What do I give that makes the relationship important and alive? And what does the other person contribute to the friendship?" If I find that I'm not honoring the relationship, or that it's not mutual, I simply let it go. In the future, the friendship may or may not revitalize, depending upon the needs of both individuals.

Here's a key question to ask yourself about any relationship: *What would I do differently if permanency wasn't an assumed part of the relationship?*

You would appreciate every moment together. You would honor one another. You would look for the best and you would share it.

Love Love, as a life force, should be permanent, because it is central to life. If love is not a permanent factor, everything else becomes transient. When you're filled with love, you are in touch with your true nature. You simply see things as they are. Through love comes reconciliation. Love heals.

Health People tend to think they're healthy if they haven't been diagnosed with a clinically recognized disease. That's a mistake, because if you're making unwise lifestyle choices, you could be well on your way to developing a serious condition that just hasn't reached a crisis stage yet. You're going down the wrong road, but you think you're on the right one just because there are no obvious signposts saying WRONG ROAD. Sometimes there aren't any until it's too late; when it comes to your health you have to be a very savvy traveler.

Security   We look for permanent security and then become dependent on it. Then we start dishonoring our true nature. People who assume the government owes them a living, or lifelong welfare, people afraid to take risks, want permanent security. As a result, they will not challenge their inner demons or unjust authorities. Maintaining security is more important. We become prisoners when we seek permanent security.

Your Appearance   The first time you look in the mirror and see yourself aging, you don't accept it. You believe the first wrinkle and first gray hair will go away. It's a way of denying what is happening.

Transcending the need to disguise your appearance involves accepting it and allowing yourself to feel happy with who and what you are at this point in your life. Both men and women suffer angst about their appearance and the aging process. Accept your appearance as temporary.

Passion   Although you need not feel passionately all the time, it is possible to find passion in everything. You can feel passion as you see someone's face looking through a little bag of belongings, which is all they have in the world. Suddenly you sense injustice in the way we live; some have so little and others so much. In that moment, you feel humility. You realize that you've ignored those who have nothing, and complained at not having enough. The passion of the moment connects you to what is real and right about life. Passion is an immediate bridge between the superficiality of our conditioning and the essence of life.

Is your need for absolute security blinding you?

If you grow up insecure, then you are going to look for things that are absolute and provide you with absolute security. In so doing, you will tend not to look at the contradictions and the limitations. Rather, you will accept something because it provides you with a secure place.

Insecurity does not become secure because it has found a safe haven. It merely has a respite before it is confronted with additional insecurity. It's better to go through the insecurity and at least be free. Then you can grow.

People stagnate when they hold on to security, even as they go through the motions of growth. They tell me, for instance, that they are going to come to my lectures and change their lives. Well, they come to my lectures, but they change nothing. They are so much a part of other belief systems that they can't let go of them.

These individuals are neither here nor there. They are in a psychic spasm. They are the spiritual materialists, the people who think they are growing because they experience something. Experience, however, does not equal knowledge or growth. You can go to a million workshops. You can even sit at the feet of Buddha, Christ, or Confucius. It means nothing unless it is done with an open-ended consciousness. Then the experience can be used as a way of growing. Otherwise, it's just another experience.

Are you too quick to generalize from one experience?

Sometimes we make our experiences more important than they should be. Our experiences directly affect our beliefs. Here's how this works: Let's say you go to a vegetarian, macrobiotic restaurant. They give you a lump of brown rice, some overcooked beans, some toasted sesame seeds, and soy sauce. You try this and think it is tasteless and terrible. From this experience, you form a belief that vegetarian food is boring and limited. Now you allow your experience to affect your beliefs. But that was just a one-time experience.

Or you go out with a woman, assuming the two of you are going to have a lot in common. Then you find out that you and the woman really have nothing to share. Not only that, you argue. That night, you think, "I don't want to go out with any other women for a long time. If this is what I'm going to find, I don't need it." You've allowed one experience with one woman to affect your beliefs about women and relationships in general. This is unfair to women and to yourself.

Think of how many times we make judgments and form beliefs based on limited experience. If I were to judge vegetarian eating based on my experience eating in vegetarian restaurants, I'd be a meat-eater. Luckily, I've allowed myself to discover the potential of home-cooked vegetarian meals, which go way beyond restaurant fare in variety and tastiness. Don't close yourself off to things without exploring all their facets.

What beliefs do you accept unquestioningly?

We like to think we wake up each day feeling how we want to

feel. This is only partially true. We may adhere to a clean, vegetarian diet but be around emotionally toxic people. We're taking in pure food, but we're also ingesting negative thoughts from people. One's going to undo the benefits of the other.

One reason we may be taking in negative thoughts is because our belief system has taught us to be tolerant of other people. We just accept things as they are instead of questioning them. Think of the rituals you engage in just because your mother or father did them. There's a classic example: Every time a woman made a rump roast she would cut the end of it off before placing it in the roasting pan and into the oven. When asked why she did that she said it was because her mother and grandmother did it that way. One day the grandmother was over, and the husband asked her, "Why did you cut off the end of the rump roast?" She said, "One day I had a rump roast that didn't fit in the pan, so I had to cut off the end of it."

How many things do we do that really make no sense? Realize that you've got a choice. Ask yourself, "Is my old belief system serving me, or do I create a new reality?" Creating a new reality can be scary. So most people rely upon the old belief system and hence the old pattern of behavior. If your mother was used to dealing with people by just turning off, the likelihood is that you've learned to turn off, too. But you're not going to acknowledge that she was the reason for this. It will simply be a natural part of your life. It's almost like a congenital defect. We're practically born with it, so it's natural to us. We didn't acquire it through a crisis or accident in life. That would have been traumatizing.

Many of these things weren't traumatizing while we were growing up. We were simply little kids watching our mother and father. We watched how they dealt and adapted. We observed a pattern of behavior. And now we begin as adults to take on the same pattern. Of course as adults, we think that we've created this and this is normal. It's not. This behavior, however, will control how you feel.

Here's an example: Let's say you used to see that your mother didn't like waking up early in the morning; she couldn't get out of bed. So after awhile you yourself start your days thinking, "Maybe I can stay in bed a few more minutes," and then you turn the alarm on and off ten times. Now as an adult you could get out of bed, but you choose to stay in bed as long as possible. It's become a normal part of your existence. You don't feel good if you have to get up early. When you've got to get up early, you're grumpy, and you're late for appointments or work. "Oh, I hate getting up," you say. So now you're starting your days on a negative footing. And it all stems from an inherited belief system. It has nothing to do with the moment. You could be completely rested, but you're going to allow an old, unquestioned assumption to affect your whole day.

Did you ever wake up and realize that something is still missing?

You don't know what it is. You're eating right, you're exercising, you're trying to do everything right, but it just doesn't feel as if it's come together. There seems to be something missing. The question is—what? Let's look at that big question mark.

When we do everything we were taught we were supposed to do to gain acceptance and we still don't feel that we are acceptable, then doing more of the same is not going to make a difference. You've got to start doing it differently or doing something different. Here's a medical example: Think of all the surgeons out there who truly believe that what you need is another coronary bypass operation. They've seen many of their patients have their arteries reocclude, or reclog, a year or two after a bypass, and so they're given another operation. I know people who have had three, four, or even five coronary bypass. Not once have they been told, in a really meaningful way, about major lifestyle changes. It's as if there's only one way to approach the problem.

How many times in life have you repeated patterns of behavior only to find yourself right back where you started? How in the world do you expect something to change if the process is never different? If I keep putting the same ingredients into a recipe and it keeps coming out bad, I've got to change the ingredients. Yet time after time I see people in bad relationship after bad relationship. They blame the relationships. It never occurs to them that maybe what they're doing in the relationships, one after the other, might be leading to problems.

How many times in interpersonal relationships have you gotten angry, and then said something to the other person knowing it was going to hurt? You knew what to do to get a response. But did you realize that what you were doing was getting the exact kind of response you did not want? At some point you're going to have to have the courage to stop everything that you're doing in life and re-evaluate the whole life process. That's not easy for most people. Think of what we have committed to our life process: our education, our knowledge, our acceptance by peers and family, our acquisitions, our homes, our position in society, our standing. Men, in particular, live with hierarchical order that is always there from childhood that they're always honoring. What if you said, "I'm in the wrong program? I've got to start all over again"?

We can choose to change, or we will be forced to change by accident, death, firing, illness, or other loss.

Change is part of life. When we feel the need for change, we can be in control of it, or we can wait and let circumstances force change upon us. An example: You feel the need to get out of your relationship, but you don't. The stress results in disease. Or you feel that you have outgrown your job but remain there instead of moving on. You get fired and are unprepared for a transition.

When you procrastinate and say, "I'll make a change later," you're saying, in effect, that you do not want to be in control of the changes that occur. You are saying that you will let them happen to you. Isn't it better to just deal with the moment? Learn to make needed changes.

Do you engage in integral thinking?

We have 28 million Americans living in gated, well-manicured, guarded communities. These generally have a lake and a country club. It takes anywhere from $300,000 to $3 million to live in them. There's very little crime, but there's a lot of dysfunction. There's no less anger inside those communities than there is in the ghetto. The difference is that the environment looks different.

Now let's take a look at life energies. At least 85 percent of people have what I call adaptive supportive energy. They work in the post office, as sanitation workers, and as secretaries. They plow your corn, milk your cows, and cut your hair. These people are the support system of the world. If they weren't doing their jobs consistently, society would dissolve into anarchy overnight. Imagine if you didn't have someone to pick up your garbage for a month. What if no one grew your food? What would you do? Would you hire someone? There would be no one to hire, because only the adaptive supportives are going to be able to do it. When we turn on the water, we don't appreciate what it means to have it come out. We have hot water because someone makes the water hot. Someone builds the elevators we ride, and someone maintains them. We can walk on lighted streets at night because someone maintains them and changes the light bulbs. These people are not being invited into the gated communities. They don't get in because they're not making the money.

You may not think about this. You may assume that anybody can live there. In reality, not everyone can live in the gated communities, or in the co-ops on Fifth or Park avenues. Not everyone can afford decent housing in more modest locales. Not everyone can afford housing of any sort.

I'm not suggesting that we all should feel guilty and move back to the inner cities. What I'm suggesting is that we may be perpetuating a problem by not taking a step back to see how we can be a part of the solution. I'm suggesting that we put our energies into committing ourselves to something. We should look at one thing that needs changing, and then focus upon that, using our intellect and resources. I'm not saying, "Change the world." We like to think that we can't help anybody because there are too many people out there who need help. Why bother at all? But that's faulty thinking. If you can help one person, do it. What if you were that person? What if that person was your brother, father, or mother? Suddenly the help becomes important. Imagine if every individual was to help one other person. Imagine if people of various life energies got together to go in and make the ghetto a safe place to live. Ghettos only become ghettos when certain life energies abandon them. They don't have dynamic energies. Without dynamic energies, all systems fail. No business can succeed without a dynamic energy.

Don't just think about yourself. Don't just ask, "What's in it for me?" Stop and think in a more integrated way. I'll give you an example of integral thinking:

My radio show is on New York's WBAI weekdays at noon. At one point, I spoke with the station manager about programming. A lot of death shows had been scheduled right after mine because my ratings are so high. The idea was to get my audience to expand its time listening to the station. By doing this, the station made more money in the short term because, at fund-raising time, my audience began to order premiums during other shows. But at the end of the year, the total listening time of the audience dropped.

Instead, I felt, a completely different show should be scheduled near mine, one that has its own subject and voice. Such a show could bring its own audience and still serve the needs of WBAI. By making every hour and every premium different, I said, you will have a healthier station in the long term, because each hour will build its own audience, just as I did. When I started my show, no one was listening. I was on the dead hour. They put me on at noon because no one else wanted it.

So the short-term idea was to make money now. Program now for crisis. But there was no long-term plan to build a stronger, more viable station, meaning that you have to sacrifice immediately in order to have a strong future. That's what we do in almost every part of our society. We want it now; we don't want to sacrifice. We don't look at long-term planning. Then we wonder why we're fat, why we get a heart attack or stroke. These things happen because we look only at immediate satisfaction, at the short term.

We keep postponing fundamental changes to integrate our life, to get away from temporary, piecemeal solutions that don't work. It takes sacrifice and commitment to change your life, as well as to change society for the better. It means that you have to acknowledge what parts are falling away and pull them back into the integrated whole.

What influences your beliefs?

In the 1960s and 1970s, American youth seemed to question everything. The generation that came of age then believed that the system was corrupt and unethical. We believed that our mothers had given away their power. We believed that they were not being treated equally, and they were not. We believed that our fathers were keeping quiet on important social issues. They weren't speaking out against racism, sexism, and corporate greed. We were right about our parents—to an extent.

At the same time, our parents sacrificed everything for us. To give us a future, they gave up a lot of theirs. That's an enormous thing to do for someone. That kind of sacrifice takes a lot of love and commitment.

In contrast, our generation has sacrificed nothing. We've been the greediest bunch in history. We want it now, not tomorrow. We have to buy it, charge it, or steal it. We have no ethics. Individuals do, but as a group we have made and spent more money on ourselves than any other group in history. And we have less to show for it. Certainly there is less happiness. We have instantaneous pleasure, but no sustained joy. Nor is there any spiritual growth.

So, while our parents didn't have control over society, they at least had some control over their own lives. They lived well within their means, and they knew how to save.

Isn't it ironic that the people who didn't go into debt or bankrupt, didn't have to give up their homes and their Armani suits, were our parents? Today, many of them are living in Florida, Texas, or California, frequently retired on small savings and small pensions. They found their meaning in smaller issues than we did. We tackled the big issues. We started our idealistically. We wanted to share the wealth and save the world. But we forgot about that when we started getting rich. Then we didn't want to give the wealth to the poor. We thought if we could make it, so could they. We forgot about our liberal views and became self-absorbed. At first we had a sense of commitment to greater ideals, but one day we woke up and we didn't believe in a whole lot.

We didn't know how to use freedom in a responsible way. Many people's idea of freedom was to get high, be promiscuous, and drop out of everything for a while. We would get angry, but not use our anger constructively. Much of the time we turned it against our own parents. Imagine the misery we put our parents through by condemning them. We were insensitive and thoughtless. How do you think they must have felt knowing they did everything they could to raise us by the conventions they respected, only to have us condemn them?

We forget now. The wound is healed. Our parents are very giving in forgiving us. But I remember clearly that many people communicated with their parents only by denigrating them. That's why I stopped joining movements. I found that people in the health movement, the anti-war movement, and the vegetarian movement hated people in other groups who weren't like them. I would think, "What's the difference between you hating someone and them hating you? None. Hate's hate."

I started to take a look at the way we were brought up. I took a respite from everyone and everything by secluding myself. I became introspective because I wanted to understand how we ended up in the mess we are in. I didn't want to be a part of that mess. I didn't want to be a victim, like my parents. And I didn't want to be antagonistic, like my friends. I wanted to be part of a healing process. So I took a look at all that my family was: the best that it was and the worst that it was. And I saw that what they believed in that allowed them to feel whole or fragmented came from their families or what they had been taught. They believed in some things that made sense and some that did not.

But they didn't know how to separate what made sense from what didn't. It was all or nothing. "This is the way it is," they said. "This is the way we eat." "This is the way we live." So, it wasn't as if we had an aunt who was a vegetarian who said to eat some vegetarian food. It was meat and potatoes and that was it. Or if you went to church, everybody went to church. Maybe you didn't want to go to church, but everyone went to church on Sunday. You sat there and you tried not to be caught falling asleep. That's just the way it was. That's the way we lived. We didn't allow for relative expression. We were tolerant, but our tolerance still honored an obedience to society until we broke through—and then we weren't obedient to anything. The trouble was, we weren't free for something greater than that which we were opposing. We were merely in a vacuum. We were angry and we expressed it in different ways—some colorful, some creative, some sadistic. Everybody had a different way of showing what they were against.

Very few people had a way of constructively showing what they were for. Small groups were more idealistic. You'd find them in Esalin, Findhorne, or down at The Farm in Tennessee, or at some of the first co-op movements or women's health collectives. These were the more positive groups that took something from all the turmoil and built on it. But most people didn't build something new. Most went right back into that old belief system. They went right back into the old nonintegrated life.

Even many of the people in the so-called alternative movements of the time weren't integrated. They would eat vegetarian foods and then do drugs. Nor were they a part of the political process. A relatively small percentage of Americans protest against any political situation. At the height of the Vietnam War, for instance, only half a million people were out there protesting. So we had many Americans angry but not constructively seeking change. They were immersed in their own lives, and their own lives were all that mattered to them.

Even many of those who did protest soon went right back into the very society they loathed and became a part of it. So they didn't learn a lot from their experience. They became what they feared. They became their parents, but with an attitude.

Where does your anger originate?

Anger starts at the point where the real self gives up its identity and takes on a false identity, the persona, in order to exist. If your father wants you to be a tough little athlete, and you take on the mantle of your father's ego, you become terrified inside. You deny your terror and your fear. But there is anger behind those. As you get older, you continue to hold on to that anger. You are living other people's images of you and losing touch with who you really are. That creates anger.

Anger does not have to be a negative emotion. I feel anger can be dealt with constructively, nonviolently, by acknowledging it. By acknowledging the anger, you're acknowledging that the repression that was there hurt you. Just show your anger, bring it out, nonlethally, in a way that allows you to acknowledge, "Yes, I've held this inside. Now I'm through with it." What was the cause of it? Express the cause and let it go. When you can forgive, past anger no longer needs to be a companion to the present.

Denial has to end sometime.

There comes a time when you've got to have some courage, to stand up, to say, "I don't like what you are. What you are is not nice. You're a murderer, an anti-Semite, a racist. You represent everything that's deadly and bad about life. The facts that you mow your lawn and pay your taxes and go to church don't mean anything. Hitler petted his dog. So what? What are you? It's what you are and how you manifest it that count."

I don't have a lot of respect for people who pride themselves on being part of a collective consciousness. "I'm a Democrat," they say. "We vote Democratic every year." Why? Why not vote for what is right and who is right on each separate occasion? Why would I want the collective mind controlling my life, telling me what to believe in? No thank you. Do I want to be controlled by a person who believes in the basic four food groups and who won't go to see an alternative therapist because if the doctor says there's no chance, they'd rather die than be cured with alternative therapies? There are people who literally would rather die than deviate from what is expected by the accepted authorities. "The doctor might get mad if I try a different approach. I don't want to alienate the doctor." I see this all the time.

We live in a lethal time and it's becoming more lethal. That's all the more reason to accelerate your growth. You need to understand the crisis around you so that you don't become enmeshed in it. It's easy to become immobilized, demoralized. That's why I have respect for many people who are self-employed. I don't usually see them sitting around complaining about how bad things are. Rather, they go out and do something about it. They trust in themselves and their own abilities.

You see, I can spend all day blaming everyone else for why something doesn't work, or I can go out and try to change something to make it work, and make my life work. My life works because I make it. If my life doesn't work, it's because I make it not work. I can't live by influencing myself negatively and expect positive results. If I go into a championship race, I can't expect to win if I haven't trained as a champion. How can I expect to live a healthy life if I continue to eat some things that are healthy and others that are garbage? When I am honoring what I do, my actions become congruent with my expectations. When what you do is also what you expect, then you have a unity between spiritual self and conscious self.

I'm integrated with all life. Therefore, it wouldn't matter to me if you were a Muslim, or black, or white, or old or young, poor or rich, educated or not. Universalist thinkers are connected to everything. Everyone, everywhere, anyplace, anytime—they are in balance. You can't shake them. They're always in the rhythm of life. The universalist thinker is the person who doesn't engage in artificial conflict and blame. Just remember, when you start to blame, you've already taken the lower position.

When you give up denial, the only things you've got are positive. Let's look at a person who is forty-five years old and in a crisis. He hasn't achieved what he thought he should have at this point. Or what he has achieved in the past. He's now lost. That, by the way, is the case for a lot of Americans. Anyway, this person feels that at this point, he should be entitled to a home, land, a family, or something that gives him a sense of gratification. So he's unhappy about where he is in life. And he's in denial that he created that situation. He'd like to blame everyone else for being a part of his problem. IBM laid him off; they're to blame. But he should have known all along that IBM was in crisis. And he should have been re-educating yourself, going to night school, taking extra classes, learning a new vocation.

He was lazy, though. He would rather go home, watch television, and complain. He'd rather indulge in his pleasures. He didn't want to go through any more of that hard stuff. He didn't want to work through his comfort zone. His brain cells hadn't been to a class in a long time. He found it difficult to even read a book, and he was impatient with everything. He was quick to judge, and critical. That's all part of the process of denial.

When will you be ready for a true healthy change?

Ask most people if they want to get healthy and they'll say, "Sure I do. I don't want heart disease, arthritis, hemorrhoids, depression, cancer. I don't need that." Fair enough. But putting a time frame on when they'll begin to make the necessary changes is another thing.

About 98 percent of the people who listen to my radio show don't actualize what I talk about. I just finished a year-and-a-half hair study to help people grow new hair and reverse graying and thinning. Seven people who completed the protocol now have new, thick hair. In addition, their skin is less wrinkled, and they have overcome all kinds of illnesses. Although 140 enrolled in the study, only seven finished. That's only 5 percent. What happened to the other 95 percent? They were unwilling to follow through because they were not willing to make true changes.

What you say is immaterial if it doesn't match what you do. What you do tells me who you are. If what you do and what you say are the same, then you're in balance. But most people say they want to be healthy, yet they do unhealthy things. Well, if you do something that's immoral, then you're not moral. If you do something that's unhealthy, then you're not healthy. We've got to stop deceiving ourselves.

Over one third of the American population is chronically ill. And that's an understatement, because that figure is based on the assumption, which we mentioned earlier, that you're only ill after you've been diagnosed with a classically defined disease. That figure doesn't take into account the idea that you can be 80 percent unwell before the first symptoms manifest. It may take twenty years for a person to develop enough tumor cells to show up on an X ray or mammogram. At the time of the diagnosis, then, you're at the end stage of a healing crisis, not the beginning. Your arteries could be 90 percent occluded before you have symptoms of angina or some other condition. It might take forty years for an occlusion to get that bad. You're told it was caught early, when, in actuality, you got it at the end. So we've got another 100 million people walking around who are processing disease that is not yet diagnosed.

In addition, we have another 50 million people—bringing us up to 90 percent of the American population—who have the early stages of disease. These are our youth. Take 100 ten-year-olds at random and you will find that 50 percent of them already have some development of the diseases of old age. They already have the beginnings of coronary heart disease, arthritis, or loss of smell, sound, or taste, due to overstimulated lives. Think back—readers who are baby boomers and older—you didn't grow up exclusively on a junk-food diet. You probably had junk foods a couple of times a week, but not at every single meal. And you exercised. Many of today's children eat junk food at every meal. Many are almost totally sedentary. And they live in an overly excited, toxic environment. That's why their health is so much worse than the health of those of us who grew up in earlier times.

To put it in an economic perspective, 90 percent of the American population contributes to a $1.3 trillion disease budget. We're increasing our health care costs at almost 13 percent per year, and the greatest single increase in our gross national product is in medicine. The trouble is, we have little to show for it as far as cures go. Most of the improvement in the heart disease situation has been due to lifestyle improvements, not medical ones. The same goes for cancer. People are making changes in their habits that are helping them to prevent the disease.

Still, only a small percentage of the American population is making those kinds of changes. Are you part of that group? If you are, you know that you have to work on health as you have to work on disease. They're both processes based upon the choices we make.

If you're not, when will you change? You'll change when you lose it all, when you realize one day that you've made the wrong choices. Have there already been times when you changed because you lost everything? Perhaps you had warning signs along the way that what you were doing wasn't right, but you didn't pay attention. You had to hit bottom before you were forced to change. Then you did so grudgingly. "Okay, I guess I'll change," you said. But there's little energy in that. That's not the best motivation.

Act. Don't wait.

A person in my health support group, whom I'll call Jim, has changed. He finally started to unclutter his life. This came after twenty years of being around me. You can listen and just be on information overload and do nothing with the information, or you can do something about your intentions. I said, "Today you've got to change, Jim. I don't want you here for another twenty years doing nothing." So, he went out and cut his beard and cut his hair. Now Jim looks twenty years younger. He has started to clean up and organize his apartment and unclutter his life. He's started acting and stopped waiting.

Breaking old patterns of behavior takes courage. You have to stop thinking about everything else that's a distraction. Otherwise, you have a thousand exits along your path. You keep looking for the exits instead of going forward.

You've got to do something, not think about it. One evening of Jim making actual, physical changes was worth more than twenty years of coming to my talks. We're a society that overthinks. We're all waiting for someone to provide us with a perfect answer instead of looking for adequate answers ourselves and then acting. It's better to act on many ideas that ultimately don't work than to wait and wait for the one ideal answer to present itself. Everything is a learning process anyway. There is no perfect answer in life. Perfection does not exist anywhere in the universe; everything is imperfect. For instance, you want to be a part of a pastoral scene in the countryside where people collect wild flowers. Well, they're probably contracting Lyme disease at the same time. There's always something to mar the picture of perfection when we get close enough, but we never allow ourselves to see that. We intentionally blur the difference between what we need to see and what is actually there. Therefore, we can always dream about what we feel is perfect when it is not.

So Jim is now in the process of changing. He has taken the first step, and that gives him confidence to take the second step. Before, he was stepping in his mind, but he never actualized it. Now he is. He's moving forward.

When are you ready to learn?

When is the right time to learn? Right now. When do most people learn? Later. What happens between learning and being where you're at now? What's in between? Sameness. There's a familiarity with what you know. You don't know how you're going to feel about something new. If the new is different enough, you may have to make so many changes to accommodate the new knowledge that it's going to change everything you feel. There will be no certainty.

People spend their whole lives trying to guard against uncertainty. We insure ourselves against uncertainty. That's why we want only certain people in our lives, certain communities to live in. We want very predictable patterns of behavior from people. We don't want people saying anything that makes us feel uncomfortable. We exclude anyone who challenges us intellectually, emotionally, spiritually, sexually, nutritionally, and ecologically. We'll give them a name that discredits them, and thus excludes them from the dialogue. We'll call them extremists or we'll call them radicals, or pseudo-scientific. That immediately means we no longer have to engage with them. We can continue to engage only with people of a like mind. But what if people of a like mind have a mind that is locked into beliefs that are no longer beneficial to themselves or anyone else?

I grew up in a small town in West Virginia. I remember once going to the country club a friend's father owned. A group of people were sitting around playing cards, including local town doctors and a judge. I was sixteen years old, and I went over to them. I said to one man, "I don't understand something. You're all educated. Why are you still racist?" There was dead silence.

I used to do that kind of thing. I was the only person in my home town who held a strike to protest local corruption. I walked right around the high school one day with a little plaque saying, THIS

TOWN'S POLITICIANS ARE CORRUPT. I was told by everyone not to do this because it would embarrass people. But I did it anyhow. None of my friends would join in because their parents advised them not to. My dad said, "I hope you don't do it, but if you do, that's fine, too. But understand that once you do it, no one in this town will ever think the same of you." That did not seem like a negative to me. I've always been an idealist who protested corruption on any level.

After that incident, that seemed to be all people talked about for a year. Sometimes I wonder if any of those people, later in life, said, "Yes, I should have been there, too." The likelihood is, they'll spend their lives hiding behind the protective barriers of their conformist belief system, watching corruption, knowing it exists, and denying responsibility.

Those people still aren't willing to learn. When I went back for my high school reunion, I spoke with people I'd grown up with. Nothing had changed. They were still doing the same things over and over and over again. They ate the same foods, they wore the same clothes, they did the same things on Wednesday nights. Nothing had changed. I asked, "Why not?" "Well," they said, "we're kind of comfortable. We got what we want." They're disconnected from everything else.

When you really begin to learn, you connect with everything and everyone else. Suddenly a whole window opens up and you see people whom you never knew. When I was jogging through Riverside Park, I saw two people on a bench who were not quite sitting up; they seemed to be sleeping. I saw other joggers run by, oblivious, and I thought, "How could they not at least pay some attention to the fact that those are human beings?" Had they been white, upper-middle-class people sitting there, someone would have stopped and asked them what was wrong. But these were people from South America who simply didn't have any money. You could tell because their clothes were neatly folded and stacked. Their shoes were shined, and one of their shoes had a little plastic bag in it with a toothbrush and toothpaste. They were just surviving as best they could.

It's very easy in our society not to care about anyone but yourself. We're conditioned to do that. We're very moralistic, which I'm absolutely opposed to. I've never met a moralistic person who was a humane person. Moralistic people are self-righteous, mean-spirited, condescending, judgmental, and always establishing criteria that even Christ, Buddha, or Mohammed couldn't meet. Then they condemn you for not meeting these standards! What's lacking is humanistic value, compassion, sensitivity, and joy. Have you ever met a moralistic person who knows how to laugh?

Do you understand the value of surrender?

We must surrender the old in order to let in the new. But many people are too inflexible to understand this. Egotistical people, in particular, don't like to surrender. They use control as a way to measure their lives, their values, their worth, their position, and their power. Look at how many people in positions of power in corporate America and in government refuse to take responsibility for having harmed individuals. The Pentagon doesn't feel responsible for anything; nor does the White House. Nobody takes responsibility for anything in America. You never see a CEO standing up to say, "Yes, we did it wrong." And if they are proven guilty of some conspiracy, they will never come forward to apologize.

None of that allows you to grow. Whenever you're not willing to surrender, you're keeping yourself in the same place. You stay fragmented. If you're fragmented you're not integrated. If you're not integrated, you're not harmonized. Without harmony you open yourself up to chronic conflict and discontent.

We must surrender old beliefs and old patterns of behavior. We need to say, "This is how I used to think, act, and be. I'm letting this go." In effect, this is tantamount to a hero who takes a journey, embraces his fear, dies in the process, comes back, and is reborn with a new sense of awareness, a new sense of life. That's the process of surrender, and it is in the surrender that we gain.

PART VIII

AND IN CONCLUSION

18

THE VIEW FROM HERE

As I see it, the fight against aging has become an industry unto itself, crossing the lines between health and fitness; nutrition and exercise; traditional and alternative healing modalities. In fact, advances in anti-aging technology are being made at such a rapid pace that, by the time you read this book, the volume of new scientific research supporting this process will have doubled.

Historically, one of the dilemmas of either physician, nutritionist, or holistic nurse, the primary directors of this information and health care in this country, has been the lack of quality, scientific studies that could support an alternative healing modality. Orthodox practitioners would note that claims that vitamin C has an antiviral effect and ask, "Where's the proof?"

In response, people within the health movement—which, until relatively recently, generally meant the health-food store movement, would look to the advice of its leaders, such as Dr. Carlton Fredericks, Adele Davis, Paul Bragg, Linda Clark, Gaylord Hauser, Pablo Irola, and about fifteen other lesser-known pioneers in nutritional and other alternative healing modalities. They used the anecdotal evidence of these health movement pioneers to validate their claims, to which the traditionalists, who happen to represent the regulatory agencies controlling the practice and dissemination of information about these protocols, responded, "Where's your proof? Where're the data on your double-blind studies?"

The result of these challenges left the holistic health movement with a battle for acceptance, despite masses of evidence of healing successes. Standards of proof differed on either side of the healing sciences. While holistic or alternative practitioners could point to countless incidences of healing, or at least improved health and vitality, orthodox scientists demanded stringent reports from sterile, double-blind, placebo-controlled studies. We must remind these traditional scientists who are crying for laboratory reports and evaluations that there were no double-blind studies, for example, for coronary by-pass surgery.

And look at antibiotics, and influenza and emphysema. There is no double-blind control evidence that antibiotics cure either condition. Annually, 5 million people are given prescriptions for antibiotics for these diseases when, for approximately 33 percent of them, these medications are worthless. Influenza, for example, is viral in nature; antibiotics target bacteria.

Dr. Fredericks and his cohorts responded to challenges to their science by saying, "If we have a large number of people using a vegetarian diet, with lots of fiber and juicing, exercising and taking large amounts of broad-spectrum vitamins, why are we living longer? Why do we have less cancer?"

If anecdotal data is invalid, why is it that every time you go into a doctor's office, the first thing the physician asks is how you are feeling? Based on your response, the practitioner adjusts the medical procedure or course of treatment. In virtually every single case in medicine, input from the patient is essential in guiding the doctor in planning treatment. The practice of medicine *is* anecdotal.

It is not possible to do a double-blind, placebo-controlled study on every patient every time you see that patient. A health practitioner must trust that every patient knows what he or she is feeling. When a person sees an alternative physician and the doctor says, "I gave you 400 mg of St. John's wort for depression and bitter melon for your high titers—hepatitis. How are you feeling?" and the patient replies, "I feel much better. I don't have so many mood swings, and I have lots more stamina . . ." *that's* anecdotal medicine.

The difference is that orthodox Western medicine's anecdotes are accepted. The same case study, with the same results and conclusions, reported by a physician who employed alternative treatment, would be rejected. There is clearly a case of double standards. At the risk of sounding flippant, validation of evidence garnered in the course of creating viable health-care protocols—including those directed to reverse aging—boils down to whose anecdotes have the most impact, the most credibility.

Since 1849, when the American Medical Association wrested control of homeopathy, the prevailing health and healing climate has been medically based. Medical procedures and drug technology have superseded the power of the patient to participate in his own healing process. There would be room for only one voice to champion curing in the circle of knowledge in the twenty-first century, and that would be the proprietary process fostered by the drug culture of the medical technology innovators.

Nature, and the power of the individual to create or participate in his or her treatment, was not merely denied, it was denigrated. The ridicule heaped upon those who sought to prevent disease was based on bias, fear of loss of control, and the economic and political agendas of special-interest groups. Science/medicine became so orthodox that virtually nothing was offered in the way of prevention of disease and the promotion of wellness.

In the midst of this, we had a new phenomenon—iatrogenic, or drug- and doctor-induced illness and death. The numbers are staggering: more than half of the drugs prescribed, x-rays or tests taken, are defensively motivated strictly to protect the doctor from malpractice. Such overtesting, overmedicating, and overdiagnosing has resulted in a cottage industry, accounting for more than $500 million per year. The fraud in medicine is higher than organized crime, making doctors, hospitals—the medical industry—the number-one criminals in America today. Unnecessary procedures and medications often have side effects, making medical malpractice the number-one cause of death and disability.

When patients sought to take control of their healing process, or at least become equal partners, doctors went ballistic. The argument was given in the media and at the Food and Drug Administration and the American Medical Association that no one can dispense alternative health-care treatments as they are unproven and prevent people from getting *proven* treatment.

To this, I—and the new generation of health-care practitioners and consumers—ask: "What, pray tell, can you prove by double-blind placebo studies about which procedures will work better than a natural approach? You have no controlled studies for pertussis and tetanus procedures, or for anthrax and botulism vaccines that were given to our soldiers in the Gulf War, or in most surgeries, or, in fact, most of medicine that is traditionally practiced."

However, there *had* been a serious error in the generations of Dr. Fredericks and his successors. They had looked to validate alternative healing modalities by examining any work done in this field by the same standards employed to assess allopathic, or orthodox, medical procedures. This is an invalid measure. The two approaches are not comparable.

Alternative methods rely on the mind as the power in the healing process. This is backed up by studies in psychoneuroimmunology.

What I found was that we had missed the mother lode. There is incredible, overwhelming, *scientific* evidence to support alternative therapies, certainly in regard to nutrients and botanicals. It rests within orthodox *science,* but not within orthodox *medicine.* Therefore, we have taken a great deal of effort to collect and analyze over five thousand studies—from respected, recognized scientific journals that support the safety and efficacy of the nutrients listed in this book as part of the anti-aging protocols.

APPENDICES

APPENDICES

SPECIFIC APPLICATIONS OF VITAMINS, NUTRIENTS, AND HERBS

NOTE: Dosages are noted where useful and appropriate to the reader. In some instances, the dosage information is so similar to previously noted studies on the same condition that it has been left off to avoid repetition. In other instances, the dosage information stated was suited to laboratory conditions only and has been left out to avoid confusion.

ACETYL L-CARNITINE

Aging

Cipolli, C. and Chiari, G. 1990. [Effects of L-acetylcarnitine on mental deterioration in the aged: Initial results]. *Clin Ter,* 132 (6Suppl), Mar. 31, 479–510.
Dose: 1500 mg/day.

Salvioli, G. and Neri, M. 1994. L-acetylcarnitine treatment of mental decline in the elderly. *Drugs Exp Clin Res,* 20 (4), 169–176.
Dose: 1500 mg/day for 90 days.

Bella, R. et al. 1990. Effect of acetyl-L-carnitine on geriatric patients suffering from dysthymic disorders. *Int J Clin Pharmacol Res,* 10 (6), 355–360.
Dose: 3 gm/day for 30–60 days.

Passeri, M. et al. 1990. Acetyl-L-carnitine in the treatment of mildly demented elderly patients. *Int J Clin Pharmacol Res,* 101 (1–2), 75–79.
Dose: 2 gm/day for 3 months.

Franceschi, C. et al. 1990. Immunological parameters in aging: Studies on natural immunomodulatory substances. *Int J Clin Pharmacology Res,* 10 (1–2), 53–57.

Alcoholism

Tempesta, E. et al. 1990. Role of acetyl-L-carnitine in the treatment of cognitive deficit in chronic alcoholism. *Int J Clin Pharmacology Res,* 10 (1–2), 101–107.

Alzheimer's disease

Sano, M. et al. 1992. Double-blind parallel design pilot study of acetyl levo-carnitine in patients with Alzheimer's disease. *Arch Neurol,* 49 (11), Nov., 1137–1141.
Dose: 2.5 gm/day for 3 months.

Spagnoli, A. et al. 1991. Long-term acetyl-L-carnitine treatment in Alzheimer's disease. *Neurology,* 41 (11), Nov., 1726–1732.

Rai, G. et al. 1990. Double-blind, placebo controlled study of acetyl-L-carnitine in patients with Alzheimer's dementia. *Curr Med Res Opin,* 11 (10), 638–647.
Dose: 2 gm/day for 24 weeks.

Parnetti, L. et al. 1992. Pharmacokinetics of IV and oral acetyl-L-carnitine in a multiple dose regimen in patients with senile dementia of Alzheimer type. *European J Clin Pharmacology,* 42 (1), 89–93.

Pettegrew, J. W. et al. 1995. Clinical and neurochemical effects of acetyl-L-carnitine in Alzheimer's disease. *Neurobiol Aging,* 16 (1), Jan.–Feb., 1–4.

Amenorrhea

Genazzani, A. D. et al. 1991. Acetyl-L-carnitine as possible drug in the treatment of hypothalamic amenorrhea. *Acta Obstet Gynecol Scand,* 70 (6), 487–492.
Dose: 2 gm/day for 6 months.

Cardiovascular/Coronary heart disease

Adembri, C. et al. 1994. Ischemia-reperfusion of human skeletal muscle during aortoiliac surgery: Effects of acetylcarnitine. *Histol Histopathol,* 9 (4), Oct., 683–690.
Dose: 3 mg/day iv prior to surgery.

Dementia

Sinforiani, E. et al. 1990. Neuropsychological changes in demented patients treated with acetyl-L-carnitine. *Int J Clin Pharmacology Res,* 10 (1–2), 69–74.

Bonavita, E. 1986. Study of the efficacy and tolerability of L-acetylcarnitine therapy in the senile brain. *Int J Clin Pharmacol Ther Toxicol*, 24 (9), Sept., 511–516.
Dose: 1,000 mg/day.

Depression

Garzya, G. et al. 1990. Evaluation of the effects of L-acetylcarnitine on senile patients suffering from depression. *Drugs Exp Clin Res*, 16 (2), 101–16.
Dose: 1,500 mg/day.

Neurological function

Mezzina, C. et al. 1992. Idiopathic facial paralysis: New therapeutic prospects with acetyl-L-carnitine. *Int J Clin Pharmacology Res*, 12 (5–6), 299–304.
Dose: 3 gm/day for 14 days.

Mazzocchio, R. et al. 1990. Enhancement of recurrent inhibition by intravenous administration of L-acetylcarnitine in spastic patients. *J Neurol Neurosurg Psychiatry*, 53 (4), Apr., 321–326.

Parkinson's disease

Puca, F. M. et al. 1990. Clinical pharmodynamics of acetyl-L-carnitine in patients with Parkinson's disease. *Int J Clin Pharmacol Res*, 10 (1–2), 139–143.
Dose: 1 or 2 gm/day for 7 days.

Stroke

Arrigo, A. et al. 1990. Effects of acetyl-L-carnitine on reaction times in patients with cerebrovascular insufficiency. *Int J Clin Pharmacol Res*, 10 (1–2), 133–137.

Postiglione, A. et al. 1990. Cerebral blood flow in patients with chronic cerebrovascular disease: Effect of acetyl-L-carnitine. *Int J Clin Pharmacology Res*, 10 (1–2), 129–132.
Dose: 1.5 gm iv.

Rosadini, G. et al. 1990. Acute effects of acetyl-L-carnitine on regional cerebral blood flow in patients with brain ischaemia. *Int J Clin Pharmacol Res*, 10 (1–2), 123–128.
Dose: 1,500 mg iv.

Postiglione, A. et al. 1991. Effect of acute administration of L-acetyl carnitine on cerebral blood flow in patients with chronic cerebral infarct. *Pharmacology Res,* 23 (3), Apr., 241–246.
Dose: 1.5 gm iv.

ALOE

Cardiovascular/Coronary Heart Disease

Agarwal, O. P. 1985. Prevention of atheromaous heart disease. *Angiology,* 36 (8), Aug., 485–492.

Constipation

Odes, H. A. and Madar, Z. 1991. A double-blind trial of a celandin, Aloe vera and psyllium laxative preparation in adult patients with constipation. *Digestion,* 49 (2), 65–71.

Diabetes

Ghannam, N. et al. 1986. The antidiabetic activity of aloes: Preliminary clinical and experimental observations. *Hormone Res,* 24 (4), 288–294.
Dose: ¹/₂ tsp/day for 4–14 weeks.

Ghannam, N. et al. 1986. The antidiabetic activity of aloes. *Hormone Res,* 24, 288–294.
Dose: ¹/₂ tsp 4x/day for 14 weeks.

Skin Damage

Syed, T. A. et al. 1996. Management of psoriasis with aloe vera extract in a hydrophilic cream: A placebo-controlled, double-blind study. *Trop Med Int Health,* 1 (4), Aug., 505–509.
Dose: 0.5% aloe vera extract in a hydrophilic cream.

Wound Healing

Fulton Jr., J. E. The stimulation of postdermabrasion wound healing with stabilized aloe vera gel-polyethylene oxide dressing. *J Dermatol Surg Oncology,* 16 (5), May, 460–467.
Dose: stabilized aloe vera.

Visuthiokosol, V. et al. 1995. Effect of aloe vera gel to healing of burn wound: a clinical and histologic study. *J Med Assoc Thailand,* 78 (8), Aug., 403–409.
Dose: aloe vera gel.

ALPHA LIPOIC ACID

Diabetes

Kahler, W. et al. 1993. Diabetes Mellitus-A free radical-associated disease. Results of adjuvant supplementation. Z. *Gesante Inn Med,* 48 (5), May, 223–232.
Dose: 600 mg/day for 3 months.

Jacob, S. et al. 1995. Enhancement of glucose disposal in patients with type 2 diabetes by alpha-lipoic acid. *Arzneimittelforschung,* 45 (8), Aug., 872–874.
Dose: 1000 mg.

Ziegler, D. et al. 1995. Treatment of symptomatic diabetic peripheral neuropathy with anti-oxidant alpha-lipoic acid. A 3-week multicentre randomized controlled trial. *Diabetologia,* 38 (12), Dec., 1425–1433.
Dose: 600 mg/day over a 3 week period.

Klein, W. 1975. [Treatment of diabetic neuropathy with oral alpha-lipoic acid]. *MMW Munch Med Wochenschr,* 117 (22), May 30, 957–958.
Dose: 2x50 mg or 2x100 mg/day.

General

Barbirolli, B. et al. 1995. Lipoic (thiotic) acid increases brain energy availability and skeletal muscle performance as shown by an in vivo 31P-MRS in a patient with mitochondrial cytopathy. *J Neurology,* 242 (7), July, 472–477.
Dose: 600 mg/day for 1 month.

Glaucoma

Filina, A. A. et al. 1995. Lipoic acid as a means of metabolic therapy of open-angle glaucoma. *Vestn Oftalmol,* 111 (4), Oct.–Dec., 6–8.
Dose: 0.15 gm/day for 1 month.

APPLE PECTIN

Acute Intestinal Infections

Potievskii, E. G. et al. 1994. [Experimental and clinical studies of the effect of pectin on the causative agents of acute intestinal infections]. *Zh Mikrobiol Epidemiol Immunobiol,* Suppl 1, Aug., 106–109
Dose: 5% pectin solution.

Diarrhea

de la Motte, S. et al. 1997. [Double-blind comparison of an apple pectin-chamomile extract preparation with placebo in children with diarrhea]. *Arzneimittelforschung*, 47 (11), Nov., 1247–1249
Dose: apple pectin and chamomile.

Hypercholesterolemia

Biesenbach, G. et al. 1993. [The lipid lowering effect of a new guar-pectin fiber mixture in type II diabetic patients with hypercholesterolemia]. *Leber Magen Darm*, 23 (5), Sept., 204.
Dose: 1 package of 17 gm (with about 5.9 gm water-soluble fiber) dissolved in 250 ml water for the next 9 weeks: during the first 3 weeks 2 portions per day, the next 3 weeks twice ½ portion and the last 3 weeks one ½ portion daily. The fiber mixture had to be consumed 30 minutes before taking a main meal.

Pirich, C. et al. 1992. [Lowering cholesterol with Anticholest—a high fiber guar-apple pectin drink]. *Wien Klin Wochenschr*, 104 (11), 314–316.
Dose: (group 1) at dosages of 1 cup (17 gm) every second day, or (group 2) of 1 cup a day or (group 3) of 2 cups a day.

Hyperlipidemia

Grudeva-Popova, J. and Sirakova, I. 1998. Effect of pectin on some electrolytes and trace elements in patients with hyperlipoproteinemia. *Folia Med (Plovdiv)*, 40 (1), 41–45
Dose: 15 gm/day high-esterified pectin for 3 months.

Grudeva-Popova, J. et al. 1997. Application of soluble dietary fibres in treatment of hyperlipoproteinemias. *Folia Med (Plovdiv)*, 39 (1), 39–43.

Satiety

Tiwary, C. M. et al. 1997. Effect of pectin on satiety in healthy US Army adults. *J Am Coll Nutr*, 16 (5), Oct., 423–428
Dose: 5, 10, 15, 20g.

ARGININE

Cancer

Brittenden, J. et al. 1994. L-arginine stimulates host defenses in patients with breast cancer. *Surgery*, 115 (2), Feb., 205–212.
Dose: 30 gm/day for 3 days.

Cardiovascuar/Coronary heart disease

Rector, T. S. et al. 1996. Randomized, double-blind, placebo controlled study of supplemental oral L-arginine in patients with heart failure. *Circulation,* 93 (12), June 15, 2135–2141.

Dose: 5.6 to 12.6 gm/day over 6 weeks.

Koifman, B. et al. 1995. Improvement of cardiac performance by intravenous infusion of L-arginine in patients with moderate congestive heart failure. *J Am Coll Cardiol,* 26 (5), Nov. 1, 1251–1256.

Dose: 20 gm iv.

Clarkson, P. et al. 1996. Oral L-arginine improves endothelium-dependent dilation in hypercholesterolemic young adults. *J Clin Investigation,* 97 (8), Apr. 15, 1989–1994.

Dose: 7 gm 3x/day over 4 weeks.

McCaffrey, M. J. et al. 1995. Effect of L-arginine infusion on infants with persistent pulmonary hypertension on the newborn. *Biol Neonate,* 6794, 240–243.

Dose: 500 mg/kg infused over 30 minutes.

Hishikawa, K. et al. 1992. L-arginine as a antihypertensive agent. *J Cardiovascular Pharmacol,* 20 (suppl 12), S196–S197.

Kilbourn, R. G. et al. 1995. NG-methyl-L-arginine, an inhibitor of nitric oxide synthase, reverses interleukin-2-induced hypotension. *Crit Care Med,* 23 (6), June, 1018–1024.

Dose: 12 mg/kg followed by 4mg/kg every 4 hours.

General

Pittari, A. M. et al. 1993. Therapy with arginine chlorohydrate in children with short constitutional stature. *Minerva Pediatr,* 45 (1–2), Jan.–Feb., 61–65.

Dose: 4 gm/day.

Hepatitis

Rizzo, S. 1986. Clinical trial with arginine tidiacicate in symptomatic chronic persistent hepatitis. *Int J Clin Pharmacol Res,* 6 (3), 225–230.

Dose: 80 ml of 10% L-arginine HCL daily per os over 6 months.

Pain

Harima, A. et al. 1991. Analgesic effect of L-arginine in patients with persistent pain. *European Neuropsychopharmacol,* 1 (4), Dec., 529–533.

Dose: iv 10% solution, 300ml (30g)/patient over a 60–70 minute period.

Wound healimg

Lu, S. L. 1993. Effect of arginine supplementation on T-lymphocyte function in burn patients. *Chung Hua Cheng Hsing Shao Shang Wai Ko Tsa Chih,* 9 (5), Sept., 368–371.

B-COMPLEX

B₁

Alzheimer's disease

Mimori, Y. et al. 1966. Thiamine therapy in Alzheimer's disease. *Metab Brain Disease,* 11 (1), Mar., 89–94.
   Dose: 100 mg/day, 12 weeks.

Cardiovascular/Coronary Heart Disease

Shimon, I. et al. 1995. Improved left ventricular function after thiamine supplementation in patients with congestive heart failure receiving long-term Furosemide therapy. *Am J Med,* 98 (5), 485–490.
   Dose: 200 mg day.

Freye and Hartung, E. 1982. The potential use of thiamine in patients with cardiac insufficiency. *Acta Vitamino Enzymol,* 4 (4), 285–290.
   Dose: 50 mg/kg.

Epilepsy

Botez, M. I. et al. 1993. Thiamine and folate treatment of chronic epileptic patients: A controlled study with the Wechsler IQ scale. *Epilepsy Res,* 16 (2), Oct., 157–163.

Fatigue

Suzuki, M. and Itokawa, Y. 1996. Effects of thiamine supplementation on exercise-induced fatigue, *Metabolic Pr Brain Dis.,* 11 (1), Mar., 95–106.

Febrile Lymphadenopathy

Lonsdale, D. 1980. Recurrent febrile lymphadenopathy treated with large doses of vitamin B₁: Report of two cases. *Dev Pharmacol Ther.,* 1 (4), 254–264.

General

Meador, K. J. et al. 1993. Evidence for a clinical cholinergic effect of high-dose thiamine. *Ann Neurol,* 34 (5), Nov., 724–726.

Smidt, L. J. et al. 1991. Influence of thiamin supplementation on the health and general well-being of an elderly Irish population with marginal thiamin deficiency. *J Gereontology,* 46 (1), Jan., M16–22.
Dose: 10 mg/day.

Lactic Acidosis

Klein, G. et al. 1990. [Life-threatening lactic acidosis during total parenteral nutrition. Successful therapy with thiamine]. *Dtsch Med Wochenschr,* 115 (7), Feb., 254–256.
Dose: 400 mg.

Liver Disease

Hassan, R. et al. 1991. Effect of thiamine on glucose utilization in hepatic cirrhosis. *J Gastroenterology Hepatology,* 6 (1), Jan.–Feb., 59–60.
Dose: 50 mg/day for 30 days.

Rossouw, J. E. et al. 1978. Red blood cell transketolase activity and the effect of thiamine supplementation in patients with chronic liver disease. *Scandinavian J Gastroenterology,* 13 (2), 133–138.
Dose: 200 mg/day.

Seasonal Ataxia

Adamolekun, B. et al. 1994. A double-blind, placebo-controlled study of the efficacy of thiamine hydrochloride in a seasonal ataxia in Nigerians. *Neurology,* 44 (3 Pt 1), Mar., 549–551.

Surgical Stress

Vinogradov, V. V. et al. 1981. [Thiamine prevention of the corticosteroid reaction after surgery]. *Probl Endokrinol,* 27 (3), May–June, 11–16.
Dose: IV administration of 0.12 g one day and 1.5–2 hours prior to surgery.

B_2

Congenital Methaemoglobinaemia

Hirano, M. et al. 1981. Congenital methaemoglobinaemia due to NADH methaemoglobin reductase deficiency: Successful treatment with oral riboflavin. *British J Haematology,* 47 (3), Mar., 353–359.
Dose: 120 mg/day.

Depression

Bell, I. R. et al. 1992. Brief communication. Vitamin B_1, B_2, and B_6 augmentation of tricyclic antidepressant treatment in geriatric depression with cognitive dysfunction. *J Am Coll Nutr.*, 11 (2), Apr., 159–163.

Dose: 10 mg B_1, B_2 and B_6 each with antidepressants.

Migraine

Schoenen, J. et al. 1994. High-dose riboflavin as a prophylactic treatment of migraine: Results of an open pilot study. *Cephalalgia*, 14 (5), Oct., 328–329.

Dose: 400 mg for at least 3 months.

Sickle Cell Disease

Ajayi, O. A. et al. 1993. Clinical trial of riboflavin in sickle cell disease. *East African Med J*, 70 (7), 418–421.

Dose: 5 mg 2x/day for 8 weeks.

B_6

Anemia

Toriyama, T. et al. 1993. Effects of high-dose vitamin B_6 therapy on microcytic and hypochromic anemia in hemodialysis patients. *Nippon Jinzo Gakkai Shi*, 35 (8), Aug., 975–980.

Dose: 180 mg for 20 weeks.

Asthma

Collipp, P. J. et al. 1975. Pyridoxine treatment of childhood bronchial asthma. *Ann Allergy*, 35 (2), Aug., 93–97.

Dose: 200 mg/day.

Cardiovascular/Coronary Heart Disease

van den Berg, M. et al. 1994. Combined vitamin B_6 plus folic acid therapy in young patients with arteriosclerosis and hyperhomocysteinemia. *J Vascular Surg.*, 20 (6), Dec., 933–940.

Dose: 250 mg for 6 weeks.

Ellis, J. M. and McCully, K. S. 1995. Prevention of myocardial infarction by vitamin B_6. *Res Commun Mol Pathol Pharmac*, 89 (2), Aug., 208–220.

Carpal Tunnel Syndrome

Ellis, J. et al. 1979. Clinical results of a cross-over treatment with pyridoxine and placebo of the Carpal Tunnel Syndrome. *Am J Clin Nutr,* 32 (10), Oct., 2040–2046.
Dose: 100 mg/day.

Kasdan, M. L. and Janes, C. 1987. Carpal Tunnel Syndrome and vitamin B_6. *Plastic Reconstructive Surgery,* 79 (3), Mar., 456–462.
Dose: 100 mg/day.

Stransky, M. et al. 1989. Treatment of Carpal Tunnel Syndrome with vitamin B_6: A double-blind study. *Southern Med J,* 82 (7), July, 841–842.

Ellis, J. M. 1987. Treatment of Carpal Tunnel Syndrome with vitamin B_6. *Southern Med J,* 80 (7), July, 882–884.
Dose: 100 mg to 200 mg/day for 12 weeks.

Guzman, F. J. L. et al. 1989. Carpal Tunnel Syndrome and vitamin B_6. *Klin Wochenschr,* 67 (1), Jan. 4, 38–41.
Dose: 150 mg/day for 3 months.

Ellis, J. et al. 1981. Therapy with vitamin B_6 with and without surgery for treatment of patients having the Idiopathic Carpal Tunnel Syndrome. *Res Commun Pathol Pharmacol,* 33 (2), Aug., 331–344.

Diabetes

Bennink, H. J. and Schreurs, W. H. 1975. Improvement of oral glucose tolerance in gestational diabetes by pyridoxine. *Br Med J,* 3 (5974), 13–15.

Immune Function

Casciato, D. A. et al. 1984. Immunologic abnormalities in hemodialysis patients: Improvement after pyridoxine therapy. *Nephron,* 38 (1), 9–16.
Dose: 50 mg/day for 3–5 weeks.

Primary Hyperoxaluria

Milliner, D. S. et al. 1994. Results of long-term treatment with orthophosphate and pyridoxine in patients with primary hyperoxaluria. *NEJM,* 331 (23), Dec. 8, 1553–1558.

B_{12}

Anemia

Samson, D. et al. 1977. Reversal of ineffective erythropoiesis in pernicious anaemia following vitamin B_{12} therapy. *Br J Haematology,* 35 (2), Feb., 217–224.

Kafetz, K. 1985. Immunoglobulin deficiency responding to vitamin B_{12} in two elderly patients with megaloblastic anemia. *Postgrad Med J,* 61 (722), Dec., 1065–1056.

Kubota, K. et al. 1987. Restoration of decreased suppressor cells by vitamin B_{12} therapy in a patient with pernicious anemia. *Am J Hematol,* 24 (2), Feb., 221–223.

Kubota, K. et al. 1992. Restoration of abnormally high CD4/CD8 ratio and low natural killer cell activity by vitamin B_{12} therapy in a patient with post-gastrectomy megaloblastic anemia. *Internal Med,* 31 (1), Jan., 125–126.

Aphthae

Wray, D. et al. 1975. Recurrent aphthae: Treatment with vitamin B_{12}, folic acid, and iron. *British Med J,* 2 (5969), May 31, 490–493.

Bronchial Squamous Metaplasia

Heimburger, D. C. et al. 1988. Improvement in bronchial squamous meta-plasia in smokers treated with folate and vitamin B_{12}. Report of a pre-liminary randomized, double-blind intervention trial. *JAMA,* 259 (10), Mar. 11, 1525–1530.
Dose: 500 mcg for 4 months.

Dementia

Regland, B. et al. 1991. Vitamin B_{12}-induced reduction of platelet mono-amine oxidase activity in patients with dementia and pernicious anae-mia. *Eur Arch Psychiatry Clin Neurosci,* 240 (4–5), 288–291.

General

Newbold, H. L. 1989. Vitamin B_{12}: Placebo or neglected therapeutic tool? *Med Hypothesis,* 28 (3), May, 155–164.

Hepatitis

Iwarson, S. and Lindberg, J. 1977. Coenzyme-B_{12} therapy in acute viral hepatitis. *Scandinavian J Infectious Dis,* 9 (2), 157–158.

Komar, I. V. 1982. [Use of vitamin B_{12} in the combined therapy of viral hepatitis]. *Vopr Pitan,* (1), Feb., 26–29.
Dose: 100 mcg every other day.

Imerslund-Grasbeck Syndrome

Salameh, M. M. et al. 1991. Reversal of severe neurological abnormalities after vitamin B_{12} replacement in the Imerslund-Grasbeck Syndrome. *J Neurology,* 238 (6), Sept., 349–350.

Methylmalonic Acidemia

Gordon, B. A. and Carson, R. A. 1976. Methylmalonic acidemia controlled with oral administration of vitamin B_{12}. *Canadian Med Assoc J,* 115 (3), Aug. 7, 233–236.

Dose: Continuous intramuscular supplements in doses of 1 mg on alternate days followed by 15 mg/day taken orally.

Multiple Sclerosis

Kira, J. et al. 1994. Vitamin B_{12} metabolism and massive-dose methyl vitamin B_{12} therapy in Japanese patients with multiple sclerosis. *Internal Med,* 33 (2), Feb., 82–86.

Dose: 60 mg/day for 6 months.

Sleep

Honma, K. et al. 1992. Effects of vitamin B_{12} on plasma melatonin rhythm in humans: Increased light sensitivity phase-advances the Circadian Clock? *Experentia,* 48 (4), Aug. 15, 716–720.

Dose: 3 mg/day.

Ohta, T. et al. 1991. Treatment of persistent sleep-wake schedule disorders in adolescents with methylcobalamin (vitamin B_{12}). *Sleep,* 14 (5), Oct., 414–418.

Dose: 3,000 mcg/day.

Okawa, M. et al. 1990. Vitamin B_{12} treatment for sleep-wake rhythm disorders. *Sleep,* 13 (1), Feb., 15–23.

Dose: 1.5 mg /day tid.

Vitiligo

Montes, L. F. et al. 1992. Folic acid and vitamin B_{12} in vitiligo: A nutritional approach. *Cutis* 50, (1), July, 39–42.

BEE POLLEN

Climacteric Symptoms

Szanto, E. et al. 1994. [Placebo-controlled study of melbrosia in treatment of climacteric symptoms]. *Wien Med Wochenschr,* 144 (7), 130–133.

Memory Function

Iversen, T. et al. 1997. The effect of Nao Li Su on memory functions and blood chemistry in elderly people. *J Ethnopharmacol*, 56 (2), Apr., 109–116.

Sclerosis

Iarosh, A. A. 1990. [Changes in the immunological reactivity of patients with disseminated sclerosis treated by prednisolone and the preparation *Proper-Myl*].

Syringomyelia

Ludianskii, E. A. 1991. [The use of apiotherapy and radon baths in treating syringomyelia]. *Zh Nevropatol Psikhiatr Im S Korsakova*, 91 (3), 102–103.

CALCIUM

Calcium Pancreatitis

Kaur, N. et al. 1996. Chronic calcific pancreatitis associated with osteomalacia and secondary hyperparathyroidism. *Indian J Gastroenterology*, 15 (4), Oct., 147–148.

Calcium absorption

Harvey, J. A. et al. 1990. Superior calcium absorption from calcium citrate than calcium carbonate using external forearm counting. *J Am Coll Nutr*, 9 (6), Dec., 583–587.

Cancer

Duris, I. et al. Calcium chemoprevention in colorectal cancer. *Hepatogastroenterology*, 43 (7), Jan.–Feb., 152–154.

Dental health

Gupta, S. K. et al. 1994. Reversal of clinical and dental fluorosis. *Indian Pediatr*, Apr., 439–443.
  Dose: 250 mg/day for 44 days.

Hip fracture

Meunier, P. 1996. Prevention of hip fractures by correcting calcium and Vitamin D insufficiencies in elderly people. *Scand J Rheumatology,* 103 (Suppl), 75–78.

Dose: 1.2 gm/day for a 3 year study.

Hypertension

Wimalawansa, S. J. 1993. Antihypertensive effects of oral calcium supplementation may be mediated through the potent vasodilator CGRP. *Am J Hypertension,* 6 (12), Dec., 996–1002.

Dose: 1.4 gm/day.

Osteoporosis

Adachi, J. D. et al. 1996. Vitamin D and calcium in the prevention of corticosteroid induced osteoporosis: A 3-year follow-up. *J Rheumatology,* 23 (6), June, 995–1000.

Dose: 1000 mg/day.

Leyes-Vence, M. et al. 1996. Transient osteoporosis of the hip. Presentation of a case and literature review. *Acta Orthop Belg,* 62 (1), Mar., 56–59.

Prince, R. et al. 1995. The effects of calcium supplementation (milk powder of tablets) and exercise on bone density in postmodern women. *J Bone Mineral Res,* 10 (7), July, 1068–1075.

Dose: 1 gm/night over a period of 2 years.

Haines, C. J. et al. 1995. Calcium supplementation and bone mineral density in postmenopausal women using estrogen replacement therapy. *Bone,* 16 (5), May, 529–531.

Warady, B. D. 1994. Effects of nutritional supplementation and bone mineral status of children with Rheumatic diseases receiving corticosteroid therapy. *J Rheumatology,* 21 (3), Mar., 530–535.

Vestibulitis

Solomons, C. C. et al. 1991. Calcium citrate of vulvar vestibulitis. A case report. *J Reproductive Med,* 36 (12), Dec., 879–882.

CHOLINE/LECITHIN

Head Injury

Levin, H. S. 1991. Treatment of postconcussional symptoms with CDP-choline. *J Neurol Sci,* 103 Suppl, July, S39–S42.

Dose: 1 gm of CDP-choline.

Maldonado, V. C. et al. 1991. Effects of CDP-choline on the recovery of patients with head injury. *J. Neurol Sci,* 103 Suppl, July, S15–S18.

Hemiplegia

Hazama, T. et al. 1980. Evaluation of the effect of CDP-choline on post-stroke hemiplegia employing a double-blind controlled trial. Assessed by a rating scale for recovery in hemiplegia. *Int J Neurosci,* 11 (3), 211–215.
Dose: ranging from 250–1000 mg over an 8 week period.

Hepatic Steatosis

Buchman, A. L. et al. 1995. Choline deficiency: A cause of hepatic steatosis during parenteral nutrition that can be reversed with intravenous choline supplementation. *Hepatology,* 22 (5), Nov., 1399–1403.
Dose: 1–4 g choline chloride over a period of 4 weeks.

Neurological Function

Fernandez, R. L. 1983. Efficacy and safety of oral CDP-choline. Drug surveillance study in 2817 cases. *Arzeimittelforschung,* 33 (7A), 1073–1080.
Dose: 6 ml/day mean dose of CDP-choline.

Seizures

McNamara, J. O. et al. 1980. Effects of oral choline on human complex partial seizures. *Neurology,* 30 (12), 1334–1336.
Dose: 12–16 g/day.

Stroke

Tazaki, Y. et al. 1988. Treatment of acute cerebral infarction with a choline precursor in a multicenter double-blind placebo-controlled study. *Stroke,* 19 (2), Feb., 211–216.
Dose: 1000 mg iv CDP-choline/day for 14 days.

Tardive Dyskinesia

Gelenberg, A. J. et al. 1979. Choline and lecithin in the treatment of tardive dyskinesia: Preliminary results from a pilot study. *Am J Psychiatry,* 136 (6), June, 772–776.

Growdon, H. et al. 1977. Oral choline administration to patients with tardive dyskinesia. *NEJM* 297 (10), Sept. 8, 524–527.

Arranz, J. and Ganoza, G. 1983. Treatment of chronic dyskinesia with CDP-choline. *Arzneimittelforschung,* 33 (&a), 1071–1073.

Dose: 500–1200 mg CDP-choline/day.

Nasrallah, H. A. et al. 1984. Variable clinical response to choline in tardive dyskinesia. *Psychol Med,* 14 (3), Aug., 697–700.

CHRYSANTHEMUM

Yu, X. Y. 1993. [A prospective clinical study on reversion of 200 precancerous patients with hua-sheng-ping]. *Chung Kuo Chung Hsi I Chieh Ho Tsa Chih,* 13 (3) Mar., 147–149.

Zhou, Y. L. 1987. [Chrysanthemum morifolium in the treatment of hypertension]. *Chung Hsi I Chieh Ho Tsa Chih,* 7 (1) Jan., 18–20.

COENZYME Q_{10}

Cancer

Lockwood, K. et al. 1995. Progress therapy on breast cancer with vitamin Q_{10} and the regression of metastases. *Biochem Biophys Res Commun,* 212 (1), July 6, 172–177.

Dose: 390 mg/day for 3–5 years.

Lockwood, K. et al. 1994. Partial and complete regression of breast cancer in patients in relation to dosage of Coenzyme Q_{10}, *Biochem Biophys Res Commun,* 199 (3), Mar. 30, 1504–1508.

Dose: 390 mg/day after 1 month tumor no longer palpable, after 2 months mammagrophy indicated no tumor.

Tsubaki, K. et al. 1984. [Investigation of the preventive effect of CoQ_{10} against the side effects of anthracycline antineoplastic agents], *Gan To Kagaku Ryoho,* 11 (7) July, 1420–1427.

Dose: 1 mg/kg/day iv.

Okuma, K. et al. 1983. [Protective effect of Coenzyme Q_{10} in cardiotoxicity induced by adriamycin], *Gan To Kagaku Ryoho,* 11 (3), Mar., 502–508.

Cardiovascular/Coronary heart disease

Kamikawa, T. et al. 1985. Effects of Coenzyme Q_{10} on exercise tolerance in chronic stable angina pectoris. *Am J Cardiology,* 56 (4), Aug. 1, 1985, 247–251.

Dose: 150 mg/day for 4 weeks.

Tanaka, J. et al. 1983. Coenzyme Q_{10}: The prophylactic effect on low cardiac output following cardiac valve replacement. *Annals Thoracic Surg.*, 33 (2), Feb., 145–151.
Dose: 30–60 mg/day orally for 6 days.

Chello, M. et al. 1994. Protection by Coenzyme Q_{10} from myocardial reperfusion injury during coronary artery bypass grafting. *Annals Thoracic Surg.*, 58 (5), Nov., 1427–1432.
Dose: 150 mg/day for 7 days before surgery.

Chen, Y. F. et al. 1994. Effectiveness of Coenzyme Q_{10} in myocardial preservation during hypothermic cardioplegic arrest. *J Thoracic Cardiovascular Surg.*, 107 (1), Jan., 242–247.

Greenberg, S. M. and Frishman, W. H. 1988. Coenzyme Q_{10}: A new drug for myocardial ischemia? *Med Clin North America*, 72 (1), Jan., 243–258.

Nishikawa, Y. et al. 1989. Long-term Coenzyme Q_{10} therapy for a mitochondrial encephalomyopathy with cytochrome C oxidase deficiency: A 31P NMR study. *Neurology*, 39 (3), Mar., 399–403.

Ogasahara, S. et al. 1985. Improvement of abnormal pyruvate metabolism and cardia conduction defect with Coenzyme Q_{10} in Kearns-Sayre syndrome, *Neurology*, 35 (3), Mar., 372–373.
Dose: 60–120 mg/day for 3 months.

Folkers, K. et al. 1992. Therapy with Coenzyme Q_{10} of patients in heart failure who are eligible or ineligible for a transplant. *Biochem Biophys Res Commun*, 182 (1) Jan. 15, 247–253.

Sunamori, M. et al. 1991. Clinical experience of Coenzyme Q_{10} to enhance intraoperative myocardial protection in coronary artery revascularization, *Cardiovasc Drugs Ther*, 5 Suppl 2, Mar., 297–300.
Dose: pretreatment with 5mg/kg iv.

Baggio, E. et al. 1993. Italian multicenter study of the safety and efficacy of Coenzyme Q_{10} as adjunctive therapy in heart failure (interim analysis). The CoQ_{10} drug surveillance investigators. *Clin Investigations*, 71 (8 Suppl), S145–149.
Dose: 50–100 mg/day for 3 months.

Langsjoen, P. H. et al. 1993. Isolated diastolic dysfunction of the myocardium and its response to CoQ_{10} treatment. *Clin Investigations*, 71 (8 Suppl), S140–144.

Morisco, C. et al. 1993. Effect of Coenzyme Q_{10} therapy in patients with congestive heart failure: A long-term multicenter randomized study. *Clin Investigations,* 71 (8 Suppl), S134–146.
Dose: 2 mg/kg/day for 1 year.

Lampertico, M. and Conis, S. 1993. Italian multicenter study on the efficacy and safety of Coenzyme Q_{10} as adjuvant therapy in heart failure. *Clin Investigations,* 71 (8 Suppl), S129–S133.
Dose: 50 mg/day for 4 weeks.

Mortensen, S. A. 1993. Perspectives on therapy of cardiovascular diseases with Coenzyme Q_{10} (Ubiquinonq). *Clin Investigations,* 71 (8 Suppl), S116–S123.

Mortensen, S. A. et al. 1985. Long-term Coenzyme Q_{10} therapy: A major advance in the management of resistant myocardial failure. *Drugs Exp Clin Res,* 11 (8), 581–593.
Dose: 100 mg/day.

Langsjoen. P. H. et al. 1985. Effective treatment with Coenzyme Q_{10} of patients with chronic myocardial disease. *Drugs Exp Clin Res,* 11 (8), 577–579.

Oda, T. 1985. Effect of Coenzyme Q_{10} on stress-induced cardiac dysfunction in paediatric patients with mitral valve prolapse: A study by stress echocardiography. *Drugs Exp Clin Res,* 11 (8), 557–576.
Dose: 3–3.4 mg/day.

Suzuki, H. et al. 1984. Cardiac performance and Coenzyme Q_{10} levels in thyroid disorders. *Endocrinol Japan,* 31 (6), Dec., 755–761.

Kato, T. et al. 1990. Reduction in blood viscosity by treatment with Coenzyme Q_{10} in patients with ischemic heart disease. *Int J Clin Pharmacol Ther Toxicol,* 28 (3), Mar., 123–126.
Dose: 60 mg/day for 2 months.

Manzoli, U. et al. 1990. Coenzyme Q_{10} in dilated cardiomyopathy. *Int J Tissue React,* 12 (3), 173–178.
Dose: 100 mg/day orally.

Langsjoen, P. H. et al. 1990. A six-year clinical study of therapy of cardiomyopathy with Coenzyme Q_{10}. *Int J Tissue React,* 12 (3), 168–171.

Langsjoen, P. H. et al. 1990. Pronounced increase of survival of patients with cardiomyopathy when treated with Coenzyme Q_{10} and conventional therapy. *Int J Tissue React,* 12 (3), 163–168.

Diabetes

Suzuki, Y. et al. 1995. A case of Diabetic amyotrophy associated with 3243 mitochondrial tRNA (leu: UUR) Mutation and successful therapy with Coenzyme Q_{10}, *Endocr J*, 42 (2), Apr., 141–145.

Immune enhancement

Folkers, K. et al. 1993. The activities of Coenzyme Q_{10} and vitamin B_6 for immune responses. *Biochem Biophys Res Commun*, 193 (1), May 28, 88–92.

Lung disease

Fujimoto, S. et al. 1993. Effects of Coenzyme Q_{10} administration on pulmonary function and exercise performance in patients with chronic lung diseases. *Clin Investigations*, 71 (8 Suppl), S126–S166.
Dose: 90 mg/day for 8 weeks.

Muscular Injury

Folkers, K. and Simonsen, R. 1995. Two successful double-blind trials with Coenzyme Q_{10} (vitamin Q_{10}) on muscular dystrophies and neurogenic atrophies. *Biochim Biophys Acta*, 127 (1), May 24, 281–286.

CRUCIFEROUS VEGETABLES

Cancer

Yuan, J. M. et al. 1998. Cruciferous vegetables in relation to renal cell carcinoma. *Int J Cancer*, 77 (2), Jul. 17, 211–216.

Rosen, C. A. 1998. Preliminary results of the use of indole-3-carbinol for recurrent respiratory papillomatosis. *Otolaryngol Head Neck Surg*, 118 (6), Jun., 810–815.
Dose: oral indole-3-carbinol and had a minimum follow-up of 8 months and a mean follow-up of 14.6 months.

DeMarini, D. M. et al. 1997. Pilot study of free and conjugated urinary mutagenicity during consumption of pan-fried meats: possible modulation by cruciferous vegetables, glutathione S-transferase-M1, and N-acetyltransferase-2. *Mutat Res*, 381 (1), Nov. 19, 83–96.
Dose: Ingestion of cruciferous vegetables.

Witte, J. S. et al. 1996. Relation of vegetable, fruit, and grain consumption to colorectal adenomatous polyps. *Am J Epidemiol*, 144 (11), Dec. 1, 1015–1025.

Steinmetz, K. A. and Potter, J. D. 1996. Vegetables, fruit, and cancer prevention: a review. *J Am Diet Assoc*, 96 (10), Oct., 1027–1039.

General

Michnovicz, J. J. et al. 1997. Changes in levels of urinary estrogen metabolites after oral indole-3-carbinol treatment in humans. *J Natl Cancer Inst*, 89 (10), May 21, 718–723.

Dose: Oral ingestion of I3C (6–7 mg/kg/day). Men received for 1 week, women received for 2 months.

Chen, L. et al. 1996. Decrease of plasma and urinary oxidative metabolites of acetaminophen after consumption of watercress by human volunteers. *Clin Pharmacol Ther*, 60 (6), Dec., 651–660.

Dose: Watercress homogenates (50 gm).

Smokers

Taioli, E. et al. 1997. Effects of indole-3-carbinol on the metabolism of 4-(methylnitrosamino)-1-(3-pyridyl)-1-butanone in smokers. *Cancer Epidemiol Biomarkers Prev*, 6 (7), Jul., 517–522.

Dose: 400 mg of I3C on 5 consecutive days and maintained constant smoking habits during this period.

CURCUMINE (TURMERIC)

Anti-inflammatory Effects

Satoskar, R. R. et al. 1986. Evaluation of anti-inflammatory property of curcumin (Diferuloyl Methane) in patients with postoperative inflammation. *Int J Clin Pharmacol Ther Toxicol*, 24 (12), Dec., 651–654.

Cancer

Polasa, K. et al. 1992. Effect of turmeric on urinary mutagens in smokers. *Mutagenesis*, 7 (2), Mar., 107–109.

Kuttan, R. et al. 1987. Turmeric and curcumin as topical agents in cancer therapy. *Tumori*, 73 (1), Feb. 28, 29–31.

Cariovascular/Coronary Heart Disease

Soni, K. B. and Kuttan, R. 1992. Effect of oral curcumin administration on serum peroxides and cholesterol levels in human volunteers. *Indian J Physiol Pharmacol*, 36 (4), Oct., 273–275.

Dose: 500 mg/day for 7 days.

DANDELION ROOT

Chronic Colitis

Chakurski, I. et al. 1981. [Treatment of chronic colitis with an herbal combination of *Taraxacum officinale*, Hipericum perforatum, Melissa officinaliss, Calendula officinalis and Foeniculum vulgare]. *Vutr Boles*, 20 (6), 51–54.

DHEA

Aging

Yen, S. S. et al. 1995. Replacement of DHEA in aging men and women. Potential remedial effects. *Ann NY Acad Sci*, 774, Dec. 29, 128–142.

Alzheimer's disease

Yanase, T. et al. 1996. Serum dehyfroepiandrosterone (DHEA) and DHEA-sulfate (DHEA-S) in Alzheimer's disease and in cerebrovascular dementia. *Endocr J*, 43 (1), Feb., 119–123.

Cognitive function

Friess, E. et al. 1995. DHEA administration increases rapid eye movement sleep and EEG power in the Sigma frequency range. *Am J Physiol*, 268 (1 Pt 1), Jan., E107–13.

Dose: 500 mg oral dose.

Depression

Wolkowitz, O. M. et al. 1997. Dehydroepiandrosterone (DHEA) treatment of depression. *Biol Psychiatry*, 41 (3), Feb. 1, 311–318.

Dose: 30–90 mg/day for 4 weeks.

General

Khorram, O. 1996. DHEA: A hormone with multiple effects. *Curr Opin Obstet Gynecol,* 8 (5), Oct., 351–354.

Lupus

Van Vollenhoven, R. F. and McGuire, J. L. 1996. Studies of dehydroepiandrosterone (DHEA) as a therapeutic agent in systemic lupus erythematosus. *Ann Med Interne,* 147 (4), 290–296.

DMAE

Hemiballismus-hemichorea

Jameson, H. D. et al. 1977. Hemiballismus-hemichorea treated with dimethylaminoethanol. *Dis Nerv Syst,* 38 (11), Nov., 931–932.

EVENING PRIMROSE OIL

Arthritis

Jantti, J. et al. 1989. Evening primrose oil in rheumatoid arthritis: Changes in serum lipids and fatty acids. *Ann Rheum Disease,* 48 (2), Feb., 124–127.
Dose: 20 ml evening primrose oil (EPO) containing 9% of gamma-linolenic acid for 12 weeks.

Brzeski, M. et al. 1991. Evening primrose oil in patients with rheumatoid arthritis and side-effects of non-steroidal anti-inflammatory drugs. *British J Rheumatology,* 30 (5), Oct., 370–372.
Dose: 6 gm/day.

Eczema

Schlin-Karrila, M. et al. Evening primrose oil in the treatment of atopic eczema: Effect on clinical status, plasma phospholipid fatty acids and circulating blood prostaglandins. *British J Dermatology,* 117 (1), July, 11–19.

Biagi, P. L. et al. 1988. A long-term study on the use of evening primrose oil (Efamol) in atopic children. *Drugs Exp Clin Res,* 14 (4), 285–290.

Diabetes

Uccella, R. et al. [Action of evening primrose oil on cardiovascular risk factors in insulin-dependent diabetics]. *Clin Ter,* 129 (5), June 15, 381–388.
Dose: 3 gm/day.

Takahashi, R. et al. 1993. Evening primrose oil and fish oil in non-insulin-dependent diabetes. *Prostaglandins Leukot Essent Fatt Acids,* 49 (2), Aug., 569–571.

Dose: 4 gm/day for 4 weeks.

FOLIC ACID

Anemia

Raphael, J. C. et al. 1975. [Myelopathy and macrocytic anemia associated with a folate deficiency. Cure by folic acid]. *Ann Med Interne,* 126 (5), May, 339–348.

Arthritis

Morgan, S. L. et al. 1994. Supplementation with folic acid during methotrexate therapy for rheumatoid arthritis. A double-blind, placebo-controlled trial. *Annals Intern Med,* 121 (11), Dec. 1, 833–841.

Dose: 5 mg or 27.5 mg at weekly doses.

Morgan, S. L. et al. 1990. The effect of folic acid supplementation on the toxicity of low dose methotrexate in patients with rheumatoid arthritis. *Arthritis Rheum,* 33 (1), Jan., 9–18.

Dose: 1 mg folic acid/day.

Flynn, M. A. et al. 1994. The effect of folate and cobalamin on osteoarthritic hands. *J American Colle Nutr,* 13 (4), Aug., 351–356.

Dose: 6400 mcg folate/day.

Cancer

Saito, M. et al. 1994. Chemoprevention effects on bronchial squamous metaplasia by folate and vitamin B_{12} in heavy smokers. *Chest,* 106 (2), Aug., 496–499.

Jennings, E. 1995. Folic acid as a cancer-preventing agent. *Med Hypotheses,* 45 (3), Sept., 297–303.

Cardiovascular/Coronary Heart Disease

Landgren, F. et al. 1995. Plasma homocysteine in acute myocardial infarction: Homocysteine-lowering effect of folic acid. *J Intern Med,* 237 (4), Apr., 381–388.

Dose: 2.5 mg or 10mg over a 6 week period.

van den Berg, M. et al. 1994. Combined vitamin B$_6$ plus folic acid therapy in young patients with arteriosclerosis and hyperhomocysteinemia. *J Vascular Surgery,* 20 (6), Dec., 933–940.

Dose: 5 mg folic acid/day.

Morrison, H. I. et al. 1996. Serum folate and risk of fatal coronary heart disease. *JAMA,* 275 (24), June 26, 1893–1896.

Wilcken, D. E. et al. 1988. Folic acid lowers elevated plasma homocysteine in chronic renal insufficiency: Possible implications for prevention of vascular disease. *Metabolism,* 37 (7), July, 697–701.

Dose: 5 mg folic acid/day for average of 15 days.

Arnadottir, M. et al. 1993. The effect of high-dose pyridoxine and folic acid supplementation on serum lipid and plasma homocysteine concentrations in dialysis patients. *Clinical J Nephrol,* 40 (4), Oct., 236–240.

Dose: 5 mg/day.

Cervical Dysplasia

Butterworth, Jr. C. E. 1982. Improvement of cervical dysplasia associated with folic acid therapy in users of oral contraceptives. *Am J Clin Nutr,* 35 (1), Jan., 73–82.

Dose: 10 mg folic acid/day for 3 months.

Fragile X Syndrome

Brown, W. T. et al. Folic acid therapy in the Fragile X Syndrome. *Am. J Med Genetics,* 17 (1), Jan., 289–297.

Hagerman, R. J. et al. 1986. Oral folic acid versus placebo in the treatment of males with the Fragile X Syndrome. *Am. J Med Genetics,* 23 (1–2), Jan.–Feb., 241–262.

Dose: 10 mg/day.

Lejeune, J. et al. 1984. [Trial of folic acid treatment in Fragile X Syndrome]. *Ann Genet,* 27 (4), 230–232.

Dose: 0.5 mg/kg per day of folic acid.

Gingival Health

Vogel, R. I. et al. 1976. The effect of folic acid on gingival health. *J Periodontology,* 47 (11), Nov., 667–668.

Dose: 4 mg/day for 30 days.

Homocystinuria

Takenaka, T. et al. 1993. [Effect of folic acid for treatment of homocystinuria due to 5,10-methylenetetrahydrofolate reductase deficiency]. *Rinsho Shinkeigaku,* 33 (11), Nov., 1140–1145.

Dose: 400 mcg/day of folic acid over approx 70 days.

Kidney Damage

Chauveau, P. et al. 1996. Long-term folic acid (but not pyridoxine) supplementation lowers elevated plasma homocysteine level in chronic renal failure. *Miner Electrolyte Metab,* 22 (1–3), 106–109.

Dose: 10 mg/day folate for 3 months.

Lithium Prophylaxis

Coppen, A. et al. 1986. Folic acid enhances lithium prophylaxis. *J Affective Disorders,* 10 (1), Jan.–Feb., 9–13.

Dose: 200 mcg/day folic acid.

Multiple Sclerosis

Kanevskaia, S. A. et al. 1990. [Folic acid in the combined treatment of patients with disseminated sclerosis and chronic gastritis]. *Vrach Delo,* (4), Apr. 96–97.

Dose: 200–300 mcg/day.

Zinc Absorption

Milne, D. B. et al. 1984. Effect of oral folic acid supplements on zinc, copper, and iron absorption and excretion. *Am J Clin Nutr,* 39 (4), Apr., 535–539.

Dose: 400 mcg folic acid every other day for 16 weeks.

GARLIC

Cancer

You, W. C. et al. 1989. Allium vegetables and reduced risk of stomach cancer. *J National Cancer Inst,* 81 (2), Jan. 18, 162–164.

Cardiovascular/Coronary Heart Disease

Gadkari, J. V. and Joshi, V. D. 1991. Effect of ingestion of raw garlic on serum cholesterol level, clotting time and fibrinolytic activity in normal subjects. *J Postgrad Med,* 37 (3), July, 128–131.

Dose: 10 gm/day for 2 months.

Bordia, A. 1981. Effect of garlic on blood lipids in patients with coronary heart disease. *Am J Clin Nutr*, 34 (10), Oct., 2100–2103.

Jain, A. K. et al. 1993. Can garlic reduce levels of serum lipids? A controlled clinical study. *Am J Med*, 94 (6), June, 632–635.
Dose: 300 mg 3x/day.

Warhafsky, S. et al. 1993. Effect of garlic on total serum cholesterol. A meta-analysis. *Annals Int Med*, 119 (7 Pt 1), Oct. 1, 599–605.

Vorberg, G. and Schneider, B. 1990. Therapy with garlic: Results of a placebo-controlled, double-blind study. *British J Clin Pract Symp Suppl*, 69, Aug., 7–11.
Dose: 900 mg garlic powder for 4 months.

Auer, W. et al. 1990. Hypertension and hyperlipidaemia: Garlic helps in mild cases. *British J Clin Pract Symp Suppl*, 69, Aug., 3–6.

McMahon, F. G. and Vargas, R. 1993. Can garlic lower blood pressure? A pilot study. *Pharmacotherapy*, 13 (4), July–Aug., 406–407.
Dose: 1.3% allicin at 2400mg.

Ali, M. and Thomson, M. 1995. Consumption of a garlic clove a day could be beneficial in preventing thrombosis. *Prostaglandins Leukot Essent Fatty Acids*, 53 (3), Sept., 211–212.
Dose: 1 fresh clove of garlic/day for 16 weeks.

Kieswetter, H. et al. 1993. Effect of garlic on platelet aggregation in patients with increased risk of juvenile ischaemic attack. *European J Pharmacology*, 45, 333–336.
Dose: 800 mg powdered garlic over 4 weeks.

Silagy, C. A. and Neil, A. W. 1994. A meta-analysis of the effect of garlic on blood pressure. *J Hypertension*, 12, 463–468.
Dose: 600–900 mg/day of dried garlic powder for 12 weeks.

Hepatopulmonary Syndrome

Caldwell, S. H. et al. 1992. Ancient remedies revisited: Does Allium Sativum palliate the hepatopulmonary syndrome? *J Clin Gastroenterology*, 15 (3), Oct., 248–250.

Meningitis

Davis, L. E. et al. 1990. Antifungal activity in human cerebrospinal fluid and plasma after intravenous administration of Allium Sativum. *Antimicrob Agents Chemother*, 34 (4), Apr., 651–653.

GINKGO BILOBA

Aging

Taillandier, J. et al. 1986. [Treatment of cerebral aging disorders with Ginkgo Biloba extract. A longitudinal multicenter double-blind drug vs. placebo study]. *Presse Med,* 15 (31), Sept. 25, 1583–1587.

Allard, M. 1986. [Treatment of the disorders of aging with Ginkgo Biloba extract. From pharmacology to clinical medicine]. *Presse Med,* 15 (31), Sept. 25, 1540, 1545.

Anti-Clastogenic Effects

Emerit, I. et al. 1995. Clastogenic factors in the plasma of Chernobyl accident recovery workers: Anticlastogenic effect of Ginkgo Biloba extract. *Radiat Res,* 144 (2), Nov., 198–205.
Dose: 120 mg/day for 2 months.

Brain Function/Injury

Hofferberth, B. 1989. [The effect of Ginkgo Biloba extract on neurophysiological and psychometric measurement results in patients with psychotic organic brain syndrome. A double-blind study against placebo]. *Arzneimittelforschung,* 39 (8), Aug., 918–922.
Dose: 120 mg/day for 8 weeks.

Hopfenmuller, W. 1994. [Evidence for a therapeutic effect of Ginkgo Biloba special extract. Meta-analysis of 11 clinical studies in patients with cerebrovascular insufficiency in old age]. *Arzneimittelforschung,* 44 (9), Sept., 1005–1013.
Dose: 150 mg/day.

Gessner, B. et al. 1985. Study of the long-term action of a Ginkgo Biloba extract on vigilance and mental performance as determined by means of quantitative pharmaco-EEg and psychometric measurements. *Arzneimittelforschung,* 35 (9), 1459–1465.
Dose: 120 mg/day.

Kleijnen, J. and Knipschild, P. 1992. Ginkgo Biloba for cerebral insufficiency. *British J Clin Pharmacology,* 34 (4), Oct., 352–358.
Dose: 120 mg/day for 4–6 weeks.

Allain, H. et al. 1993. Effect of two doses of Ginkgo Biloba extract (EGb 761) on the dual coding test in elderly subjects. *Clin Ther,* 15 (3), May–June, 549–558.
Dose: 320 or 600 mg.

Rai, G. S. et al. 1991. A double-blind, placebo controlled study of Ginkgo Biloba extract ('tanakan') in elderly outpatients with mild to moderate memory impairment. *Curr Med Res Opin,* 12 (6), 350–355.
Dose: 120 mg/day at 12 and 24 weeks.

Grassel, E. 1992. [Effect of Ginkgo-biloba extract on mental performance: Double-blind study using computerized measurement conditions in patients with cerebral insufficiency]. *Fortschr Med,* 110 (5), Feb. 20, 73–76.

Eckmann, F. 1990. [Cerebral insufficiency—Treatment with Ginkgo-biloba extract. Time of onset of effect in a double-blind study with 60 inpatients]. *Fortschr Med,* 108 (29), Oct. 10, 557–560.
Dose: 160 mg/day.

Gerhardt, G. et al. 1990. [Drug therapy of disorders of cerebral performance: Randomized comparative study of dihydroergotoxine and Ginkgo Biloba extract]. *Fortschr Med,* 108 (19), June 30, 384–388.

Subhan, Z. and Hindmarch, I. 1984. The psychopharmacological effects of Ginkgo Biloba extract in normal healthy volunteers. *Int J Clin Pharmacology Res,* 4 (2), 89–93.
Dose: 120, 240, or 600 mg/day.

Raabe, A. et al. 1991. [Therapeutic follow-up using automatic perimetry in chronic cerebroretinal ischemia in elderly patients. prospective double-blind study with graduated dose Ginkgo Biloba treatment (EGb 761)]. *Klin Monatsbl Augenheilkd,* 199 (6), Dec., 432–438.
Dose: 160 mg/day for 4 weeks.

Lebuisson, D. A. et al. 1986. [Treatment of senile macular degeneration with Ginkgo Biloba extract. A preliminary double-blind drug vs. placebo study]. *Presse Med,* 15 (31), Sept. 25, 1556–1558.

Funfgeld, E. W. 1989. A natural and broad spectrum nootropic substance for treatment of SDAT—the Ginkgo Biloba extract. *Prog Clin Biol Res,* 317, 1247–1260.

Cardiovascular/Coronary Heart Disease

Schneider, B. 1992. [Ginkgo Biloba extract in peripheral arterial diseases. Meta-analysis of controlled clinical studies]. *Arzneimittelforschung,* 42 (4), Apr., 428–436.

Jung, F. et al. 1990. Effect of Ginkgo Biloba on fluidity of blood and peripheral microcirculation in volunteers. *Arzneimittelforschung,* 40 (5), May, 589–593.

Bauer, U. 1984. 6-month double-blind randomised clinical trial of Ginkgo Biloba extract versus placebo in two parallel groups in patients suffering from peripheral arterial insufficiency. *Arzneimittelforschung,* 34 (6), 716–720.

Schaffler, K. and Reeh, P. W. 1985. [Double blind study of the hypoxia protective effect of a standardized Ginkgo Biloba preparation after repeated administration in healthy subjects]. *Arzneimittelforschung,* 35 (8), 1283–1286.

Witte, S. et al. 1992. [Improvement of hemorheology with Ginkgo Biloba extract. Decreasing a cardiovascular risk factor]. *Fortschr Med,* 110 (13), May 10m 247–250.
Dose: 240 mg/day for 12 weeks.

Koltringer, P. et al. 1993. [Hemorheologic effects of Ginkgo Biloba extract EFb 671. Dose-dependent effect of EGb 761 on microcirculation and visoelasticity of blood]. *Fortschr Med,* 111 (10), Apr. 10, 170–172.
Dose: single injection of 50, 100, 150, 200 mg.

Bauer, U. 1986. [Ginkgo Biloba extract in the treatment of arteriopathy of the lower extremities. A 65-week trial]. *Presse Med,* 15 (31), Sept. 25, 1546–1549.

Koltringer, P. et al. 1989. [Microcirculation in parenteral Ginkgo Biloba extract therapy]. *Wien Klin Wochenschr,* 101 (6), Mar. 17, 198–200.

Claudication

Erns, E. 1996. [Ginkgo Biloba in treatment of intermittent claudication. A systematic research based on controlled studies in the literature]. *Fortschr Med,* 114 (8), Mar. 20, 85–87.

Drabaek, H. et al. 1986. [The effect of Ginkgo Biloba extract in patients with intermittent claudication]. *Ugeskr Laeger,* 158 (27), July 1, 3928–3931.
Dose: 120 mg/day for 3 months.

Diabetes

Lanthony, P. and Cosson, J. P. 1988. [The course of color vision in early diabetic retinopathy treated with Ginkgo Biloba extract. A preliminary double-blind versus placebo study]. *J Fr Ophtalmol,* 11 (10), 671–674.

Edema

Lagrue, G. et al. [Idiopathic cyclic edema. The role of capillary hyperpermeability and its correction by Ginkgo Biloba extract]. *Presse Med*, 15 (31), Sept. 25, 1550–1553.

General

Lagrue, G. et al. 1986. [Recurrent shock with monoclonal gammopathy. Treatment in the acute and chronic phases with oral and parenteral Ginkgo Biloba extract]. *Presse Med*, 15 (31), Sept. 25, 1554–1555.

Hearing Loss

Hoffman, F. et al. 1994. [Ginkgo extract EGb 761 (tenobin)/HAES versus Naftidrofuryl (Dusodril)/HAES. A randomized study of therapy of sudden deafness]. *Laryngorhinootologie*, 73 (3), Mar., 149–152.

Dubreuil, C. 1986. [Therapeutic trial in acute cochlear deafness. A comparative study of Ginkgo Biloba extract and Nicergoline]. *Presse Med*, 15 (31), Sept. 25, 1559–1561.

Hepatitis

Li, W. et al. [Preliminary study of early fibrosis of chronic hepatitis B treated with Ginkgo Biloba composita]. *Chung Kuo Chung Hsi I Chieh Ho Tsa Chih*, 15 (10) Oct., 593–595.

Neuropathy

Koltringer, P. et al. 1989. [Ginkgo Biloba extract and folic acid in the therapy of changes caused by autonomic neuropathy]. *Acta Med Austriaca*, 16 (2), 35–37.
Dose: 87.5 mg for 4 days.

Tinnitus

Meyer, B. 1986. [Multicenter randomized double-blind drug vs. placebo study of the treatment of Tinnitus with Ginkgo Biloba extract]. *Presse Med*, 15 (31), Sept. 25, 1562–1564.

Vertigo

Haguenaauer, J. P. et al. 1986. [Treatment of equilibrium disorders with Ginkgo Biloba extract. A multicenter double-blind drug vs. placebo study]. *Presse Med*, 15 (310), Sept. 25, 1569–1572.

GLUTAMINE

Cancer

Skubitz, K. M. and Anderson, P. M. 1996. Oral glutamine to prevent chemotherapy induced stomatitis: A pilot study. *J Lab Clin Med,* 127 (2), Feb., 223–228.
Dose: 4 gm swish and swallow.

Cardiovascuar/Coronary heart disease

Svedjeholm, R. et al. 1995. Glutamate and high-dose glucose-insulin-potassium (GIK) in the treatment of severe cardiac failure after cardiac operations. *Ann Thirac Surg,* 59 (2 Suppl), Feb., S23–S30.

General

Castell, L. M. et al. 1996. Does glutamine have a role in reducing infections in athletes? *Eur J Appl Physiol,* 73 (5), 488–490.

Liver damage

Santagati, G. et al. 1978. [Glutamic acid gamma-ethyl ester in high doses in the treatment of high blood ammonia levels in severe hepatic failure]. *Minerva Med,* 69 (20), Apr. 28, 1367–1374.

Neurotoxicity

Jackson, D. V. et al. 1988. Amelioration of vincristine neurotoxicity by glutamic acid. *Am J Med,* 84 (6), June, 1016–1022.
Dose: 1,500 mg/day.

Short Bowel Syndrome

Byrne, T. A. et al. 1995. A new treatment for patients with short-bowel syndrome. Growth hormone, glutamine, and a modified diet. *Annals Surg,* 222 (3), Sept., 243–254.

Tinnitus

Ehrenberger, K. and Brix, R. 1983. Glutamic acid and glutamic acid diethylester in tinnitus treatment. *Acta Otolaryngol,* 95 (5–6), May–June, 599–605.

Wound injury

Yan, R. et al. 1995. Early enteral feeding and supplement of glutamine prevent occurence of stress ulcer following severe thermal injury. *Chung Hua Cheng Hsing Shao Shang Wai Ko Tsa Chih,* 11 (3), May, 189–192.

GLUTATHIONE

Aging

Julius, M. et al. 1994. Glutathione and morbidity in a community-based sample of elderly. *J Clin Epi,* 47 (9), Sept., 1021–1026.

Cancer

Flagg, E. W. et al. 1994. Dietary glutathione intake and the risk of oral and pharyngeal cancer. *Am J Epi,* 139 (5), Mar. 1, 453–465.

Cascinu, S. et al. 1995. Neuroprotective effect of reduced glutathione on cisplatin-based chemotherapy in advanced gastric cancer: A randomized double-blind placebo-controlled trial. *J Clin Oncology,* 13 (1), Jan., 26–32.

Bowman, A. et al. 1994. Effect of adding glutathione (GSH) to cisplatin (CDDP) in the treatment of stage I-IV ovarian cancer. *British J Cancer,* 71 (Suppl 24), 14.
Dose: 3 gm/m2 for 21 days.

Spatti, G. B. et al. 1990. Cisplatin with minimal hydration and glutathione protection in the treatment of ovarian carcinoma. *Anticancer Res,* 10 (5B), 1425–1456.
Dose: 2.5–5 gm in 100–200 ml of normal saline over 15 minutes iv.

Dalhoff, K. et al. 1992. Glutathione treatment of hepatocellular carcinoma. *Liver,* 12 (5), Oct., 341–343.
Dose: 5 gm/day.

Trickler, D. et al. 1993. Inhibition of oral carcinogenesis by glutathione. *Nutr Cancer,* 20 (2), 139–144.

Smyth, J. et al. 1995. Glutathione improves the therapeutic index of cisplatin and quality of life for patients with ovarian cancer. *Proceedings Annual Meeting Am Soc Clin Oncologists,* 14, A761.

Cataracts

Sternberg Jr., P. 1993. Protection of retinal pigment epithelium from oxidative injury by glutathione and precursors. *Invest Ophthalmol Vis Sci,* 34 (13), Dec., 3661–3668.

Gastric injury

Loguericio, C. et al. 1953. Glutathione prevents ethanol induced gastric mucosal damage and depletion of sulfydryl compounds in humans. *Gut,* 34 (2), Feb., 161–165.

Liver damage

Nardi, E. A. et al. 1991. [High-dose reduced glutathione in the therapy of alcoholic hepatopathy]. *Clin Ter,* 136 (1), Jan. 15, 47–51.

Dentico, P. et al. 1995. [Glutathione in the treatment of chronic fatty liver diseases], *Recenti Prog Med,* 86 (7–8), July–Aug., 290–293.

HIBISCUS

Renal Stone Disease

Kirdpon, S. et al. 1994. Changes in urinary chemical composition in healthy volunteers after consuming roselle (Hibiscus sabdariffa Linn.) juice. *J Med Assoc Thai,* 77 (6), Jun., 314–321.
   Dose: roselle juice consumption, 16 gm/day.

L-METHIONINE

Hepatitis

Windsor, J. A. and Wynne-Jones, G. 1988. Halothane hepatitis and prompt resolution with methionine therapy: Case report. *New Zealand Med J,* 101 (851), Aug. 10, 502–503.

Neuropathy

Stacy, C. B. et al. 1992. Methionine in the treatment of nitrous-oxide–induced neuropathy and myeloneuropathy. *J Neurol,* 239 (7), Aug., 401–403.

Paracetamol Poisoning

Vale, J. A. et al. 1981. Treatment of acetaminophen poisoning. The use of oral methionine. *Arch Intern Med,* 141 (3 Spec No), Feb. 23, 394–396.

Crome, P. et al. 1976. Oral methionine in the treatment of severe Paracetamol (Acetaminophen) overdose. *Lancet,* 2 (7990), Oct. 6, 829–830.

Dose: 2–5 gm every 4 hours up to a total of 10g beginning within 10 hours of overdose.

Breen, K. J. et al. 1982. Paracetamol self-poisoning: Diagnosis, management, and outcome. *Med J Australia,* 1 (2), Jan. 23, 77–79.

MAGNESIUM

Gastrointestinal Problems

Sue, Y. J. et al. 1994. Efficacy of magnesium citrate cathartic in pediatric toxic ingestions. *Ann Emerg Med,* 24 (4), Oct., 709–712.

MELATONIN

Cancer

Lissoni, P. et al. 1992. Biological and clinical results of a neuroimmunotherapy with interleukin-2 and the pineal hormone melatonin as a first line treatment in advanced non-small cell lung cancer. *British J Cancer,* 66 (1), July, 155–158.

Dose: 10 mg/day.

Lissoni, P. et al. 1995. Modulation of cancer endocrine therapy by melatonin: A phase II study of Tamoxifen plus melatonin in metastatic breast cancer patients progressing under Tamoxifen alone. *British J Cancer,* 71 (4), Apr., 854–856.

Dose: 20 mg/day.

Neri, B. et al. 1994. Modulation of human lymphoblastoid interferon activity by melatonin in metastatic renal cell carcinoma: A phase II study. *Cancer,* 73 (12), June 15, 3015–3019.

Dose: 10 mg/day.

Lissoni, P. et al. 1994. A randomized study with the pineal hormone melatonin versus supportive care alone in patients with brain metastases due to solid neoplasms. *Cancer,* 73 (3), Feb 1, 699–701.

Lissoni, P. et al. 1989. Endocrine and immune effects of melatonin therapy in metastic cancer patients. *European J Cancer Clin Oncol,* 25 (5), May, 789–795.

Dose: 20 mg/day intramuscular, followed with 10 mg/day in patients experiencing remission.

Viviani, S. et al. 1990. Preliminary studies on melatonin in the treatment of Myelodysplastic Syndromes following cancer chemotherapy. *J Pineal Res,* 8 (4), 347–354.

Dose: 20 mg/day.

Gonzalez, R. et al. 1991. Melatonin therapy of advanced human malignant melanoma. *Melanoma Res,* 1 (4), Nov.–Dec., 237–243.

Dose: daily oral dose of 5 mg/m2 to 700 mg/m2 after 5 weeks.

Lissoni, P. et al. 1991. Clinical results with pineal hormone melatonin in advanced cancer resistant to standard antitumor therapies. *Oncology,* 48 (6), 448–450.

Dose: 20 mg/day followed with 10 mg/day orally.

Jet Lag

Petri, K. et al. 1989. Effect of melatonin of jet lag after long haul flights. *BMJ,* 298 (6675), Mar. 18, 705–707.

Dose: 5 mg 3 days prior to flight.

Petrie, K. et al. A double-blind trial of melatonin as a treatment for jet lag in internatinal cabin crew. *Biological Psychiatry,* 33 (7), Apr. 1, 526–530.

Dose: 5 mg 3 days prior to flight.

Sleep

Palm, L. et al. 1991. Correction of non-24-hour sleep/wake cycle by melatonin in a blind retarded boy. *Ann Neurol,* 29 (3), Mar., 336–339.

Zhdanova, I. V. et al. 1995. Sleep-inducing effects of low doses of melatonin ingested in the evening. *Clin Pharmacol Therapy,* 57 (5), 552–558.

Dose: 0.3 or 1.0 mg at 6, 8 or 9 P.M.

Dahlitz, M. et al. 1991. Delayed sleep phase syndrome response to melatonin. *Lancet,* 337 (8750), May 11, 1121–1124.

Dose: 5 mg for 4 weeks.

Garfinkel, D. et al. 1995. Improvement of sleep quality in elderly people by controlled-release melatonin. *Lancet,* 346 (8974), Aug. 26, 541–544.

Dose: 2 mg/night for 3 weeks.

Etzioni, A. et al. 1996. Melatonin replacement corrects sleep disturbances in a child with pineal tumor. *Neurology,* 46 (1), Jan, 261–263.
Dose: 3 mg/night for 2 weeks.

MacFarlane, J. G. et al. 1991. The effects of exogenous melatonin on the total sleep time and daytime alertness of chronic insomniacs: A preliminary study. *Biological Psychiatry,* 30 (4), Aug. 15, 371–376.
Dose: 75 mg per os/night.

Folkard, S. et al. 1993. Can melatonin improve shift workers' tolerance of the night shift? Some preliminary findings. *Chronobiol Int,* 10 (5), Oct., 315–320.
Dose: 5 mg/night.

Jan, J. E. et al. 1994. The treatment of sleep disorders with melatonin. Dev *Med Child Neurol,* 36 (2), Feb., 97–107.
Dose: 2–10 mg.

Waldhauser, F. et al. 1990. Sleep laboratory investigations on hypnotic properties of melatonin. *Psychopharmacology,* 100 (2), 222–226.

Tzischinsky, O. and Lavie, P. 1994. Melatonin possesses time-dependent hypnotic effects. *Sleep,* 17 (7), Oct., 638–645.
Dose: 5 mg.

Haimov, I. et al. 1995. Melatonin replacement therapy of elderly insomniacs. *Sleep,* 18 (7), Sept., 598–603.
Dose: 2 mg/night for 7 consecutive days. 1 mg of sustained release.

Vision

Samples, J. R. et al. 1988. Effect of melatonin on intraocular pressure. *Current Eye Res,* 7 (7), July, 649–653.

N-ACETYLCYSTEINE

Adult respiratory distress syndrome

Laurent, T. et al. 1996. Oxidant-antioxidant balance in granulocytes during ARDS. Effect of N-acetylcysteine. *Chest,* 109 (1), Jan., 163–166.

Bernard, G. R. 1990. Potential of N-acetylcysteine as treatment for the Adult Respiratory Distress Syndrome. *European Resp J Suppl,* 11 Oct., 496s–498s.

Cardiovascuar/Coronary heart disease

Reinhart, K. et al. 1995. N-acetylcysteine preserves oxygen consumption and gastric mucosal pH during hyperoxic ventilation. *Am J Resp Critical Care Med,* 151 (3 Pt 1), Mar., 773–779.
Dose: 150 mg/kg-1.

Boesgaard, S. et al. 1992. Preventive administration of intravenous N-acetylcysteine and development of tolerance to isosorbide dinitrate in patients with angina pectoris. *Circulation,* 85 (1), Jan., 143–149.
Dose: 2 gm NAC over 15 minutes iv.

Horowitz, J. D. et al. 1993. Potentiation of the cardiovascular effects of nitroglycerin by N-acetylcysteine. *Circulation,* 68 (6), Dec., 1247–1253.
Dose: 100 mg/kg of NAC iv.

Arstall, M. A. et al. 1995. N-acetylcysteine in combination with nitroglycerin and streptokinase for the treatment of evolving acute myocardial infarction. Safety and biochemical effects. *Circulation,* 92 (10), Nov. 15, 2855–2862.
Dose: 15 gm iv NAC.

Boesgaard, S. et al. 1994. Altered peripheral vasodilator profile of nitroglycerin during long-term infusion of N-acetylcysteine. *J Am Coll Cardiology,* 23 (1), Jan., 163–169.
Dose: 2 gm iv NAC followed by 5 mg/kg per hour on human veins.

Spies, C. et al. 1996. [Effect of prophylactically administered N-acetylcysteine on clinical indicators for tissue oxygenation during hyperoxic ventilation in cardiac risk patients], *Anaesthesist,* 45 (4), Apr., 343–350.
Dose: 150 mg/kg NAC.

Horowitz, J. D. et al. 1990. Nitroglycerine/N-acetylecysteine in the management of unstable angina pectoris. *European Heart J,* 9 (Suppl A) Jan., 95–100.
Dose: 5 gm 6 hourly iv.

Svendsen, J. H. et al. 1989. N-acetylcysteine modifies the acute effects of isosorbide-5-mononitrate in angina pectoris patients. *Pharmacol,* 13 (2), Feb., 320–323.

Andersen, L. W. et al. 1995. The role of N-acetylcysteine administration on the oxidative response of neutrophils during cardiopulmonary bypass. *Perfusion,* 10 (1), 21–26.
Dose: bolus of 100 mg/kg of NAC followed by a continuous infusion of 20 mg/kg.

Chronic Bronchitis

Rasmussen, J. B. and Glennow, C. 1988. Reduction in days of illness after long-term treatment with N-acetylcysteine controlled-release tablets in patients with chronic bronchitis. *European Respir J*, 1 (4), Apr., 351–355.
Dose: 300 mg bid.

Gerards, H. H. and Vits, U. 1991. [Therapy of bronchitis. Successful single-dosage treatment with N-acetylcysteine, results of an administration surveillance study in 3,076 patients]. *Fortschr Med*, 109 (34), Nov. 30, 707–710.
Dose: 600 mg/kg.

Boner, A. L. et al. 1984. A combination of cefuroxine and N-acetylcysteine for the treatment of maxillary sinusitis in children with respiratory allergy. *Int J Clin Pharmacol Ther Toxicol*, 22 (9), Sept, 511–514.
Dose: 15–25 mg/kg/day over a 10 day period.

Santagelo, G. et al. 1985. A combination of Cefuroxime and N-acetylcysteine for the treatment of lower respiratory tract infections in children. *Int J Clin Pharmacol Ther Toxicol*, 23 (5), May, 279–281.

General

Smilkstein, M. J. et al. 1991. Acetaminophen overdose: A 48-hour intravenous N-acetylcysteine treatment protocol. *Annals Emergency Med.*, 20 (10), Oct., 1058–1063.
Dose: (12) 70 mg/kg dose every 4 hours and a loading dose of 140 mg/kg.

Lund, M. E. et al. 1984. Treatment of acute methylmercury ingestion by hemodialysis with N-acetylcysteine (Mucomyst) infusion and 2,3-di-mercaptopropane sulfonate. *J Toxicol Clin Yoxicol*, 22 (1), July, 31–49.

Jensen, T. et al. 1988. Effect of oral N-acetylcyteine administration on human blood neutrophil and monocyte function. *APMIS*, 96 (1), Jan., 62–67.
Dose: 400 mg oral dose.

De Groote, J. and Van Steenbergen, W. 1995. Paracetamol intoxication and N-acetylcysteine treatment. *Acta Gastroenterol Belg*, 58 (3–4), May–Aug., 326–334.

Todisco, T. et al. 1985. Effect of N-acetylcysteine in subjects with slow pulmonary mucociliary clearance. *European J Respir Diseases Suppl*, 139, 136–141.
Dose: 0.6 gm/day.

Beckett, G. J. et al. 1990. Intravenous N-acetylcysteine, hepatoxicity and plasma glutathione S-transferase in patients with Paracetamol overdosage. *Hum Exp Toxicol,* 9 (3), May, 183–186.

Brahm, J. et al. 1992. [Paracetamol overdose: A new form of suicide in Chile and the value of N-acetylcysteine administration]. *Rev Med Chil,* 120 (4), Apr., 427–499.

Glutathione deficiency

Jan, A. et al. 1994. Effect of ascorbate or N-acetylcysteine treatment in a patient with hereditary glutathione synthetase deficiency. *J Pediatrics,* 124 (2), Feb., 229–233.

Martensson, J. et al. 1989. A therapeutic trial with N-acetylcysteine in subjects with hereditary glutathione synthetase deficiency (5-oxoprolinuria), *J Inherist Metab Dis,* 12 (2), 120–130.
Dose: 15 mg/kg/day.

Hepatitis

Hansen, R. M. et al. 1991. Gold induced hepatitis and pure red cell aplasia. Complete recovery after corticosteroid and N-acetylcysteine therapy. *J Pheumatology,* 18 (8), Aug., 1251–1253.

Liver damage

Bromley, P. N. et al. 1995. Effects of intraoperative N-acetylcysteine on orthotopic liver transplantation. *British J Anaesth,* 75 (3), Sept., 352–354.

Oh, T. E. and Shenfield, G. M. 1980. Intravenous N-acetylcysteine for Paracetamol poisoning. *Med J Australia,* 1 (13), June 28, 664–665.

Lung damage

Meyer, A. et al. 1995. Intravenous N-acetylcysteine and lung glutathione of patients with pulmonary fibrosis and normals. *Am J Respiratory Crit Care Med,* 152 (3), Sept., 1055–1060.
Dose: 1.8 gm.

Suter, P. M. et al. 1994. N-acetylcysteine enhances recovery from acute lung injury in man. A randomized, double-blind, placebo-controlled clinical study. *Chest,* 105 (1), Jan., 190–194.
Dose: 40 mg/kg/day iv over a period of 72 hours.

Eklund, A. et al. 1988. Oral N-acetylcysteine reduces selected humoral markers of inflammatory cell activity in BAL fluid from healthy smokers: Correlation to effects on cellular variables. *European Respir J,* 1 (9), Oct., 832–838.

Dose: 200 mg tid over an 8 week period.

Linden, M. et al. 1988. Effects of oral N-acetylecysteine on cell content and macrophage function in bronchoalveolar lavage from healthy smokers. *European Respiratory J,* 1 (7), July, 645–650.

Dose: 200 mg tid over an 8 week period.

Muscle fatigue

Reid, M. B. et al. 1994. N-acetylcysteine inhibits muscle fatigue in humans. *J Clin Investigations,* 94 (6), Dec., 2468–2474.

Dose: pretreatment with 150 mg/kg.

Sjogren's Syndrome

Walters, M. T. et al. 1986. A double-blind, cross-over study of oral N-acetylcysteine in Sjogren's syndrome. *Scandanavian J Pheumatol Suppl,* 61, 253–258.

NIACIN

Chojnowska-Jezierska, J. and Adamska-Dyniewska, H. 1998. Efficacy and safety of one-year treatment with slow-release nicotinic acid. Monitoring of drug concentration in serum. *Int J Clin Pharmacol Ther,* 36 (6), Jun., 326–332.

Dose: 1.5 g/d (2 months), and subsequently 2–3 g/d (10 months), on average 2.13 g/d. During the treatment with 2.0 g/d dose.

Hoogerbrugge, N. et al. 1998. The additional effects of acipimox to simvastatin in the treatment of combined hyperlipidaemia. *J Intern Med,* 243 (5), May, 151–156.

Dose: Acipimox in a daily dose of 3 X 250 mg for 12 weeks.

Brown, B. G. et al. 1998. Lipid altering or antioxidant vitamins for patients with coronary disease and very low HDL cholesterol? The HDL-Atherosclerosis Treatment Study Design. *Can J Cardiol,* Suppl A, Apr. 14, 6A–13A.

Chojnowska-Jezierska, J. and Adamska-Dyniewska, H. 1997. [Prolonged treatment with slow release nicotinic acid in patients with type II hyperlipidemia]. *Pol Arch Med Wewn,* 98 (11), Nov., 391–399.

Dose: one-year therapy with slow-release nicotinic acid.

McKenney, J. M. et al. 1998. A randomized trial of the effects of atorvastatin and niacin in patients with combined hyperlipidemia or isolated hypertriglyceridemia. Collaborative Atorvastatin Study Group. *Am J Med,* 104 (2), Feb., 137–143.
Dose: immediate-release niacin 1 g 3x/day for 12 weeks.

Brown, B. G. et al. 1998. Use of niacin, statins, and resins in patients with combined hyperlipidemia. *Am J Cardiol,* 81 (4A), Feb. 26, 52B–59B.

Fagerberg, B. et al. 1998. Mortality rates in treated hypertensive men with additional risk factors are high but can be reduced: a randomized intervention study. *Am J Hypertens,* 11 (1 Pt 1), Jan., 14–22.

Kukharchuk, V. V. et al. 1997. [The effect of long-term Enduracin monotherapy on the clinical and biochemical status of patients with ischemic heart disease]. *Ter Arkh,* 69 (9), 41–45.
Dose: enduracin in a dose 1500 mg/day.

Brown, B. G. et al. 1997. Moderate dose, three-drug therapy with niacin, lovastatin, and colestipol to reduce low-density lipoprotein cholesterol <100 mg/dl in patients with hyperlipidemia and coronary artery disease. *Am J Cardiol,* 80 (2), Jul. 15, 111–115.
Dose: initial 12-month phase, regular niacin 500 mg qid alternated with a polygel controlled-release formula.

Gardner, S. F. et al. 1997. Combination of low-dose niacin and pravastatin improves the lipid profile in diabetic patients without compromising glycemic control. *Ann Pharmacother,* 31 (6), Jun., 677–682.
Dose: low-dose niacin (1.5 g/d) over a 14 week period.

OMEGA FATTY ACIDS

Arthritis

Kremer, J. M. 1991. Clinical studies of omega-3 fatty acid supplementation in patients who have Rheumatoid arthritis. *Rheum Dis Clin North Am,* 17 (2), May, 391–402.

Geusens, P. et al. 1994. Long-term effect of omega-3 fatty acid supplementation in active Rheumatoid Arthritis. A 12-month, double-blind, controlled study. *Arthritis Rheum,* 37 (6), June, 824–829.
Dose: 2.6 gm/day for 12 months.

Cancer

Kemen, M. et al. 1995. Early postoperative enteral nutrition with arginine-omega-3 fatty acids and ribonucleic acid-supplemented diet versus placebo in cancer patients: An immunologic evaluation of impact. *Crit Care Med,* 23 (4), Apr., 652–659.

Anti, M. et al. 1992. Effect of omega-3 fatty acids on rectal mucosal cell proliferation in subjects at risk for colon cancer. *Gastroenterology,* 103 (3), Sept., 883–891.
Dose: 4 g EPA, 3.6 g DHA for 12 weeks.

Cardiovascular/Coronary heart disease

Levine, P. H. et al. 1989. Dietary supplementation with omega-3 fatty acids prolongs platelet survival in hyperlipidemic patients with atherosclerosis. *Arch Intern Med,* 149 (5), May, 1113–1116.

Illingworth, D. R. et al. 1984. Inhibition of low density lipoprotein synthesis by dietary omega-3 fatty acids in humans. Arteriosclerosis. *Arch Intern Med,* 4 (3), May–June, 270–275.
Dose: 24 gm/day for 4 weeks.

Harris, W. S. et al. 1984. Dietary omega-3 fatty acids prevent carbohydrate-induced hypertriglyceridemia. *Metabolism,* 33 (11), Nov., 1016–1019.

d'Ivernois, C. et al. [Potential value of omega-3 polyunsaturated fatty acids in the prevention of atherosclerosis and cardiovascular diseases]. *Arch Mal Coeur Vaiss,* 85 (6), June, 899–904.

Lox, C. D. 1990. The effects of dietary marine fish oils (Omega-3 fatty acids) on coagulation profiles in men. *Gen Pharmacol,* 21 (2), 241–246.
Dose: 900 mg over a period of 30 days.

Engler, M. B. 1994. Vascular effects of omega-3 fatty acids: Possible therapeutic mechanisms in cardiovascular disease. *J Cardiovascular Nurs,* 8 (3), Apr., 53–67.

Lungershausen, Y. K. et al. 1994. Reduction of blood pressure and plasma triglycerides by omega-3 fatty acids in treated hypertensives. *J Hypertension,* 12 (9), Sept., 1041–1045.

Diabetes

Landgraf-Leurs, M. M. et al. 1990. Pilot study on omega-3 fatty acids in type I Diabetes Mellitus. *Diabetes,* 39 (3), Mar., 369–375.
Dose: 5.4 gm EPA, 2.3 gm DHA.

Popp-Snijders, C. et al. 1987. Dietary supplementation of omega-3 polyunsaturated fatty acids improves insulin sensitivity in non-insulin-dependent diabetes. *Diabetes Res,* 4 (3), Mar., 141–147.
Dose: EPA and DHA 3 gm for 8 weeks.

ORNITHINE

Aging

Brocker, P. et al. 1994. A two-centre, randomized, double-blind trial or or-
nithine oxoglutarate in 194 elderly, ambulatory, convalescent subjects,
Age Ageing, 23 (4), July, 303–306.
Dose: 10 gm/day for 2 months.

Cancer

Dunzendorfer, U. 1981. Alpha-difluoromethyornithine (alpha DFMO) and
phenoxybenzamine hydrochloride in the treatment of chronic non-sup-
purative prostatitis. *Arzneimittelforschung,* 31 (2), 382–385.
Dose: 18 gm/day over 1 month.

Alberts, D. S. et al. 1996. Positive randomized, double blinded, placebo controlled study of topical difluoromethyl ornithine (DFMO) in the chemoprevention of skin cancer. *Proc Annual Meeting Am Soc Clin Oncology,* 15,
A342.
Dose: 10% w/w topical solution of DFMO applied for 6 months.

Encephalopathy

Herlong, H. F. et al. 1980. The use of ornithine salts of branched-chain
ketoacids in portal-systemic encephalopathy. *Ann Intern Med,* 93 (4),
Oct., 545–550.
Dose: 34 mmol/day over 7–10 days.

Surgical Trauma

Wernerman, J. et al. 1989. Glutamine and ornithine-alpha-ketoglutarate
but not branched-chain amino acids reduce the loss of muscle glutamine after surgical trauma. *Metabolism,* 38 (8 Suppl 1), Aug., 63–66.

PEPPERMINT

General

Gobel, H. et al. 1994. Effect of peppermint and eucalyptus oil preparations
on neurophysiological and experimental algesimetric headache parameters. *Cephalalgia,* 14 (3), June, 228–234.

Irritable Bowel Syndrome

Treating irritable bowel syndrome with peppermint oil. *British Med J*, Oct. 6, 835–836.

Dose: peppermint oil in enteric-coated capsules.

Ulcers

Meyer, J. et al. 1945. Action of oil of peppermint on the secretion and motility of the stomach in man. *Arch Int Med*, 56, 88–97.

PHOSPHATIDYL SERINE

Alzheimer's disease

Heiss, W. D. et al. 1994. Long-term effects of phosphatidylserine, pyritinol, and cognitive training in Alzheimer's Disease. A neuropsychological, EEG, and PET investigation. *Dementia*, 5 (2), Mar.–Apr., 88–98.

Dose: 400 mg/day.

Engel, R. R. et al. 1992. Double-blind cross-over study of phosphatidylserine vs. placebo in patients with early dementia of the Alzheimer type. *Eur Neuropsychopharmacol*, 2 (2), June, 1992, 149–155.

Dose: 300 mg/day for 8 weeks.

Crook, T. et al. 1992. Effects of phosphatidylserine in Alzheimer's disease. *Psychopharmacol Bull*, 28 (1), 61–66.

Dose: 100 mg/day for 12 weeks.

Brain Function

Lombardi, G. F. 1989. [Pharmacological treatment with phosphatidyl serine of 40 ambulatory patients with senile dementia syndrome]. *Minerva Med*, 80 (6), June, 599–602.

Crook, T. H. et al. 1991. Effects of phosphatidylserine in the age-associated memory impairment. *Neurology*, 41 (5), May, 644–649.

Dose: 100 mg for 12 weeks.

Delwaide, P. J. et al. 1986. Double-blind randomized controlled study of phosphatidylserine in senile demented patients. *Acta Neurol Scand*, 73 (2), Feb., 136–140.

Dose: 3x100 mg.

Maggioni, M. et al. (1990). Effects of phosphatidylserine therapy in geriatric patients with depressive disorders. *Acta Psychiatr Scand,* 81 (3), Mar., 265–270.
Dose: 300 mg/day for 30 days.

Cenacchi, T. et al. 1993. Cognitive decline in elderly: A double-blind, placebo-controlled multicenter study on efficacy of phosphatidylserine administration. *Aging,* 5 (2), Apr., 123–133.
Dose: 300 mg/day.

Sakai, M. et al. 1996. Pharmacological effect of phosphatidylserine enzymatically synthesized from soybean lecithin on brain functions in rodents. *J Nutr Sci Vitaminol,* 42 (1), Feb., 47–54.
Dose: 300 mg/day.

Epilepsy

Loeb, C. et al. 1987. Preliminary evaluation of the effect of GABA and phosphatidylserine in epileptic patients. *Epilepsy Res,* 1 (3), May, 209–212.

Parkinson's disease

Finfgeld, E. W. et al. 1989. Double-blind study with phosphatidylserine (PS) in Parkinsonian patients with senile dementia of Alzheimer's type. *Prog Clin Biol Res,* 1235–1246.

Schizophrenia

Tachik, K. H. et al. 1986. Phosphatidyleserine inhibition of monoamine oxidase in platelets of schizophrenics. *Biol Psychiatry,* 21 (1), Jan., 59–68.

Stress

Monteleone, P. et al. 1992. Blunting by chronic phosphatidylserine administration of the stress-induced activation of the hypothalamo-pituitary-adrenal axis in healthy men. *European J Clin Pharmacol,* 42 (4), 385–388.
Dose: 800 mg/day for 10 days.

Monteleone, P. et al. 1990. Effects of phosphatidylserine on the neuroendocrine response to physical stress in humans. *Neuroendocrinology,* 52 (3), 243–248.
Dose: 50 and 75 mg/day.

PREGNENOLONE

Araneo, B. A. et al. 1995. Dehydroepiandrosterone reduces progressive dermal ischemia caused by thermal injury. *J Surg Res,* 59 (2), Aug., 250–262.

Dose: Subcutaneous administration of DHEA at approximately 1 mg/kg/day achieved optimal protection against the development of progressive dermal ischemia.

PSYLLIUM

Zumarraga, L. et al. 1997. Absence of gaseous symptoms during ingestion of commercial fibre preparations. *Aliment Pharmacol Ther,* 11 (6), Dec., 1067–1072.

Dose: psyllium 3.4 gm.

McRorie, J. W. et al. 1998. Psyllium is superior to docusate sodium for treatment of chronic constipation. *Aliment Pharmacol Ther,* 12 (5), May, 491–497.

Dose: psyllium (5.1 gm b.d.).

Moran, S. et al. 1997. [Effects of fiber administration in the prevention of gallstones in obese patients on a reducing diet. A clinical trial]. *Rev Gastroenterol Mex,* 62 (4), Oct., 266–272.

Dose: psyllium 15 gm.

Rigaud, D. et al. 1998. Effect of psyllium on gastric emptying, hunger feeling and food intake in normal volunteers: a double blind study. *Eur J Clin Nutr,* 52 (4), Apr., 239–245.

Dose: psyllium 7.4 gm.

Segawa, K. et al. 1998. Cholesterol-lowering effects of psyllium seed associated with urea metabolism. *Biol Pharm Bull,* 21 (2), Feb., 184–187.

Davidson, M. H. et al. 1998. Long-term effects of consuming foods containing psyllium seed husk on serum lipids in subjects with hypercholesterolemia. *Am J Clin Nutr,* 67 (3), Mar., 367–376.

Dose: psyllium seed 3.4, 6.8, or 10.2 gm for 24 weeks.

Washington, N. et al. 1998. Moderation of lactulose-induced diarrhea by psyllium: Effects on motility and fermentation. *Am J Clin Nutr,* 67 (2), Feb., 317–321.

Dose: psyllium 3.5 gm 3x/day.

Olson, B. H. et al. 1997. Psyllium-enriched cereals lower blood total cholesterol and LDL cholesterol, but not HDL cholesterol, in hypercholesterolemic adults: results of a meta-analysis. *J Nutr,* 127 (10), Oct., 1973–1980.

Dose: 3 gm soluble fiber/day.

RED CLOVER

Cancer

Marshal, M. E. et al. 1987. Treatment of metastatic renal cell carcinoma with coumarin (1,2-benzopyrone) and cimetide: A pilot study. *J Clin Oncology,* 5f (6), June, 862–866.

Dose: 100 mg/day coumarin.

SILYBUM MARIANUM (MILK THISTLE)

Alcohol Abuse

Fintelmann, V. 1970. [Zur therapie der fettleber mit silymarin]. *Therapiewoche,* 20, 1055.

Cirrhosis

Ferenci, P. et al. 1989. Randomized controlled trial of silymarin treatment in patients with cirrhosis of the liver. *J Hepatol,* 9 (1), Jul., 105–113.

Dose: 140 mg silymarin 3x/day.

Diabetes

Velussi, M. et al. 1997. Long-term (12 months) treatment with an antioxidant drug (silymarin) is effective on hyperinsulinemia, exogenous insulin need and malondialdehyde levels in cirrhotic diabetic patients. *J Hepatol,* 26 (4), Apr., 871–879.

Dose: 600 mg silymarin/day.

Zhang. J. Q. et al. 1993. [Effects of silybin on red blood cell sorbitol and nerve conduction velocity in diabetic patients]. *Chung Kuo Chung Hsi I Chieh Ho Tsa Chih,* 13 (12), Dec., 725–726.

Dose: silybin 231 mg/day for 4 weeks.

Geller, L. I. et al. 1993. [Treatment of fatty hepatosis in diabetics]. *Probl Endokrinol (Mosk)*, 39 (5), Sept., 20–22.

Drug Abuse

Carrescia, O. et al. 1980. Silymarin in the prevention of hepatic damage by psychopharmacologic drugs. Experimental premises and clinical evaluation. *Clin Ter*, 95, 157.

Hepatitis

Buzzelli, G. et al. 1993. A pilot study on the liver protective effect of silybin-phosphatidylcholine complex (IdB1016) in chronic active hepatitis. *Int J Clin Pharmacol Ther Toxicol*, 31 (9), Sept., 456–460.

Dose: 240 mg silybin bid.

TRIMETHYLGLYCINE BETAINE

Dry Mouth

Soderling, E. et al. 1998. Betaine-containing toothpaste relieves subjective symptoms of dry mouth. *Acta Odontol Scand*, 56 (2), Apr., 65–69.

Dose: betaine-containing toothpaste.

Homocystinuria

Wilcken, D. E. et al. 1985. Homocystinuria due to cystathionine beta-synthase deficiency—the effects of betaine treatment in pyridoxine-responsive patients. *Metabolism*, 34 (12), Dec., 1115–1121.

Dose: betaine (trimethylglycine) 6 g/d.

Wendel, U. and Bremer, H. J. 1984. Betaine in the treatment of homocystinuria die to 5,10-methylenetetrahydrofolate reductase deficiency. *Europ J Pediatrics*, 142 (2), June, 147–150.

Dose: 15–20 gm/day.

VITAMIN C

Aging

Phillips, C. L. et al. 1994. Effects of ascorbic acid on proliferation and collagen synthesis in relation to the donor age of human dermal fibroblasts. *J Invest Dermatol*, 103 (2), Aug., 228–232.

Postaire, E. et al. 1995. Increase of singlet oxygen protection of erythrocytes by Vitamin E, Vitamin C and Beta Carotene intakes. *Biochem Mol Biol Int,* 35 (2), Feb., 371–375.
Dose: 30 mg/day vitamin C.

Okamoto, K et al. 1992. [The relationship between dietary ascorbic acid intake and serum lipid concentration in the aged.] *Nippon Ronen Igakkai Zasshi,* 29 (12), Dec., 908–911.

Cheraskin, E. 1994. Chronologic versus biologic age. *J Advancement Med,* 7 (1), Spring, 31–41.
Dose: 100 mg–200 mg/day vitamin C

Cheraskin, E. 1993. Vitamin C, cancer and aging. *Age,* 16, 55–58.

Delafuente, J. C. et al. 1986. Immunologic modulation by vitamin C in elderly. *Int J Immunopharmacol,* 8 (2), 205–211.

Alcohol Toxicity

Susick, R. L. and Zannoni, V. G. 1987. Effect of ascorbic acid on the consequences of acute alcohol consumption in humans. *Clin Pharmacol Ther,* 41 (5), May, 502–509.
Dose: 0.95 gm/kg body weight over 2.5 hours for 2 weeks.

Wickramasinghe, S. N. and Hasan, R. 1994. In vivo effects of vitamin C on the cytotoxicity of post-ethanol serum. *Biochem Pharmacol,* 48 (3), Aug. 3, 621–624.
Dose: 1 gm/day for 3 days.

Chen, M. F. et al. 1990. Effect of ascorbic acid on plasma alcohol clearance. *J Am Coll Nutr,* 9 (3), June, 185–189.

Arthritis

Oldroyd, K. G. and Dawes, P. T. 1985. Clinically significant vitamin C deficiency in rheumatoid arthritis. *British J Rheumatology,* 24 (4), Nov., 362–363.

Davis, R. H. et al. 1990. Vitamin C influence of localized adjuvant arthritis. *J American Podiatry Med Assoc,* 80 (8), Aug., 414–418.
Dose: 150 mg/kg of subcutaneous vitamin C for 20 days.

Asthma

Hatch, G. E. 1995. Asthma, inhaled oxidants, and dietary antioxidants. *American J Clin Nutr,* 61 (3 Suppl), Mar., 625S–630S.

Anderson, R. et al. 1980. The effect of ascorbate on cellular humoral immunity in asthmatic children. *South African Med J*, 58 (24), Dec 13, 974–977.
Dose: 1 g ascorbic single daily dose for a 6-month period.

Anah, C. O. et al. 1980. High dose ascorbic acid in Nigerian asthmatics. *Trop Geogr Med*, 32 (2), June, 132–137.
Dose: 1 g of ascorbic acid daily.

Rozanov, E. M. et al. 1987. [Vitamin PP and C allowances and their correction in the treatment of bronchial asthma patients.] *Vopr Pitan*, (6), Nov–Dec, 21–24.
Dose: 275–300 mg of vitamin C.

Cancer

Block, G. et al. 1991. Epidemiologic evidence regarding vitamin C and cancer. *Am J Clin Nutr*, 54 (6 Suppl), Dec., 1310S–1314S.

Herrero, R. et al. A case-control study of nutrient status and invasive cervical cancer: I. Dietary indicators. *Am J Epi*, 134 (11), Dec. 1, 1335–1346.

Stahelin, H. B. et al. Plasma antioxidant vitamins and subsequent cancer mortality in the 12-year follow-up of the prospective based study. *Am J Epi*, 133 (8), Apr. 15, 766–775.

Knekt, P et al. 1991. Dietary antioxidants and the risk of lung cancer. *Am J Epi*, 134 (5), Sept. 1, 471–479.

Trizna, Z. et al. 1991. Effects of N-acetyl-L-cysteine and ascorbic acid on mutagen-induced chromosomal sensitivity in patients with head and neck cancers. *Am J Surgery*, 162 (4), Oct., 294–298.

Ferraroni, M. et al. 1994. Selected micronutrient intake and the risk of colorectal cancer. *British J Cancer*, 70 (6), Dec., 1150–1155.

Shibata, A. et al. 1992. Intake of vegetables, fruits, beta-carotene, vitamin C and vitamin supplements and cancer incidence among the elderly: A prospective study. *British J Cancer*, 66 (4), Oct., 673–679.

Bussey, H. J. et al. A randomized trial of ascorbic acid in polyposis coli. *Cancer*, 50 (7), Oct. 1, 1434–1439.
Dose: 3 g/day of ascorbic acid for 9 months.

Fontham, E. T. et al. 1988. Dietary vitamins A and C and lung cancer risk in Louisiana. *Cancer*, 62 (10), Nov. 15, 2267–2273.

Park, C. H. et al. 1980. Growth suppression of human leukemic cells in vitro by L-ascorbic acid. *Cancer Res,* 40 (4), 1062–1065.

Kaugars, G. et al. 1993. Serum and tissue antioxidant levels in supplemented patients with premalignant oral lesions (meeting abstract). *FASEB J,* 7 (4), A519.
Dose: 1000 mg vitamin C for 9 months.

Sobala, G. M. et al. 1989. Ascorbic acid in the human stomach. *Gastroenterology,* 97 (2), Aug., 357–363.

Paganelli, G. M. et al. 1992. Effect of vitamin A, C, and E supplementation on rectal cell proliferation in patients with colorectal adenomas. *J National Cancer Inst.,* 84 (1), Jan. 1, 47–51.

Brock, K. E. et al. Nutrients in diet and plasma and risk of in situ cervical cancer. *J National Cancer Inst.,* 80 (8), June 15, 580–585.

Potter, J. D. and McMichael, A. J. 1986. Diet and cancer of the colon and rectum: A case-control study. *J National Cancer Inst.,* 76 (4), Apr., 557–569.

Moffat, L. et al. 1983. High dose ascorbate therapy and cancer. *NFCR Cancer Res Assoc Symp.,* (2), 243–256.
Dose: 2.5 g vitamin C 4x/day.

Kaugars, G. et al. 1993. The role of antioxidants in the treatment of oral leukoplakia. CCPC-93: *Second Int Cancer Chemo Prevention Conf.,* Berlin, Germany, Apr. 28–30, 65.
Dose: 1000 mg/day of ascorbic acid for 9 months.

Greco, A. M. et al. 1982. Study of blood vitamin C in lung and bladder cancer patients before and after treatment with ascorbic acid: A preliminary report. *Acta Vitaminol Enzymol,* 4 (1–2), 155–162.
Dose: 5 g/day.

Glatthaar, B. E. et al. The role of ascorbic acid in carcinogenesis. *Adv Exp Med Biol,* 206, 357–377.

Chen, L. H. et al. 1988. Vitamin C, vitamin E and cancer. *Anticancer Res,* 8 (4), July–Aug., 739–748.

Garcia-Alejo Hernandez, R. et al. 1989. [Radioprotective effect of ascorbic acid on oral structures in patients with cancer of the head and neck]. *Av odontoestomatol,* 5 (7), Sept., 469–472.

La Vecchia, C. et al. Selected micronutrient intake and the risk of gastric cancer. *Cancer Epidemiol Biomarkers Prev.,* 3 (5), July–Aug., 393–398.

Dyke, G. W. et al. Effect of vitamin C supplementation on gastric mucosal DNA damage. *Carcinogenesis,* 15 (2), 291–295.

Slattery, M. L. et al. 1990. Dietary vitamins A, C, and E and selenium as risk factors for cervical cancer. *Epidemiology,* 1 (1), Jan., 8–15.

Reed, P. I. et al. 1991. Effect of ascorbic acid on the intragastric environment in patients at increased risk of developing gastric cancer. *IARC Sci Publ.,* 105, 139–142.

Nomura, A. M. et al. 1991. Dietary factors in cancer of the lower urinary tract. *Int. J Cancer,* 48 (2), May 10, 199–205.

Verreault, R. et al. 1989. A case-control study of diet and invasive cervical cancer. *Int J Cancer,* 43 (6), June 15, 1050–1054.

Cameron, E. 1982. Vitamin C and cancer: An overview. *Int J Vitamin Nutr Res Suppl,* 23, 115–127.

Murata, A. et al. 1982. Prolongation of survival times of terminal cancer patients by administration of large doses of ascorbate. *Int J Vitamin Nutr Res Suppl,* 23, 103–113.

Waddell, R. and Germer, R. E. 1980. Indomethacin and ascorbate inhibit desmoid tumors. *J Surg Oncol,* 15 (1), 85–90.

Ghosh, J. and Das, S. 1995. Evaluation of vitamin A and C status in normal and malignant conditions and their possible role in cancer prevention. *Japanese J Cancer Res,* 76 (12), Dec., 1174–1178.

Cameron, E. and Campbell, A. 1991. Innovation vs. quality control: An "Unpublishable" clinical trial on supplemental ascorbate in incurable cancer. *Med Hyp,* 36 (3), Nov., 185–189.

Jaffey, M. Vitamin C and cancer: Examination of the value of eleven trial results using broad inductive reasoning. *Med Hyp,* 8 (1), 49–84.
Dose: 10 g/day vitamin C.

Campbell, A. et al. 1991. Reticulum cell sarcoma: Two complete spontaneous' regressions in response to high-dose ascorbic acid therapy. A report on subsequent progress. *Oncology,* 48 (6), 495–497.

Kaminski, M. and Boal, R. 1992. An effect of ascorbate acid on delayed-onset muscle soreness. *Pain,* 50 (3), Sept., 317–321.

Raushenbakh, M. O. et al. [Effect of ascorbic acid on formation and leukemogenic activity of p-hydroxyphenyllactic acid]. *Probl Gematol Pereliv Krovi,* 27 (7), 3–6.
Dose: 8 g/day over 8–10 days before chemotherapy.

Stahelin, H. B. 1989. [Vitamins and cancer: Results of a Basel study]. *Soz Praventivmed,* 34 (2), 75–77.

Gorozhanskaia. E. G. et al. [The role of ascorbic acid in the combined pre-operative preparation of cancer patients]. *Vopr Onkol,* 35 (4), 436–441.
Dose: 1.5 g/day of ascorbic acid for 7 days.

Baikova, V. N. et al. 1982. [The effect of large doses of ascorbic acid on tyrosine metabolism and hemoblastosis course in children]. *Vopr Onkol,* 28 (9), 28–34.
Dose: 100 mg/kg/day.

Yuan, J. M. et al. 1995. Diet and breast cancer in Shanghai and Tianjin, China. *British J Cancer,* 71, 1353–1358.

Howe, G. R. et al. 1990. Dietary factors and the risk of breast cancer: Combined analysis of 12 case-controlled studies. *J National Cancer Inst.,* 82, 561–569.

Van Eenwyk, J. 1993. The role of vitamins in the development of cervical cancer. *The Nutrition Report,* 11 (1), Jan., 1–8.

Amburgey, C. F. et al. 1993. Undernutrition as a risk factor for cervical intraepithelial neoplasia: A case control analysis. *Nutrition and Cancer,* 20 (1), 51–60.

Cardiovascular/Coronary Heart Disease

Salonen, J. T. et al. 1991. Effects of antioxidant supplementation on platelet function: A randomized pair-matched, placebo-controlled, double-blind trial in men with low antioxidant status. *Am J Clin Nutr.,* 53 (5), May, 1222–1229.
Dose: 600 mg of ascorbic acid/day.

Trout, D. L. 1991. Vitamin C and cardiovascular risk factors. *Am J Clin Nutr,* 53 (1 Suppl), Jan., 322S–325S.

Sisto, T. et al. 1995. Pretreatment with antioxidants and allopurinol diminishes cardiac onset events in coronary artery bypass grafting. *Ann Thorac Surg,* 59 (6), June, 1519–1523.

Khaw, K. T. and Woodhouse, P. 1988. Interrelation of vitamin C, infection, haemostatic factors and cardiovascular disease. *British Med J,* 310 (6994), June 17, 1559–1563.
Dose: 60 mg.

Brox, A. G. et al. 1988. Treatment of idiopathic thrombocytopenic purpura with ascorbate. *British J Haematology,* 70 (3), Nov., 341–344.

Singh, R. B. et al. 1995. Effect of antioxidant-rich foods on plasma ascorbic acid, cardiac enzyme, and lipid peroxide levels in patients hospitalized with acute myocardial infarction. *J Am Dietetic Assoc.,* 95 (7), July, 775–780.

Singh, R. B. et al. 1994. Plasma levels of antioxidant vitamins and oxidative stress in patients with acute myocardial infarction. *Acta Cardiol,* 49 (5), 441–452.

Riemersma. R. A. et al. 1989. Low plasma vitamins E and C. Increased risk of angina in Scottish men. *Annals NY Academy Sci.,* 570, 291–295.

Gey, K. F. et al. 1987. Relationship of plasma level of vitamin C to mortality from ischemic heart disease. *Annals NY Academy Sci.,* 498, 110–123.

Cordova, C, et al. 1982. Influence of ascorbic acid on platelet aggregation in vitro and in vivo. *Atherosclerosis,* 41 (1), Jan., 15–19.
Dose: 2 g of ascorbic acid.

Bordia, A. K. 1980. The effect of vitamin C on blood lipids, fibrinolytic activity and platelet adhesiveness in patients with coronary artery disease. *Atherosclerosis,* 35 (2), Feb., 181–187.
Dose: 2 g/day vitamin C.

Li, C. C. 1990. [Changes on creatine phosphokinase and malondialdehyde in the serum and clinical use of large doses of vitamin C following open heart surgery]. *Chung Hua Wai Ko Tsa Chih,* 28 (1), Jan., 16–17, 60–61.
Dose: 250 mg/kg vitamin C prior to heart surgery.

Bordia, A. and Verma, S. K. 1985. Effect of vitamin C on platelet adhesiveness and platelet aggregation in coronary artery disease patients. *Clinical Cardiology,* 8 (10), Oct., 552–554.
Dose: 1 g and 1 g every 8 hours over 10 days.

Yoshioka, M. et al. 1984. Inverse association of serum ascorbic acid level and blood pressure or rate of hypertension in male adults aged 30–39 years. *Int J Vitamin Nutr Res.,* 54 (4), 343–347.

Simon, J. A. 1992. Vitamin C and cardiovascular disease: A review. *J Am Coll Nutr.,* 11 (2), Apr., 107–125.

Mostafa, S. et al. 1989. Beneficial effects of vitamin C on risk factors of cardiovascular diseases. *J Egyptian Public Health Assoc.,* 64 (1–2), 123–133.
Dose: 500 mg/day of vitamin C.

Fujimura, I. et al. [Correlation between hypercholesterolemia and vitamin C deficient diet]. *Rev Hosp Clin Fac Med Sao Paulo,* 46 (1), Jan.–Feb., 14–18.

Dobson, H. M. et al. 1984. The effect of ascorbic acid on the seasonal variations in serum cholesterol levels. *Scottish Med J,* 29 (3), July, 176–182.
Dose: 1 g of ascorbic acid for 2 months.

Gey, K. F. et al. [Essential antioxidants in cardiovascular diseases-Lessons
for Europe]. *Ther Umsch,* 51 (7), July, 475–482.

Dingchao, H. et al. 1994. The protective effects of high-dose ascorbic acid
on myocardium against reperfusion injury after cardiopulmonary bypass. *Thorac Cardiovasc Surg,* 42 (5), Oct., 276–278.
Dose: 250 mg/kg.

Cataracts

Jacques, P. F. and Chylack Jr., L. T. Epidemiologic evidence of a role for the
antioxidant vitamins and carotenoids in cataract prevention. *Am J Clin
Nutr,* 53 (1 Suppl), Jan., 352S–355S.

Robertson, J. M. et al. 1991. A possible role for vitamins C and E in cataract
prevention. *Am J Clin Nutr.,* 53 (1 Suppl), Jan., 346S–351S.

Jacques, P. F. et al. 1988. Antioxidant status in persons with and without
senile cataract. *Arch Ophthalmol,* 106 (3), Mar., 337–340.

Gerster, H. 1989. Antioxidant vitamins in cataract prevention. *Z Ernahrungswiss.,* 28 (1), Mar., 56–75.

Cervical Dysplasia

Wassertheil-Smoller, S. et al. 1981. Dietary vitamin C and uterine cervical
Dysplasia. *Am J Epi,* 114 (5), No., 714–724.

Romney, S. L. et al. 1985. Plasma vitamin C and uterine cervical dysplasia.
Am J Obstetrics Gynecology, 151 (7), Apr. 1, 976–980.

Common Cold

Hemila, H. 1994. Does vitamin C alleviate the symptoms of the common
cold? A review of current evidence. *Scandanavian J Infect Dis,* 26 (1), 1–6.
Dose: 1 g Vitamin C.

Diabetes

Johnson, C. S. and Yen, M. F. 1994. Megadose of vitamin C delays insulin
response to a glucose challenge in normoglycemic adults. *Am J Clin
Nutr,* 60 (5), Nov., 735–738.
Dose: 2 g/day for 2 weeks.

Paolisso, G. et al. 1994. Plasma vitamin C affects glucose homeostasis in healthy subjects and in non-insulin-dependent diabetics. *Am J Physiol,* 266 (2 Pt 1), Feb., E261–268.

Davie, S. J. et al. Effect of vitamin C on glycosylation of proteins. *Diabetes,* 41 (2), Feb., 167–173.
Dose: 1 g/day of vitamin C for 3 months.

Vinson, J. A. et al. 1989. In vitro and in vivo reduction of erythrocyte sorbitol by ascorbic acid. *Diabetes,* 38 (8), Aug., 1036–1041.
Dose: 500 mg/day for 2 weeks.

Yue, D. K. et al. 1990. Abnormalities of ascorbic acid metabolism and diabetic control: Differences between diabetic patients and diabetic rats. *Diabetes Res Clin Pract.,* 9 (3), July, 239–244.

Kodama, M. et al. 1993. Diabetes mellitus is controlled by vitamin C treatment. *In vivo,* 7 (6A), Nov.–Dec., 535–350.

Cunningham, J. J. et al. 1994. Vitamin C: An aldose reductase inhibitor that normalizes erythrocyte sorbitol in insulin-dependent diabetes mellitus. *J Am Coll Nutr.,* 13 (4), Aug., 344–350.
Dose: 100–600 mg/day of vitamin C for 58 days.

Cunningham, J. J. et al. Reduced mononuclear leukocyte ascorbic acid content in adults with insulin-dependent diabetes mellitus consuming adequate dietary vitamin C. *Metabolism,* 40, 146–149.

Fatigue

Cheraskin, E. et al. 1976. Daily vitamin C consumption and fatigability. *J Am Geriatric Soc.,* 24 (3), 136–137.

Glaucoma

Jampel, H. D. 1990. Ascorbic acid is cytotoxic to dividing human Tenon's capsule fibroblasts: A possible contributing factor in glaucoma filtration surgery success. *Arch Ophthalmol.,* 108 (9), Sept., 1323–1325.

Glutathione Deficiency

Jain, A. et al. 1994. Effect of ascorbate or N-acetylcysteine treatment in a patient with hereditary glutathione synthetase deficiency. *J Pediatrics,* 124 (2), Feb., 229–233.
Dose: 0.7 mmol/kg/day for 1–2 weeks.

Herpes

Fitzherbert, J. 1979. Genital herpes and zinc. *Med J Aust,* 1, 399.
Dose: 250 mg vitamin C 2x/day.

Terezhalmy, G. T. et al. 1978. The use of water-soluble bioflavonoid-ascorbic acid complex in the treatment of recurrent herpes labialis. *Oral Surgery,* 45, 56–62.
Dose: 200 mg vitamin C for 3–5 times/day for 3 days beginning after onset of symptoms.

Immune enhancement

Anderson, R. et al. 1980. The effects of increasing weekly doses of ascorbate on certain cellular and humoral immune functions in normal volunteers. *Am J Clin Nutr.,* 33 (1), Jan., 71–76.
Dose: 2–3 g/day.

Penn, N. D. et al. 1991. The effect of dietary supplementation with vitamins A, C and E on cell-mediated immune function in elderly long-stay patients: A randomized controlled trial. *Age Ageing,* 20 (3), May, 169–174.

Kodama, M. et al. 1994. Autoimmune disease and allergy are controlled by vitamin C treatment. *In vivo,* 8 (2), Mar.–Apr., 251–257.

Delafuente, J. C. et al. 1986. Immunologic modulation by vitamin C in the elderly. *Int J Immunopharmacol,* 8 (2), 205–211.
Dose: 2 g/day for 3 weeks.

Menopause

Horoschak, A. 1959. Nocturnal leg cramps, easy bruisability and epistaxis in menopausal patients: Treated with Hesperidin and ascorbic acid. *Delaware State Med J.,* 19–22.
Dose: 200 mg of vitamin C following each meal and at bedtime for 2 weeks plus another 100 mg of both 4x/day for 4 weeks.

Neutrophil Dysfunction

Rebora, A. et al. 1980. Neutrophil dysfunction and repeated infections: Influence of levamisole and ascorbic avid. *British J Dermatology,* 102 (1), Jan., 49–56.

Levy, R. and Schlaeffer, F. 1993. Successful treatment of a patient with recurrent furunculosis by vitamin C: Improvement of clinical course and of impaired neutrophil functions. *Int J Dermatology*, 32 (11), Nov., 832–834.

Dose: 500 mg/day of vitamin C for 30 days.

Obesity

Naylor, G. J. et al. 1985. A double blind placebo controlled trial of ascorbic acid in obesity. *Nutr Health*, 4 (1), 25–28.

Dose: 3 g/day for 6 weeks.

Paget's Disease

Smethurst, M. et al. 1981. Combined therapy with ascorbic acid and calcitonin for the relief of bone pain in Paget's disease. *Acta Vitaminol Enzymol*, 3 (1), 8–11.

Pancreatitis

Scott, P. et al. 1993. Vitamin C status in patients with acute pancreatitis. *British J Surgery*, 80 (6), June, 750–754.

Parkinson's disease

Fahn, S. 1992. A pilot trial of high-dose alpha-tocopherol and ascorbate in early Parkinson's disease. *Annals Neurology*, (32 Suppl), S128–S132.

Reilly, D. K. et al. 1983. On-off effects in Parkinson's disease: A controlled investigation of ascorbic acid therapy. *Advanc Neurol*, 37, 51–60.

Linazasoro, G. and Gorospe, A. [Treatment of complicated Parkinson disease with a solution of levodopa-carbidopa and ascorbic acid]. *Neurologia*, 10 (6), June–July, 220–223.

Yapa, S. C. 1992. Detection of subclinical ascorbate deficiency in early Parkinson's Disease. *Public Health*, 106 (5), Sept., 393–395.

Periodontal Disease

Leggott, P. J. et al. 1991. Effects of ascorbic acid depletion and supplementation of periodontal health and subgingival microflora in humans. *J Dental Res*, 70 (12), Dec., 1531–1536.

Leggott, P. J. et al. 1986. The effect of controlled ascorbic acid depletion and supplementation on periodontal health. *J Periodonotal*, 57 (8), Aug., 480–485.

Respiration

Peters, E. M. et al. 1993. Vitamin C supplementation reduces the incidence of postrace symptoms of upper-respiratory-tract infection in ultramarathon runners. *Am J Clin Nutr.*, (2), Feb., 170–174.
Dose: 600 mg/day vitamin C.

Mohsenin, V. 1987. Effect of vitamin C on NO2-induced airway hyperresponsiveness in normal subjects: A randomized double-blind experiment. *Am Rev Resp Dis,* 136 (6), Dec., 1408–1411.
Dose: 500 mg 4x/day of ascorbic acid for 3 days.

Bucca, C. et al. 1990. Effect of vitamin C on histamine bronchial responsiveness of patients with allergic rhinitis. *Ann Allergy,* 65 (4), Oct., 311–314.
Dose: 2 g of vitamin C.

Bucca, C. et al. 1989. Effects of vitamin C on airway responsiveness to inhaled histamine in heavy smokers. *European Respir J,* 2 (3), Mar., 229–233.
Dose: 2 g of vitamin C.

Schizophrenia

Sandyk, R. and Kanofsky, J. D. 1993. Vitamin C in the treatment of schizophrenia. *Int J Neuroscience,* 68 (1–2), Jan., 67–71.

Sickle Cell Anemia

Jain, S. K. et al. 1985. Reduced levels of plasma ascorbic acid (vitamin C) in sickle cell disease patients: Its possible role in the oxidant damage to sickle cells in vivo. *Clin Chim Acta,* 149 (2–3), July 15, 257–161.

Smoking Cessation

Levin, E. D. et al. 1993. Clinical trials using ascorbic acid aerosal to aid smoking cessation. *Drug Alcohol Depend,* 33 (3), Oct., 211–223.

Stroke

Gale, C. R. et al. 1995. Vitamin C and risk of death from stroke and coronary heart disease in cohort of elderly people. *British Med J,* 310 (6994), June 17, 1563–1566.

Tetanus

Jahan, J. K. et al. 1985. Effect of ascorbic acid in the treatment of tetanus. *Bangladesh Med Res Council Bull,* 10 (1), June, 24–28.
Dose: 1000 mg/day iv.

Wound healing

Ringsdorf Jr., W. M. and Cheraskin, E. 1982. Vitamin C and human wound healing. *Oral Surg Med Oral Pathol,* 53 (3), Mar., 231–236.
Dose: 500–3000 mg/day.

Goode, H. F. et al. 1992. Vitamin C depletion and pressure sores in elderly patients with femoral neck fractures. *British Med J,* 305 (6859), Oct. 17, 925–927.

VITAMIN E

Abetalipoproteinemia

Illingworth, D. R. et al. 1980. Abetalipoprotein. Report of two cases and review of therapy. *Arch Neurol,* 37 (10), Oct., 659–662.

Bishara, S. et al. 1982. Combined vitamin A and therapy prevents retinal electrophysiological deterioration in abetalipoprotein. B*ritish J Ophthalmology,* 66 (12), Dec., 767–770.

Muller, D. P. et al. 1983. Vitamin E and neurological function: Abetalipoproteinaemia and other disorders of fat absorption. *Ciba Found Symp,* 101, 106–121.

Hegele, R. A. and Angel, A. 1985. Arrest of neuropathy and myopathy in abetalipoproteinemia with high-dose Vitamin E therapy. *Canadian Med Assoc J,* 132 (1), Jan., 41–44.
Dose: 3200 mg/day over 7 years.

Aging

Courtiere, A. et al. 1989. [Lipid peroxidation in aged patients. Influence of an antioxidant combination (vitamin C-vitamin E-rutin)]. *Therapie,* 44 (1), Jan.–Feb., 13–17.

Alzheimer's disease

Adams, Jr., J. D. et al. 1991. Alzheimer's and Parkinson's Disease. Brain levels of glutathione, glutathione disulfide, and vitamin E. *Mol Chem Neuropathol.,* 14 (3), June, 213–226.

Anemia

Ono, K. 1985. Effects of large dose of vitamin E supplementation on anemia in hemodialysis patients. *Nephron,* 40 (4), 440–445.
Dose: 600 mg/day for 30 days.

Arthritis

Honkanen, V. E. et al. 1990. Serum cholesterol and vitamins A and E in juvenile chronic arthritis. *Clin Exp Pheumatol,* 8 (2), Mar.–Apr., 187–191.

Honkanen, V. E. et al. 1989. Vitamins A and E, retinol binding protein and zinc in Rheumatoid Arthritis. *Clin Exp Pheumatol,* 7 (5), Sept.–Oct., 465–469.

Ataxia

Rayner, R. J. et al. 1993. Isolated vitamin E deficiency and progressive ataxia. *Arch Dis Child,* 69 (5), Nov., 602–603.

Brain injury

Dzandzhgava, T. G. and Shakarishvili, R. R. 1991. [Effect of alpha-tocopherol and selenium on the activity of antioxidant enzymes and level of lipid peroxidation products in erythrocytes of patients with cerebral ischemia]. *Vopr Med Khim,* 37 (5), Sept.–Oct. 79–82.

Cancer

Kneky, P. et al. 1991. Vitamin E and cancer prevention. *Am J Clin Nutr,* 53 (1 Suppl), Jan., 283S–286S.

Kneky, R. et al. 1988. Serum vitamin E and risk of cancer among Finnish men during a 10-year follow-up. *Am J Epidemiology,* 127 (1), Jan., 28–41.

Knekt, P. et al. 1991. Dietary antioxidants and the risk of lung cancer. *Am J Epidemiology,* 134 (5), Sept. 1, 471–479.

Garewal, H. S. and Schantz, S. 1995. Emerging role of beta-carotene and antioxidant nutrients in prevention of oral cancer. *Arch Otalaryngol Head Neck Surg,* 121 (2), Feb., 141–144.

Wald, N. J. et al. 1984. Plasma retinol, beta-carotene and vitamin E levels in relation to the future risk of breast cancer. *British J Cancer,* 49 (3), Mar., 321–324.

Wald, N. J. et al. 1987. Serum vitamin E and subsequent risk of cancer. *British J Cancer,* 56 (1), July, 69–72.

Salonen, J. T. et al. 1985. Risk of cancer in relation to serum concentrations of selenium and vitamins A and E: Matched case-control analysis of prospective data. *British Med J,* 290 (6466), Feb. 9, 417–420.

London, R. S. et al. 1981. Endocrine parameters and alpha-tocopherol therapy of patients with mammary dysplasia. *Cancer Res,* 41 (9 Pt 2), Sept., 3811–3813.
Dose: 600 units/day.

Taylor, P. R. et al. 1994. Prevention of esophageal cancer: The nutrition intervention trials in Linxian, China: Linxian nutrition intervention trials study group. *Cancer Res,* 54 (7 Suppl), April 1, 2029s–2031s.
Dose: 30–60 IU/day for 5.25 years.

Bostick, R. M. et al. 1993. Reduced risk of colon cancer with high intake of vitamin E: The Iowa Women's Health Study. *Cancer Res,* 53 (18), Sept. 15, 4230–4237.

Zheng, W. et al. 1993. Serum micronutrients and the subsequent risk of oral and pharyngeal cancer. *Cancer Res,* 53 (4), Feb. 15, 795–798.

Menkes, M. J. 1986. Vitamin A, E, Selenium and risk of lung cancer. *Dissertation Abstracts Int.,* 46 (11), 3807.

Longnecker, M. P. et al. 1992. Serum alpha-tocopherol concentration in relation to subsequent colorectal cancer: Pooled data from five cohorts. *J National Cancer Inst.,* 84 (6), Mar. 18, 430–435.

Menkes, M. S. et al. 1986. Serum beta-carotene, vitamins A and E, selenium, and the risk of lung cancer. *NEJM,* 315 (20), Nov. 13, 1250–1254.

Wei, Q. et al. 1993. Vitamin supplementation has a protective effect on basal cell carcinoma. *Am Soc Preventive Oncology,* 17th Annual Meeting, Mar. 20–23, Tuscon, AR.
Dose: greater than 100 IU/day.

Knekt, P. 1993. Vitamin E and smoking and the risk of lung cancer. *Annals NY Acad Sci.,* 686, May 28, 280–287.

London, S. J. et al. 1992. Carotenoids, retinol, and vitamin E and risk of proliferative benign breast disease and breast cancer. *Cancer Causes Control,* 3 (6), Nov., 503–512.

Benner, S. F. et al. 1994. Reduction in oral mucosa micronuclei frequency following alpha-tocopherol treatment of oral leukoplakia. *Cancer Epidemiol Biomarkers Prev.,* 3 (1), Jan.–Feb., 73–76.
Dose: 400 IU.

de Vries, N. and Snow, G. B. 1990. Relationships of vitamins A and E and beta-carotene serum levels to head and neck cancer patients with and without second primary tumors. *Eur Arch Otorhinolaryngol,* 247 (6), 368–370.

Garewal, H. 1982. Chemoprevention of oral cancer: Beta-carotene and vitamin E in leukoplakia. *European J Cell Biology,* 28 (1), Aug., 92–97.

Knekt, P. et al. 1988. Serum vitamin E, serum selenium and the risk of gastrointestinal cancer. *Int J Cancer,* 42 (6), Dec. 15, 846–850.

Knekt, P. 1988. Serum vitamin E level and risk of female cancers. *Int J Epidemiology,* 17 (2), June, 281–286.

Prasad, K. N. and Edwards-Prasad, J. 1992. Vitamin E and cancer prevention: Recent advances and future potentials. *J Am College Nutr.,* 11 (5), Oct. 487–500.

Torun, M. et al. 1995. Serum vitamin E level in patients with breast cancer. *J Clin Pharm Ther.,* 20 (3), June, 173–178.

Lockwood, K. et al. Apparent partial remission of breast cancer in 'high risk' patients supplemented with nutritional antioxidants, essential fatty acids and Coenzyme Q$_{10}$. *Mol Aspects Med.,* 15 (Suppl), 231–240.
Dose: 2500 IU.

Palan, R. R. et al. 1991. Plasma levels of antioxidant beta-carotene and alpha-tocopherol in uterine cervix dysplasias and cancer. *Nutr Cancer,* 15 (1), 13–20.

LeGardeur, B. Y. et al. 1990. A case-control study of serum vitamins A, E, and C in lung cancer patients. *Nutr Cancer,* 14 (2), 133–140.

Wadleigh, R. et al. 1990. Vitamin E in the treatment of chemotherapy-induced mucosisitis. *Proceedings Annual Meeting Am Soc Clin Oncologists,* 9, A1237.
Dose: 400 mg/ml applied to lesions for 1 week.

Dimery, I. et al. 1992. Reduction in toxicity of high dose 13-CIS-Retinoic acid (13-CRA) with alpha-tocopherol. *Proc Annual Meeting Am Soc Clin Oncologists,* 11, A399.
Dose: 800, 1200, 1600, 2000 IU/day 4 week cycle.

Sukolinskii, V. N. and Morozkina, T. S. 1989. [Prevention of postoperative complications in patients with stomach cancer using an antioxidant complex]. *Vopr Onkol,* 35 (10), 1242–1245.

Gorozhanskaia, E. G. et al. 1995. [The role of alpha-tocopherol and retinol in correcting disorders of lipid peroxidation in patients with malignant liver neoplasms]. *Vopr Onkol,* 41 (1), 47–51.
Dose: 600 mg for 7 days prior to surgery.

Cardiovascular/Coronary heart disease

Salonen, J. T. et al. 1991. Effects of antioxidant supplementation on platelet function: A randomized pair-matched, placebo-controlled, double-blind trial in men with low antioxidant status. *Am J Clin Nutr,* 53 (5), May, 1222–1229.

Dose: 300 mg/day for 5 months.

Bellizz, M. C. et al. 1994. Vitamin E and coronary heart disease: The European paradox. *Eur J Clin Nutr.,* 48 (11), Nov., 822–831.

Dose: 1 capsule of palmvitee/day for 30 days.

Tan, D. T. et al. 1991. Effect of a palm-oil-vitamin E concentrate on the serum and lipoprotein lipids in humans. *Am J Clin Nutr.,* 53 (4 Suppl), Apr., 1027S–1030S.

Qureshi, A. A. et al. 1991. Lowering of serum cholesterol in hypercholesterolemic humans by tocopherols (Palmvitee). *Am J Clin Nutr.,* 53 (4 Suppl), Apr., 1021S–1026S.

Dose: 200 mg palmvitee capsules/day or 200mg gamma-tocotrienol/day for 4 weeks.

Paolisso, G. et al. 1995. Chronic intake of pharmacological doses of vitamin E might be useful in the therapy of elderly patients with coronary heart disease. *Am J Clin Nutr.,* 61 (4), Apr., 848–852.

Dose: 900 mg/day for 4 months.

Brown, K. M. et al. 1994. Vitamin E supplementation suppresses indexes of lipid peroxidation and platelet counts in blood of smokers and non-smokers but plasma lipoprotein concentrations remain unchanged. *Am J Clin Nutr.,* 60 (3), Sept., 383–387.

Dose: 280 mg/day for 10 weeks.

Steiner, M. et al. 1995. Vitamin E plus aspirin compared with aspirin alone in patients with transient ischemic attacks. *Am J Clin Nutr,* 62 (6 Suppl), Dec., 1381S–1384S.

Dose: 400 IU/day for up to 2 years.

Chan, A. C. et al. 1986. Transitory stimulation of human platelet 12-lipoxygenase by vitamin E supplementation. *Am J Clin Nutr.,* 44 (2), Aug., 278–282.

Dose: 400 IU/day of either D- or DL- alpha-tocopherol for 4 weeks.

Guetta, V. et al. 1995. Effect of combined 17 beta-estradiol and vitamin E on low-density lipoprotein oxidation in postmenopausal women. *Am J Clin Cardiology,* 75 (17), June 15, 1274–1276.

Knekt, P. et al. 1994. Antioxidant vitamin intake and coronary mortality in a longitudinal population study. *Am J Epidemiology*, 139 (12), June 15, 1180–1189.

Sisto, T. et al. 1995. Pretreatment with antioxidants and Allopurinol diminishes cardiac onset events in coronary artery bypass grafting. *Ann Thorac Surg*, 59 (6), June, 1519–1523.

Princen, H. M. et al. 1992. Supplementation with vitamin E but not beta-carotene in vivo protects low density lipoprotein from lipid peroxidation in vitro: Effect of cigarette smoking. *Arteriosclerosis Thrombosis*, 12 (5), May, 554–562.
Dose: 100 IU/day of DL-alpha-tocopherol.

Reaven, P. D. and Witzum, J. L. 1993. Comparisons of supplementation of RRR-alpha-tocopherol and racemic alpha-tocopherol in humans. Effects on lipid levels and lipoprotein susceptibility to oxidation. *Arterioscler Thromb*, 13 (4), Apr., 601–608.

Reaven, P. D. et al. 1993. Effect of dietary antioxidant combinations in humans: Protection of LDL by vitamin E but not by beta-carotene. *Arterioscler Thromb*, 13 (4), Apr., 590–600.

Kritchevsky, S. B. et al. Dietary antioxidants and carotid artery wall thickness: The ARIC study. Atherosclerosis risk in communities study. *Circulation*, 92 (8), Oct. 15, 2142–2150.

Jialal, I. and Grundy, S. M. 1993. Effect of combined supplementation with alpha-tocopherol, ascorbate, and beta-carotene on low-density lipoprotein oxidation. *Circulation*, 88 (6), Dec., 2780–2786.
Dose: 800 IU/day.

Luoma, P. V. et al. 1995. High serum alpha-tocopherol, albumin, selenium and cholesterol, and low mortality from coronary heart disease in Northern Finland. *J Internal Med*, 237 (1), Jan., 49–54.

Haglund, O. et al. 1991. The effects of fish oil on triglycerides, cholesterol, fibrinogen and malondialehyde in humans supplemented with vitamin E. *J Nutr.*, 121 (2), Feb., 165–169.

Hodis, H. N. et al. 1995. Serial coronary angiographic evidence that antioxidant vitamin intake reduces progression of coronary artery atherosclerosis. *JAMA*, 273 (23), June 21, 1849–1854.
Dose: 100 IU/day or more.

Fuenmayor, A. J. et al. Vitamin E and ventricular fibrillation threshold in myocardial ischemia. *Japanese Circulation J*, 53 (10), Oct., 1229–1232.

Riemersma, R. A. et al. 1991. Risk of angina pectoris and plasma concentrations of vitamins A, C, and E and Carotene. *Lancet,* 337 (8732), Jan. 5, 1–5.

Kardinaal, A. F. et al. Antioxidants in adipose tissue and risk of myocardial infarction: The EURAMIC study. *Lancet,* 342 (8884), Dec. 4, 1379–1384.

Rimm, E. B. et al. 1993. Vitamin E consumption and the risk of coronary heart disease in men. *NEJM,* 328 (20), May 20, 1450–1456.
Dose: 60 IU/day or more.

Stampfer, M. J. et al. 1993. Vitamin E consumption and the risk of coronary disease in women. *NEJM,* 328 (20), May 20, 1444–1449.

Singh, R. B. et al. 1994. Diet, antioxidant vitamins, oxidative stress and risk of coronary artery disease: The Peerzada prospective study. *Acta Cardiol,* 49 (5), 453–467.

Knight, J. A. et al. 1993. The effect of vitamins C and E on lipid peroxidation in stored erythrocytes. *Ann Clin Lab Sci,* 23 (1), Jan.–Feb., 51–56.

Postaire, E. et al. 1995. Increase of singlet oxygen protection of erythrocytes by vitamin E, vitamin C, and beta-carotene intakes. *Biochem Mol Biol Int,* 35 (2), Feb., 371–374.
Dose: 15 mg/day for 15 days.

Kleijnen, J. et al. 1989. Vitamin E and cardiovascular disease. *European J Clin Pharmacol,* 37 (6), 541–544.

Gey, K. F. 1989. Inverse correlation of vitamin E and ischemic heart disease. *Int J Vitamin Nutr Res Suppl,* 30, 224–231.

Dmoszynska-Giannopoulou, A. et al. 1987. Alpha-tocopherol: Effect of sulphinpyrazone and alpha-tocopherol on platelet activation and function in haemodialysed patients. *Int Urol Nephrol,* 22 (6), 561–566.

Cloarec, M. J. et al. Alpha-tocopherol: Effect on plasma lipoproteins in hypercholesterolemic patients. *Israeli J Med Sci,* 23 (8), Aug., 869–872.
Dose: 500 IU/day for 3 months.

Rifici, V. A. and Khachadurian, A. K. 1993. Dietary supplementation with vitamins C and E inhibits in vitro oxidation of lipoproteins. *J Am Coll Nutr,* 12 (6), Dec., 631–637.
Dose: 800 IU/day.

Lenzhofer, R. et al. 1983. Acute cardian toxicity in patients after Doxorubucin treatment and the effect of combined tocopherol and Nifedipine pretreatment. *J Cancer Res Clin Oncol,* 106 (2), 143–147.

Yukawa, S. et al. 1992. Prevention of aortic calcification in patients on hemodialysis by long-term administration of vitamin E. *J Nutr Sci Vitaminol,* Spec No, 187–190.
Dose: 600 mg/day for 2 weeks.

Gey, K. F. et al. 1994. [Essential antioxidants on cardiovascular diseases—Lessons for Europe]. *Ther Unsch,* 51 (7), July, 475–482.
Dose: 100 mg/day.

Steiner, M. 1993. Effect of alpha-tocopherol administration on platelet function in man. *Thromb Haemost,* 49 (2), Apr. 28, 73–77.
Dose: 400–1200 IU/day over 6 weeks.

Cataracts

Jacques, P. F. et al. 1988. Antioxidants status in persons with and without senile cataract. *Arch Ophthalmol,* 106 (3), Mar., 337–340.

Knekt, P. et al. 1992. Serum antioxidant Vitamins and risk of cataract. *British Med J,* 305 (6866), Dec. 5, 1392–1394.

Robertson, J. M. et al. 1989. Vitamin E intake and risk of cataracts in humans. *Ann NY Acad Sci,* 570, 372–382.

Cystic Fibrosis

Sitrin, M. D. et al. 1987. Vitamin E deficiency and neurologic disease in adults with cystic fibrosis. *Annals Int Med,* 107 (1), July, 51–54.

Sung, J. H. et al. 1980. Axonal dystrophy in the gracile nucleus in congenital biliary atresia and cystic fibrosis (mucoviscidosis): Beneficial effect of vitamin E therapy. *J Neuropathol Exp Neurol,* 39 (5), Sept., 584–597.

Cynamon, H. A. et al. 1988. Effect of vitamin E deficiency on neurologic function in patients with cystic fibrosis. *J Pediatrics,* 113 (4), Oct., 637–640.

Elias, E. et al. 1981. Association of spinocerebellar disorders with cystic fibrosis or chronic childhood cholestasis and very low serum vitamin E. *Lancet,* 2 (8259), Dec. 12, 1319–1321.

James. D. R. et al. 1991. Increased susceptibility to peroxide-induced haemolysis with normal vitamin E concentrations in cystic fibrosis. *Clin Chim Acta,* 204 (1–3), Dec. 31, 279–290.

Diabetes

Colette, C. et al. 1988. Platelet function in Type I diabetes: Effects of supplementation with large doses of vitamin E. *Am J Clin Nutr*, 47 (2), Feb., 256–261.
Dose: 1 gm/day for 35 days.

Paolisso, G. et al. Pharmacologic doses of vitamin E improve insulin action in healthy subjects and non-insulin-dependent diabetic patients. *Am J Clin Nutr*, 57 (5), May, 650–656.
Dose: 900 mg/day for 4 months.

Salonen, J. T. et al. 1995. Increased risk of non-insulin dependent Diabetes Mellitus at low plasma vitamin E concentrations: A four year follow-up study in men. *British Med J*, 311 (7013), Oct. 28, 1124–1127.

Karpen, C. W. et al. 1984. Interrelation of platelet vitamin E and thromboxane synthesis in type I Diabetes Mellitus. *Diabetes*, 33 (3), Mar., 239–243.

Watanabe, J. et al. 1984. Effect of vitamin E on platelet aggregation in Diabetes Mellitus. *Thromb Haemost*, 51 (3), July 29, 313–316.

Karpen, C. W. et al. 1985. Production of 12-hydroyeicosatetraenoic acid and VItamin E status in platelets from type I human diabetic subjects. *Diabetes*, 34 (6), June, 526–531.

Caballero, B. 1993. Vitamin E improves the action of insulin. *Nutr Rev*, 51 (11), Nov., 339–340.

Kunisaki, M. et al. 1990. Effects of vitamin E administration on platelet function in Diabetes Mellitus. *Diabetes Res*, 14 (1), May, 37–42.
Dose: 600 mg/day.

Dmoszynska-Giannopoulou, A. et al. 1989. [Effect of vitamin E on the function of blood platelets in patients with Diabetes Mellitus], *Pol Tyg Lek*, 44 (21–22), May 22–29, 496–498.
Dose: 1000 mg/day.

Dzhavad-zade, M. D. et al. 1992. [Disorders of pulmonary hemodynamics in patients with Diabetic Nephroangiopathy and its correction with antioxidants], *Probl Endokrinol*, 38 (2), Mar.–Apr., 20–22.
Dose: 8 mcg/kg/day for 2 weeks.

Mamedgasanov, R. M. and Rakhmani, S. A. [Dynamics of lipid peroxidation in patients with noninsulin-dependent Diabetes Mellitus], *Probl Endokrinol*, 35 (1), Jan.–Feb., 19–21.

Balabolkin, M. I. et al. 1994. [Effect of high doses of tocopherol on the process of lipid peroxidation and insulin secretion in patients with non-insulin-dependent Diabetes Mellitus], *Probl Endokrinol,* 40 (3), May–June, 10–12.
Dose: 600–1200 mg/day.

Kuznetsov, N. S. et al. 1993. [The use of antioxidants (alpha-tocopherol acetate) in the treatment of Diabetes Mellitus]. *Probl Endokrinol,* 39 (2), Mar.–Apr., 9–11.
Dose: 300 mg/day.

Watanabe, J. et al. 1984. Effect of vitamin E in platelet aggregation in Diabetes Mellitus. *Tohoku J Exp Med,* 143 (2), June, 161–169.

Splavskii, O. I. 1982. [Effectiveness of vitamin E in the combined therapy of the hepatobiliary system lesions in Diabetes Mellitus]. *Vopr Pitan,* (6), Nov.–Dec., 36–39.

Gerster, H. et al. 1993. Prevention of platelet dysfunction by vitamin E in diabetic athersclerosis. *Z Ernahrungswiss,* 32 (4), Dec., 243–261.

Disseminated Granuloma Anulare

Goldstein, R. K. et al. [Local treatment of disseminated granuloma anulare with a vitamin E emulsion]. *Hautarzt,* 42 (3), Mar., 176–178.

Epilepsy

Ogunmekan, A. O. and Hwang, P. A. 1989. A randomized, double-blind, placebo-controlled, clinical trial of D-alpha-tocopherol acetate (vitamin E), as add-on therapy, for epilepsy in children. *Epilepsia,* 30 (1), Jan.–Feb., 84–89.

Kovalenko, V. M. et al. 1984. [Alpha-tocopherol in the complex treatment of several forms of epilepsy]. *Zh Nevropatol Psikhiatr,* 84 (6), 892–897.
Dose: 600 mg/day

Megrabian, A. A. et al. 1986. [Use of lithium carbonate and vitamin E in the complex treatment of epileptics]. *Zh Nevropatol Psikhiatr,* 86 (9), 1407–1410.

Gastrointestinal Disease

Beno, I. et al. 1994. The activity of Cu/Zn-superoxide dismutase and catalase of gastric mucosa in chronic gastritis, and the effect of alpha-tocopherol. *Bratisl Lek Listy,* 95 (1), Jan., 9–14.

Feher, J. and Pronai, L. 1993. [Role of free radical scavengers in gastrointestinal diseases], *Orv Hetil,* 34 (13), Mar. 28, 693–696.

General

Wartanowicz, W. et al. 1984. The effect of alpha-tocopherol and ascorbic acid on the serum lipid peroxide level in elderly people. *Anna Nutr Metab,* 28 (3), 186–191.

Dose: 200 mg/day for 4 months.

Regnault, C. et al. 1993. Influence of beta carotene, vitamin E, and vitamin C on endogenous antioxidant defenses in erythrocytes. *Ann Pharmacother,* 27 (11), Nov., 1349–1350.

Denzlinger, C. et al. 1995. Modulation of the endogenous leukotriene production by fish oil and vitamin E. *J Lipid Mediat Cell Signal,* 11 (2), Mar., 119–132.

Dose: 800 IU/day.

Hearing loss

Romeo, G. 1985. The therapeutic effect of vitamins A and E in neurosensory hearing loss. *Acta Vitaminol Enzymol,* (7 Suppl), 85–92.

Romeo, G. and Giorgetti, M. 1985. [Therapeutic effects of vitamin A associated with vitamin E in perceptual hearing loss]. *Acta Vitaminol Enzymol,* 7 (1–2), 139–143.

Hemodialysis

Giardini, O. et al. 1984. Effects of alpha-tocopherol administration on red blood cell membrane lipid peroxidation in hemodialysis patients. *Clin Nephrol,* 21 (3), Mar., 174–177.

Hemolysis

Prussick, R. et al. 1992. The protective effect of vitamin E on the hemolysis associated with dapsone treatment in patients with dermatitis herpetiformis. *Arch Dermatol,* 128 (2), Feb., 210–213.

Dose: 800 IU/day for 4 weeks.

Hafez, M, et al. 1986. Improved erythrocyte survival with combined vitamin E and selenium therapy in children with glucose-6-phosphate dehydrogenase deficiency and mild chronic hemolysis. *J Pediatrics,* 108 (4), Apr., 558–561.

Dose: 800 IU/day for 2 months.

Corash, L. et al. 1980. Reduced chronic hemolysis during high-dose vitamin E administration in Mediterranean-type glucose-6-phosphate dehydrogenase deficiency. *New England J Med,* 303 (8), Aug. 12, 416–420.

Yalcin, A. S. et al. 1989. The effect of vitamin E therapy on plasma and erythrocyte lipid peroxidation in chronic hemodialysis patients. *Clin Chim Acta,* 185 (1), Oct. 31, 109–112.
Dose: 300 mg/day for 1 month.

Hepatitis

Han, Y. C. 1993. [Study of anti-lipid peroxidation of vitamin E in human body]. *Chung Hua Yu Fang I Hsueh Tsa Chih,* 27 (3), May, 132–134.
Dose: 200 mg/day after 10 days.

Immune enhancement

Meydani, S. N. et al. 1990. Vitamin E supplementation enhances cell-mediated immunity in healthy elderly subjects. *Am J Clin Nutr,* 52 (3), Sept., 557–563.
Dose: 800 mg/day for 30 days.

Kowdley, K. V. et al. 1992. Vitamin E deficiency and impaired cellular immunity related to intestinal fat malabsorption. *Gastroenterology,* 102 (6), June, 2139–2142.

Penn, N. D. et al. 1991. The effect of dietary supplementation with vitamins A, C and E on cell-mediated immune function in elderly long-stay patients: A randomized controlled trial. *Age Ageing,* 20 (3), May, 169–174.

Taccone-Gallucci, M. et al. 1986. Vitamin E supplementation in hemodialysis patients: Effects on peripheral blood mononuclear cells lipid peroxidation and immune response. *Clin Nephrol,* 25 (2), Feb., 81–86.

Gaidova, O. S. et al. 1990. [The immunomodulating properties of vitamin E in surgery involving artificial circulation]. *Grud serdechnososudistaia Khir,* (12), Dec., 30–33.
Dose: 40 mg/kg 3.5 hours prior to open heart surgery.

Kidney disease/damage

Bilenko, M. V. et al. 1983. [Use of antioxidants to prevent damage during acute ischemia and reperfusion of the kidneys]. *Bull Eksp Biol Med,* 96 (9), Sept., 8–11.

Leg cramps

Roca, A. O. et al. 1992. Dialysis leg cramps: Efficacy of quinine versus vitamin E. *ASAIO J*, 38 (3), July–Sept., M481–485.
Dose: 400 IU/day.

Mucositis

Wadleigh, R. G. et al. 1992. Vitamin E in the treatment of chemotherapy-induced Mucositis. *Am J Med.*, 92 (5), May, 481–484.

Myotonic dystrophy

Orndahl, G. et al. 1986. Myotonic dystrophy treated with selenium and vitamin E. *Acta Med Scand*, 219 (4), 407–414.
Dose: 600 mg.

Neurological function

Muller, D. P. et al. 1983. Vitamin E and neurological function. *Lancet*, 1 (8318), Jan. 29, 225–228.

Muller, D. P. 1986. Vitamin E—Its role in neurological function. *Postgraduate Med J*, 62 (724), Feb., 107–112.

Lloyd, B. W. and Dubowitz, V. 1992. Progressive neurological disorders associated with obstructive jaundice and vitamin E deficiency. *Neuropediactrics*, 13 (3), Aug., 155–157.

Davidai, G. et al. 1986. Hypovitaminosis E induced neuropathy in exocrine pancreatic failure. *Arch Dis Child*, 61 (9), Sept., 901–903.

Palmucci, L. et al. 1988. Neuropathy secondary to vitamin E deficiency in acquired in acquired intestinal malabsorption. *Italian J Neurol Sci*, 9 (6), Dec., 599–602.

Neutrophil

Chai, J. et al. 1995. [Protective effects of vitamin E on impaired neutrophil phagocytic function in patients with severe burn]. *Chung Hua Cheng Hsing Shao Shang Wai Ko Tsa Chih*, 11 (1), Jan., 32–35.

Osteoarthritis

Blankenhorn, G. 1986. [Clinical effectiveness of Spondyvit (vitamin E) in activated arthroses: A multicenter placebo-controlled double-blind study]. *Z Orthop*, 124 (3), May–June, 340–343.
Dose: 400 IU/day for 6 weeks.

Scherak, O. et al. 1990. [High dose vitamin E therapy in patients with acti-vated arthrosis]. *Z Rheumatol,* 49 (6), Nov.–Dec., 369–373.
  Dose: 400 IU/day for 3 weeks.

Machtey, I. and Ouaknine, L. 1978. Tocopherol in osteoarthritis: A con-trolled pilot study. *J Am Geriatric Soc,* 26 (7), July, 328–330.
  Dose: 600 mg/day for 10 days.

Parkinson's disease

Fahn, S. 1992. A pilot trial of high-dose alpha-tocopherol and ascorbate in early Parkinson's disease. *Ann Neurol,* 32 (Suppl), S128–S132.

Dexter, D. T. et al. 1994. Nigrostriatal function in vitamin E deficiency: Clinical, experimental, and positron emission tomographic studies. *Ann Neurol,* 35 (3), Mar., 298–303.

Peripheral neuropathy

Traber, M. G. et al. 1987. Lack of tocopherol in peripheral nerves of vitamin E–deficient patients with peripheral neuropathy. *NEJM,* 317 (5), July 30, 262–265.

Physical Performance

Simon-Schnass, I. and Pabst, H. 1988. Influence of vitamin E on physical performance. *Int J Vitam Nutr Res,* 58 (1), 49–54.
  Dose: 2x200 mg dl-alpha-tocopherol acetate for 10 weeks.

Pulmonary health

Mohsenin, V. 1991. Lipid peroxidation and antielastase activity in the lung under oxidant stress: Role of antioxidant defenses. *J Appl Physiology,* 70 (4), Apr., 1456–1462.

Respiration

Richards, G. et al. 1990. Investigations of the effects of oral administration of vitamin E and beta-carotene on the chemiluminescence responses and the frequency of sister chromatid exchanges in circulating leuko-cytes from cigarette smokers. *Am Rev Respiratory Dis,* 142 (3), Sept., 648–654.
  Dose: 900 IU for 6 weeks.

Skopinska-Rozewska, E. et al. 1987. The effect of vitamin E treatment on the incidence of OKT + 4 lymphocytes in the peripheral blood of children with chronic respiratory tract infections. *Archives Immunol Ther Exp,* 35 (2), 207–210.

Short Bowel Syndrome

Howard, L. et al. 1982. Reversible neurological symptoms caused by vitamin E deficiency in a patient with short bowel syndrome. *Am J Clin Nutr,* 36 (6), Dec., 1243–1249.

Traber, M. G. et al. 1994. Efficacy of water-soluble vitamin E in the treatment of vitamin E malabsorption in short-bowel syndrome. *Am J Clin Nutr,* 59 (6), June, 1270–1274.

Smoking

Pacht, E. R. et al. 1986. Deficiency of vitamin E in the alveolar fluid of cigarette smokers: Influence on alveolar macrophage cytotoxicity. *J Clin Invest,* 77 (3), Mar., 789–796.

Hoshino, E. et al. 1990. Vitamin E suppresses increased lipid peroxidation in cigarette smokers. *J Parenteral Enteral Nutr,* 14 (3), May–June, 300–305.
Dose: 800 mg/day for 2 weeks.

Spinocerebeller dysfunction

Brin, M. F. et al. 1985. Blind loop syndrome, vitamin E malabsorption, and spinocerebellar degeneration. *Neurology,* 35 (3), Mar., 338–342.

Spondylosis

Mahmud, Z. and Ali, S. M. 1992. Role of vitamin A and E in spondylosis. *Bangladesh Med Res Counc Bull,* 18 (1), Apr., 47–59.
Dose: 100 mg/day for 3 weeks.

Steatorrhoea

Evans, D. J. et al. 1995. Symptomatic vitamin E deficiency diagnosed after histological recognition of myometrial lipofuscinosis. *Lancet,* 346 (8974), Aug. 26, 545–546.

Stress

Meydani, M. et al. 1992. Vitamin E requirement in relation to dietary fish oil and oxidative stress in elderly. *EXS,* 62, 411–418.

Rokitzki, L. et al. 1994. Alpha-tocopherol supplementation in racing cyclists during extreme endurance training. *Int J Sport Nutr,* 4 (3), Sept., 253–264.

Hartmann, A. et al. 1995. Vitamin E prevents exercise-induced DNA damage. *Mutation Res,* 346 (4), Apr., 195–202.
Dose: 1200 mg/day for 14 days.

Tardive Dyskinesia

Egan, M. F. et al. 1992. Treatment of Tardive Dyskinesia with vitamin E. *Am J Psychiatry,* 149 (6), June, 773–777.
Dose: 1600 IU/day for 6 weeks.

Elkashef, A. M. et al. 1990. Vitamin E in the treatment of Tardive Dyskinesia. *Am J Psychiatry,* 147 (4), Apr., 505–506.

Dabiri, L. M. et al. 1994. Effectiveness of vitamin E for treatment of long-term Tardive Dyskinesia. *Am J Psychiatry,* 151 (6), June, 925–926.

Adler, L. A. et al. 1993. Vitamin E treatment of Tardive Dyskinesia. *Am J Psychiatry,* 150 (9), Sept., 1405–1407.
Dose: 1600 IU/day for 8–12 weeks.

Bischot, L. et al. 1993. Vitamin E in extrapyramidal disorders. *Pharm World Sci,* 15 (4), Aug. 20, 1993, 146–150.
Dose: 1600 IU/day.

Adler, L. A. et al. 1993. Vitamin E in Tardive Dyskinesia: Time course of effect after placebo substitution. *Psychopharmacol Bull,* 29 (3), 371–374.

Lohr, J. B. et al. 1988. Vitamin E in the treatment of Tardive Dyskinesia: The possible involvement of free radical mechanisms. *Schizophrenia Bull,* 14 (2), 291–296.

Thyroid Dysfunction

Krishnamurthy, S. and Prasanna, D. 1984. Serum vitamin E and lipid peroxides in malnutrition, hyper and hypothyroidism. *Acta Vitaminol Exzymol,* 6 (1), 17–21.

Danis, I. et al. 1990. [Vitamin E and malondialdehyde in the blood serum of thyrotoxicosis patients]. *Probl Endokrinol,* 36 (5), Sept.–Oct., 21–24.

Tuberculosis

Gur'eva, I. G. et al. [Antioxidants-Effective pathogenic agents in the combined therapy of Pulmonary Tuberculosis]. *Ter Arkh,* 59 (7), 72–74.

Ulcerative colitis

Bennet, J. D. 1986. Use of alpha-tocopherylquinone in the treatment of ulcerative colitis. *Gut,* 27 (6), June, 695–697.
Dose: 3 gm/day.

Vitiligo

Koshevenko, I. 1989. [Alpha-tocopherol in the combined treatment of Vitiligo]. *Vestn Dermatol Venerol,* (10), 70–72.

Wound healing

Haberal, M. et al. 1988. The effects of vitamin E on immune regulations after thermal injury. *Burns Incl Therm Injuries,* 14 (5), Oct., 388–393.

Yellow Nail Syndrome

Williams, H. C. et al. 1991. Successful use of topical vitamin E solution in the treatment of nail changes in Yellow Nail Syndrome. *Arch Dermatol,* 127 (7), July, 1023–1028.

ANTI-AGING RECIPES

In this chapter you will find a collection of delicious, easy-to-make recipes that will help you explore the pleasure of eating the most health-enhancing foods available. The key concept is that the food you ingest should make you feel light and more energized. It should also assist your immune system in its daily task of trying to maintain health and fight off disease, and it should provide your body with the means to counteract the increased levels of toxicity that we live with today.

The foods used in these recipes are rich in protein, complex carbohydrates, essential fatty acids, vitamins, minerals, chlorophyll, and phytochemicals—all building blocks as you start to maximize your health and improve your overall well-being. They are essential elements of the complex network of molecular events that work ceaselessly in our bodies to prevent and handle diseases such as arthritis, diabetes, and cancer and cardiovascular problems.

Protein, complex carbohydrates, and essential fatty acids can be obtained from grains, legumes, nuts, seeds, and starchy vegetables; vitamins, minerals, and chlorophyll are especially derived from juices. Fresh fruit juices are also rich in enzymes, which promote digestion and biochemical processes. Whenever possible, use organically grown fruits and vegetables. If you are unable to do so, wash your produce in a gallon of filtered water with 1/4 cup of hydrogen peroxide and 1/4 cup of apple cider vinegar to remove some of the chemicals and bacteria that are in or on them.

For juicing, some of the best vegetable combinations I like include dandelion, cucumber, kale, arugula, Swiss chard, and parsley. Generally, use only an ounce of these darker juices and dilute that with milder juices and springwater. The milder juices are made from cabbage, apple, beet, carrot, celery, and cucumber. You can also try wheat grass for its cleansing properties, but don't use more than an ounce a day of this powerful chlorophyll drink.

Carrot juice is very popular, although some people find that drinking too much of it brings the blood sugar up too high. If you have diabetes, hypoglycemia, or candida, you should be especially careful of drinking too much carrot or fruit juice. Focus instead on juices made mostly of green vegetables and aloe vera, as well as vitamin C and garlic.

Some of my favorite fruit juice combinations include pear, kiwi, pineapple, and tangerine; fresh gingerroot and apple; celery and apple; and lemon, cucumber, and apple. For the digestive system, eat blueberries, strawberries, and cinnamon. Papaya also helps with digestion. Pears are a wonderful cleanser, as are prunes for helping to eliminate constipation. Apples are an extraordinary colon cleanser and an overall tonic as well. Watermelon is an excellent blood purifier and a natural diuretic.

Once you are familiar with a new way of cooking and juicing, you can have fun and create your own favorite combinations. Remember, the choices you make in your kitchen are going to have a profound impact on your overall level of health and vitality.

APPETIZERS

Cucumber Cocktail
SERVES 2

1 cucumber
1 small onion, cut into thin slices,
   about ¼ cup
Pinch of salt
1 teaspoon rice wine vinegar
½ teaspoon honey

1 teaspoon finely chopped fresh dill
Pinch of pepper
1 tablespoon minced green bell
   pepper
1 tablespoon alfalfa sprouts
Dash of paprika

1. Slice the cucumber in half lengthwise and scoop out the seeds. Then slice the cucumber halves crosswise into thin strips. In a bowl, combine it with the onion. Stir in the remaining ingredients except for the sprouts and paprika.

2. Serve on toasted bread triangles or use as a filling for a sandwich. Top with the alfalfa sprouts and paprika.

Banana Farofa
SERVES 2

Canola oil for sautéing
3 just-ripe bananas, peeled and cut
   into thick slices
1 medium Vidalia onion, cut into
   rings

1 tablespoon grated ginger
2 tablespoons wheat germ

1. Heat the canola oil in a large skillet. Over medium heat, sauté the bananas until golden, then remove them and set aside.

2. Using the same canola oil, sauté the onion rings.

3. Return the bananas to the pan with the onions, add the ginger, and gently stir in the wheat germ. Lightly brown the mixture on medium-low heat, adding more oil if necessary. Serve hot.

Cumin Chickpeas

SERVES 2

12 ounces or one 16-ounce can
   chickpeas
1 cup water
3 tablespoons sesame oil
½ cup finely chopped onion
4 cloves garlic
1 scallion, finely chopped

⅛ teaspoon freshly grated gingerroot
3 tablespoons lemon juice
¼ cup roasted pecans
4 tablespoons finely ground cumin
1 teaspoon salt, or to taste
Radicchio for garnish

1. Simmer the chickpeas in the water with the sesame oil, onion, garlic, scallion, ginger, and lemon juice for 15 to 30 minutes, until the chickpeas are soft.

2. Add the pecans, cumin, and salt and let cook 5 more minutes. Be careful not to overcook to the point of mushiness. Drain.

3. Garnish with the radicchio and serve.

BREAKFAST DISHES

Apple and Millet Delight
SERVES 2

6 apples
1 cup water
½ cup millet
¼ cup mashed banana

2 tablespoons chopped dates
1 tablespoon unsweetened flaked
   coconut
½ teaspoon almond extract

1. Juice the apples. Set aside 1½ cups of the juice.

2. In a large saucepan, combine the 1 cup water and 1½ cup apple juice and bring to a boil over high heat.

3. Reduce the heat to medium-low and stir in the millet. Cook, uncovered, until the liquid is absorbed, about 10 minutes.

4. Add the remaining ingredients and stir.

5. Serve hot with unsweetened soy milk, rice milk, or juice.

A cup of burdock root tea is both tasty and immune-boosting when drunk 1 hour before or after this (or any) meal.

Orange and Apple Barley Cereal
SERVES 2

4 oranges
2 apples
½ cup water
⅓ cup pearl barley

⅓ cup whole dried apricots
3 tablespoons pure maple syrup
½ teaspoon ground cinnamon

1. Separately juice the oranges and the apples. Set aside 1 cup of the orange juice and ½ cup of the apple pulp.

2. In a medium saucepan, combine the 1 cup orange juice and ½ cup water and bring to a boil over high heat.

3. Reduce the heat to medium-low and stir in the barley. Cook, uncovered, for 10 to 15 minutes, stirring occasionally.

4. Add the ½ cup apple pulp and the remaining ingredients and cook for an additional 5 to 10 minutes, stirring occasionally.

5. Serve hot with unsweetened soy milk or juice.

Carob-Cocoa Kasha with Bananas
SERVES 2

4 apples
1 cup water
½ cup unsweetened soy milk or rice
   milk
⅓ cup kasha

½ cup mashed banana
½ teaspoon raw unsweetened cocoa
   or roasted carob powder
¼ cup pure maple syrup
Dash of ground cinnamon

1. Juice the apples. Set aside 1 cup of the juice.
2. In a medium saucepan, combine the 1 cup apple juice, 1 cup water, and ½ cup soy or rice milk and bring to a boil over high heat.
3. Reduce the heat to medium-low and stir in the kasha. Stir in the remaining ingredients and cook, uncovered, for 3 to 4 minutes, stirring occasionally.
4. Serve hot with unsweetened soy milk or rice milk or juice.

Sunflower Carob Granola
SERVES 2

2 tablespoons roasted carob powder
1 cup rolled oats
½ cup unsalted whole almonds
¼ cup raisins
¼ cup unsalted hulled sunflower
   seeds

½ cup pure maple syrup
2 teaspoons almond extract
½ teaspoon ground cinnamon

1. Preheat the oven to 375 degrees F.
2. In a large mixing bowl, combine all of the ingredients, mixing well.
3. Spread the mixture on a greased cookie sheet and bake for 15 minutes, or until the top of the mixture turns brown.
4. Serve the granola hot over Rice Dream or cold with unsweetened soy milk or rice milk.

A cup of ginger tea is refreshing and immune-boosting when drunk 1 hour after eating.

Banana Pecan Pancakes
SERVES 2

6 apples
1 cup carrot
2 eggs, or the equivalent egg
   substitute
¼ cup pure maple syrup
½ cup water
1 cup whole spelt flour
2 teaspoons baking powder
½ cup toasted rice germ

½ cup sliced banana
¼ cup unsalted halved or chopped
   pecans
2 tablespoons raisins
½ teaspoon ground cinnamon
2 tablespoons cold-pressed flavorless
   oil (sunflower, safflower, or
   canola)

1. Separately juice the apples and the carrot. Set aside 1½ cups of the apple juice and ¼ cup of the carrot pulp.

2. In a large mixing bowl, combine the apple juice, eggs or egg substitute, maple syrup, water and mix well.

3. Stir in the flour, baking powder, and rice germ and mix well.

4. Stir in the carrot pulp, banana, pecans, raisins, and cinnamon.

5. Heat 1 tablespoon of the oil in a small frying pan over medium-high heat, then cover the bottom with about half of the batter. Cook for 3 to 4 minutes, or until underside is brown. Flip the pancake over and reduce the heat to low. Cut into wedges to allow the center to cook. Cook for an additional 2 minutes, or until the center is done. Repeat the process with the other half of the batter.

6. Serve hot with unsweetened soy milk or rice milk or juice.

Soups

Mock Sour Cream

(To use with soup recipes)

MAKES 3 OUNCES

¼ of 12-ounce package silken tofu
1 teaspoon freshly squeezed lemon
  juice

Blend the tofu and the juice.

Green Split Pea Soup

SERVES 2

2½ cups water
¼ pound dried split green peas
1 large onion, chopped
2 scallions, chopped
2 cloves garlic, finely chopped
3 sprigs flat-leaf parsley, chopped
½ green bell pepper
½ teaspoon ground cumin

¼ teaspoon curry powder
¼ teasooon powdered ginger
1 tablespoon olive oil
3 ounces celery, chopped
Salt to taste
Freshly ground black or pink
  peppercorns to taste

1. In a medium saucepan, bring the water to a boil. Add the peas and reduce the heat to low. Should the mixture become too thick, add water for the desired consistency. Cook the peas for 1 hour, or until they begin to disintegrate.

2. Add the remaining ingredients, except the salt and pepper, and cook over low heat for ½ hour. Season with salt and freshly ground pepper to taste.

Pureed Plantain Soup

SERVES 2

One 16-ounce can chickpeas with
   liquid
3 cups water
Pinch of white pepper
Pinch of salt

Pinch of cumin
1 cup salted plantain chips, ground in
   a food processor
2 lime slices

1. Combine the chickpeas and their liquid, water, pepper, salt, and cumin in a large saucepan at room temperature. Transfer three-quarters of the mixture to a blender or a food processor and puree until smooth.

2. Return the puree to the saucepan.

3. Whisk the ground plantain chips into the soup and heat to a simmer before serving.

4. Garnish with the lime slices.

Mulligatawny Soup

SERVES 2

2 tablespoons walnut oil
1 small onion, chopped
1 scallion, chopped
1 clove garlic, chopped
½ cup chopped apple
½ cup shredded carrot
½ cup chopped celery
¼ cup unsweetened coconut milk, or
   4 ounces coconut cream
1 teaspoon mild curry powder

¼ teaspoon ground turmeric
¼ teaspoon ground cumin
1 tablespoon chopped arugula
1 tablespoon rice flour
1 teaspoon arrowroot powder
3 cups vegetable broth, or 3 cups
   water plus 2 vegetable bouillon
   cubes
1 Gardenburger (or other veggie
   burger), cut into cubes

1. In a large soup pot, heat the oil and sauté the onion, scallion, garlic, apple, carrot, and celery for about 5 minutes.

2. Stir in the coconut milk and cook for 2 more minutes. Add the remaining ingredients except for the vegetable broth and Gardenburger and cook, stirring, an additional 3 minutes.

3. Slowly add in the vegetable broth and bring to a boil. Cover, lower heat, and simmer for 15 minutes.

4. Cool half the soup, put into a blender, and puree. Return the puree to the pot and add the cubed Gardenburger. Cook for an additional 3 minutes. Serve hot.

Three-Potato Soup
SERVES 2

1 tablespoon canola oil
2 leeks, white part only, sliced
2 tablespoons minced shallots
1 small Vidalia onion, chopped
2 large baking potatoes, peeled and
diced
1 medium sweet potato, peeled and
diced

2 cups water or clear vegetable broth
1 tablespoon orange-blossom honey
¼ teaspoon dried sage
1 dried chile, crushed
½ cup soy or rice milk
Sea salt to taste
Freshly ground black pepper to taste
2 tablespoons chopped chives for
garnish

1. Heat the oil in a heavy saucepan over medium heat. Sauté the leeks, shallots, and onion until very soft, approximately 8 minutes.

2. Add the potatoes and cook for 2 minutes. Stir in the water and honey, bring to a boil, and reduce the heat. Simmer for about 20 minutes, or until the potatoes are tender. Cool the mixture.

3. Puree the soup in a blender until very smooth. Return the puree to the saucepan and add the sage, chile, and soy milk and reheat on low, stirring constantly with a wire whisk.

4. Season with salt and pepper to taste. Serve garnished with the chives.

Chickpea and Yellow Split Pea Soup
SERVES 2

½ cup dried yellow split peas
½ cup dried chickpeas
2 cups plus 4 cups water
1 tablespoon hazelnut or olive oil
½ cup finely minced yellow onion
¼ teaspoon saffron
1 teaspoon cumin

¼ teaspoon curry powder
Pinch of dried peppermint leaves
1 tablespoon tamari
2 tablespoons uncooked white
jasmine or basmati rice
Mock sour cream or 1 tablespoon soy
margarine
2 croutons

1. Combine the yellow split peas and chickpeas. Soak the pea mixture overnight in the 2 cups water. Discard the liquid and simmer chickpeas in the 4 cups water for 1½ hours until soft. Strain and reserve the broth. Refrigerate the chickpeas for garnish and another use.

2. In a saucepan, heat the oil and sauté the onion. Add the chickpea broth, saffron, cumin, curry powder, peppermint, tamari. Add the rice and simmer. When the rice is tender, put the mixture through a food mill.

3. Serve hot with a dollop (heaping tablespoon) of mock sour cream or soy margarine, some chickpeas, and a crouton on top of each serving.

Spring Stew
SERVES 2

6 medium baby red potatoes
2 large Vidalia onions, thinly sliced
  and slices divided into thirds
½ teaspoon cumin
½ teaspoon fresh Italian parsley
Sea salt to taste

Black pepper to taste
1 sprig fresh dill
1 sprig fresh thyme
2 cups water
¼ cup dried beans (red mung or red
  kidney beans), soaked overnight

1. Peel all the potatoes and thinly slice 2 of them; leave the rest whole.

2. Place a layer of the sliced potatoes in a heavy saucepan, then add one-third of the onions. Sprinkle with the cumin, parsley, and salt and pepper. Add the dill, thyme, and another third of the sliced onions. Cover with the whole potatoes.

3. Add the water, beans, and the remaining onions, and cover the pot with a tight-fitting lid. Simmer gently on the stovetop for about an hour, or until the beans are cooked (mung beans cook much faster than potatoes). The thinly sliced potatoes will thicken the sauce.

Black Bean Soup
SERVES 2

¼ cup olive oil
2 cloves garlic, minced
1½ yellow onions, chopped
½ teaspoon grated orange rind
½ teaspoon sea salt
½ teaspoon freshly ground pepper
½ teaspoon honey
½ teaspoon fennel seed
½ teaspoon celery seed
½ teaspoon dried basil
½ teaspoon dry mustard

¼ teaspoon allspice
½ cup cubed firm tofu
1 cup canned black beans
Optional seasonings to taste: paprika,
  chili powder, black pepper, onion
  powder, marjoram, oregano,
  cayenne
¾ cup tomato sauce
3 tablespoons freshly squeezed lemon
  juice

1. Heat the oil in a medium saucepan over medium heat and sauté the garlic, onions, and all of the seasonings.

2. Add the tofu and beans, cover, and simmer for 15 to 20 minutes. Use the optional seasonings if desired.

3. Add the tomato sauce and lemon juice and serve hot.

Borscht

SERVES 2

2 cups peeled and chopped fresh beets   ½ cup chopped yellow onion
5 cups water   2 cups diced small red potatoes
1 tablespoon lemon juice   1 bunch lemongrass, minced
4 tablespoons lime juice   2 tablespoons finely chopped parsley
¼ cup spelt flour   3 tablespoons minced mint
3 tablespoons olive oil   Mock sour cream for garnish

1. In a medium saucepan, simmer the beets in the water, lemon juice, and lime juice for ½ hour.

2. Add the flour, olive oil, onions, and potatoes and simmer for 10 minutes, stirring continuously.

3. Season with the lemongrass, parsley, and mint. Serve hot, garnished with a dollop of mock sour cream.

Roasted garlic or garlic browned in olive oil is an excellent complement to this dish as well as an immune booster.

Kale and Potato Soup

SERVES 2

½ bunch kale or Swiss chard   Sea salt to taste
1 medium potato, peeled   Freshly ground black pepper to taste
4 cups water   Pinch of nutmeg
2 tablespoons full-bodied extra virgin   3 teaspoons spearmint leaves
   olive oil

1. Wash the kale and cut off the stems. Twist the leaves tightly in a circular fashion and cut into very thin slices. Set aside.

2. Place the potato, water, oil, salt, and pepper in a large soup pot and bring to a boil. Reduce heat to a simmer. Cover and cook slowly for about 25 minutes, or until the potato is tender.

3. Cool the soup, then puree in a food processor or blender. Return the puree to the soup pot and add the kale strips, nutmeg, and spearmint. Cook about 15 minutes more, or until the kale is tender. Serve hot.

Add a sprinkle of turmeric and wakame seaweed, for added immune boosting.

Gazpacho
SERVES 2

1 yellow pepper
1 red bell pepper
½ cucumber
3 ripe medium tomatoes, peeled and
    seeded
1 small onion
2 cloves garlic, crushed
1 tablespoon balsamic vinegar

¼ cup olive oil
2 cups cold water
Sea salt to taste
¼ teaspoon crushed red pepper
¼ pound tempeh
Finely chopped onion, red bell pepper,
    and cucumber for garnish

1. Dice the peppers, cucumber, tomatoes, onion, and garlic; combine them in a bowl with the vinegar, oil, water, salt, and crushed red pepper. In a blender or food processor, puree the mixture until smooth. Refrigerate for 2 hours.

2. Slice the tempeh into chunks and pour the puree over it. Garnish each serving with the onion, pepper, and cucumber.

In addition to the garlic, a dandelion and alfalfa sprouts salad with this dish is immune-boosting.

SALADS

Endive Salad

SERVES 2

¼ pound endive
¼ pound Granny Smith apples
1 cup small button mushrooms
⅓ cup tofu cream cheese (see Note)
¼ cup chopped hazelnuts

Pinch of sea salt
Freshly ground black pepper to taste
¼ cup chopped cooked beets
Fresh lemon juice

1. Trim the endive and cut it into thick slices.
2. Peel and core the apples and cut into small chunks.
3. Slice the mushrooms.
4. Place the endive, apples, and mushrooms in a salad bowl.
5. In a separate bowl, combine the tofu cream cheese with the hazelnuts and season with the salt and pepper. Pour the mixture over the salad and toss together.
6. Sprinkle the beets over the salad, then sprinkle with lemon juice to taste.

NOTE: To prepare the tofu cream cheese, blend the tofu with rice milk to form a liquid the consistency of heavy cream.

Mixed Dark Green Salad

SERVES 2

2 beets (for ½ cup pulp)
1 cup chopped radicchio
1 cup chopped Belgian endive
1 cup chopped arugula

1 cup chopped Swiss chard
1 cup unsalted walnut halves
Olive oil and lemon juice as a dressing

1. Juice the beets. Set aside ½ cup of the pulp.
2. In a large mixing bowl, toss the ½ cup beet pulp with the radicchio, endive, arugula, chard, and walnuts.
3. Toss the salad with the desired amount of olive oil and lemon juice. Serve cold or at room temperature with whole-grain bread.

Green Bean Salad with Almond and Dill
SERVES 2

Small bunch of fresh dill or ¼ cup dill pulp plus ¼ cup additional fresh dill sprigs, for garnish
¼ cup soy mayonnaise
2 cups steamed green beans
¼ cup slivered blanched almonds
1 tablespoon poppy seeds

1. Blend the dill and soy mayonnaise until smooth, 2 to 3 minutes.
2. In a medium-size mixing bowl, toss the beans with the dill mayonnaise.
3. Sprinkle the almonds and poppy seeds over the bean mixture.
4. Serve cold or at room temperature, garnished with dill sprigs.

Tabouli Salad
SERVES 2

1 cup boiling water
3 cups bulgur wheat
3 carrots
2 lemons
½ cup raisins
½ cup finely chopped unsalted cashews
¼ cup sliced scallions
2 to 3 tablespoons tamari sauce

1. In a large mixing bowl, pour the boiling water over the bulgur wheat. Cover the bowl with a towel and let stand for 30 minutes. Drain off any excess liquid.
2. Separately juice the carrots and lemons. Set aside ¾ cup of the carrot pulp and ¼ cup of the lemon juice.
3. In a large mixing bowl, combine the ¾ cup of carrot pulp, ¼ cup of lemon juice, and bulgur wheat with the remaining ingredients. Mix well, then drain excess liquid thoroughly.
4. Serve cold or at room temperature, with whole-grain bread.

Drinking a cup of ginseng or ginger tea 1 hour after eating this salad is both refreshing and immune-boosting.

Coleslaw with Fresh Dill

SERVES 2

1 carrot
2 lemons
2 cups shredded green cabbage
3 tablespoons soy mayonnaise
1 tablespoon chopped fresh dill

1 teaspoon lemon juice
½ teaspoon sea salt
¼ teaspoon black pepper
Dash of apple cider vinegar

1. Separately juice the carrot and lemons. Set aside ¼ cup of the carrot pulp and 3 tablespoons of the lemon juice.

2. In a medium-size mixing bowl, toss the carrot pulp and lemon juice with the remaining ingredients.

3. Serve cold as a salad or a sandwich filling.

Summer Fruit Salad

SERVES 2

½ apple
½ lemon
1 cup diced peeled peaches
½ cup blueberries

½ cup raspberries
½ cup strawberries
½ teaspoon almond extract

1. Separately juice the apple and lemon. Set aside 2 teaspoons of the apple juice and 1½ teaspoons of the lemon juice.

2. In a medium-size mixing bowl, combine the juices with the remaining ingredients and mix well.

3. Serve cold.

SIDE AND MAIN DISHES

Olive and Rice Salad

SERVES 2

¾ cup uncooked basmati rice

1 cup distilled water

¾ teaspoon finely chopped fresh oregano, or ½ teaspoon dried

2 tablespoons finely chopped Italian parsley

1¾ tablespoons extra virgin olive oil

1 tablespoon balsamic vinegar

½ clove garlic, pressed

1 tablespoon finely chopped hazelnuts

Sea salt to taste

Freshly ground black pepper to taste

5 or 6 Greek olives, green and black, pitted and chopped

4 cups (about 6 ounces) spinach leaves, washed, dried, and steamed until just wilted

1 cup crumbled tempeh

Parsley for garnish

1. Cook the rice according to the directions on the package.

2. To make the dressing: In a glass jar, mix the water, oregano, parsley, olive oil, balsamic vinegar, garlic, hazelnuts, salt, and pepper. Cover tightly and shake well.

3. Combine the cooked rice and chopped olives in a bowl. Pour the dressing over the mixture and toss.

4. Arrange the spinach leaves on 2 plates, fill with the rice and olive mixture, and sprinkle the tempeh on top. Garnish with parsley.

A refreshing cup of ginger tea is a good immune-booster. Drink it 1 hour before or after your meal.

Zesty No-Dish Avocado

SERVES 2

1 large avocado, sliced in half
    lengthwise and pitted
1 serrano chile with seeds, diced
4 peeled crushed cloves garlic
¾ cup fresh diced cilantro leaves
2 tablespoons freshly squeezed lime
    juice

1 teaspoon sea salt
1 pound tomatillos, husked and
    chopped
Pinch of freshly ground cumin
Parsley for garnish
Slices of red and green bell pepper for
    garnish

1. With a spoon, scoop out all the avocado flesh; reserve the skins. Place the flesh with all the other ingredients, except for the garnishes (parsley and bell peppers), in a food processor and puree.

2. Fill the avocado skins with the puree. Garnish with the parsley and bell pepper slices. Chill in the refrigerator for 1 hour; serve.

Herbed Tomato Salad

SERVES 2

1 teaspoon sea salt
½ teaspoon freshly ground black
    pepper
⅛ teaspoon cayenne
2 tablespoons lime juice
2 tablespoons fresh dill

½ tablespoon chopped fresh thyme
3 ripe tomatoes
1 bunch arugula
1 bunch watercress
3 peeled crushed cloves garlic

1. To prepare the dressing: Combine the salt, black pepper, cayenne, lime juice, dill, and thyme.

2. Cut the tomatoes into thick slices; toss with the arugula and watercress. Pour the dressing over the salad and let marinate for 1 hour in the refrigerator. Serve chilled.

Spinach Sauté

SERVES 2

½ pound fresh spinach, well rinsed,
    drained, and stemmed
1½ tablespoons peanut oil
½ cup chopped Spanish or yellow
    onion

2 freshly crushed cloves garlic
1 cup skinned and chopped tomatoes
¼ cup sliced black olives
1 teaspoon basil
¼ teaspoon white pepper

1. Steam the spinach in ¼ cup water until wilted. Discard the cooking liquid or save for another recipe. Shake or press out any liquid. Set the spinach aside.

2. Heat the peanut oil in a nonstick skillet over high heat. Stir-fry the onion and garlic.

3. Add the tomatoes, olives, basil, and pepper.

4. Add the spinach and stir. Cover, reduce the heat to low, and cook for 10 minutes.

Sea Vegetable and Cabbage

SERVES 2

1 small red onion, diced
1 clove garlic, chopped
1 ounce kombu or arame seaweed,
    soaked in water for about 20
    minutes to reconstitute it
2 tablespoons olive oil
¼ teaspoon date sugar or 2
    tablespoons pure maple syrup or
    honey

½ pound green cabbage, shredded
¼ pound red cabbage, shredded
1 Granny Smith apple, diced
¼ cup white wine (Chardonnay is
    ideal)
¼ cup water
Sea salt to taste
1 tablespoon white wine vinegar

1. In a large pan over medium heat, sauté the onion, garlic, and seaweed in the oil until the onion is golden.

2. Stir in the sugar and add the cabbages and apple. Mix well, cover, and cook over low heat for 20 minutes.

3. Add the wine and water. Cover and cook for about 20 minutes more. Season with salt and vinegar.

Stuffed Grape Leaves
YIELDS 20 GRAPE LEAVES

½ yellow onion, chopped
1 clove garlic, chopped
1 carrot, chopped
1 tablespoon olive oil
1 cup tomato juice
1 cup shiitake mushrooms
½ cup cooked brown rice

¼ cup corn kernels
1 teaspoon curry powder
Sea salt to taste
Freshly ground black pepper to taste
20 grape leaves, washed thoroughly
Juice of 1 lemon

1. Preheat the oven to 300 degrees F.
2. To prepare the filling: Over medium heat, sauté the onion, garlic, and carrot in the oil until browned. In a large bowl, mix well with the tomato juice, mushrooms, rice, corn, curry powder, salt, and pepper.
3. To stuff each grape leaf: Place it—shiny side down—on a board. Place 1 teaspoon of filling in the center of the leaf. Form into a roll.
4. Pack the rolls firmly in a baking dish, sprinkle lemon juice on top, and add enough water to cover.
5. Bake for ½ hour. Serve hot.

Mushroom Stuffed Tomatoes
SERVES 2

2 large tomatoes
½ pound fresh white mushrooms,
   sliced
2 tablespoons olive oil
½ cup bread crumbs

1 teaspoon sea salt
¼ teaspoon white pepper
1 tablespoon toasted sesame seeds
1 tablespoon dried basil

1. Preheat the oven to 350 degrees F.
2. Slice the tops off the tomatoes and set aside. Scoop out the tomato seeds.
3. In a pan over medium heat, sauté the mushrooms in the oil for 5 to 10 minutes, then combine with the bread crumbs, salt, pepper, sesame seeds, and basil.
4. Fill the tomatoes with the mushroom stuffing. Cover with the tomato tops and place in a shallow greased pan. Bake for 25 to 30 minutes. Serve warm.

Yellow Bean Eggplant

SERVES 2

3 tablespoons olive oil
4 cloves garlic, crushed
1 eggplant, cut into ¼-inch slices
2 red chile peppers, seeded and
    chopped
1 tablespoon chopped fresh basil
    leaves
⅛ teaspoon dill

2 tablespoons yellow bean sauce
    (found in Asian markets)
¼ cup soy milk
1 scallion, chopped
2 tablespoons chopped green bell
    pepper
1 cup diced fresh tomatoes
4 tablespoons soy margarine
Basil for garnish

1. Heat the oil in a wok over high heat. Add the garlic and sauté until light brown.

2. Add the eggplant to the wok and cook for 5 minutes. Stir in the chile peppers, chopped basil, dill, bean sauce, soy milk, scallion, green pepper, and tomatoes. Mix well.

3. Serve immediately, topped with a dollop of soy margarine and a sprinkle of basil.

Green Pea Pilaf

SERVES 2

2 tablespoons walnut oil
2 shallots, finely chopped
1 clove garlic, minced
¾ cup white basmati or jasmine rice,
    rinsed and drained
1⅓ cups vegetable broth

⅓ cup chopped fresh spearmint
½ cup frozen peas
1 tablespoon Bragg's Liquid Aminos,
    or to taste
Spinach or arugula (optional)
Olive oil (optional)

1. In a stockpot, carefully heat the walnut oil over low heat and sauté the shallots and garlic for 3 minutes.

2. Add the uncooked rice and stir for 1 minute.

3. Add the vegetable broth, spearmint, peas, and aminos. Bring to a full boil, then reduce the heat to a simmer. Cover and cook over low heat for about 15 minutes.

4. Remove from the heat. Release steam by angling the lid away from face and hands. Cover with a towel to absorb excess water vapor without losing heat.

5. Serve on a bed of spinach or arugula, if you like, with olive oil.

Have a soothing cup of ginger or ginseng tea 1 hour before or 1 hour after this meal.

Vatapa
SERVES 2

3 slices rice bread or almond bread
   (available in health food stores)
⅓ cup unsweetened coconut milk
½ cup chopped onion
1 clove garlic, minced
½ teaspoon paprika
⅛ teaspoon cayenne
½ teaspoon chopped cilantro

½ teaspoon sea salt
½ teaspoon minced gingerroot
½ pound dulse seaweed
½ cup Brazil nuts, toasted and finely
   chopped
⅓ cup cashews, finely chopped
⅓ cup peanut oil

1. Trim the crusts from the bread and discard. Break the bread into pieces and put into a bowl.

2. Pour the ⅓ cup of the coconut milk over the bread and set aside to soften.

3. Mash the bread mixture with a fork until fine. Add the onion, garlic, paprika, cayenne, cilantro, salt, and ginger and mix well.

4. Soak the seaweed until fluffy looking; marinate with the other ingredients for 20 to 30 minutes.

5. Preheat the oven to 325 degrees F.

6. Bake for 25 minutes. Serve warm.

Zesty Cauliflower with Garlic Sauce
SERVES 2

1 cup garbanzo beans or chickpeas
   (precooked and pureed)
3 tablespoons tahini
1 cup cauliflower florets
1 cup broccoli florets
1 cup sliced red bell pepper

1 teaspoon lemon juice
¼ teaspoon turmeric
½ cup unsalted whole cashews
½ cup diced red bell pepper as garnish
4 sprigs fresh parsley, as garnish

1. Preheat the oven to 425 degrees F.

2. In a medium-size mixing bowl, combine the garbanzo puree, tahini, cauliflower, broccoli, sliced red pepper, lemon juice, turmeric, and cashews and toss to mix.

3. Pour the mixture into a greased 9 by 12-inch baking dish or other large glass or ceramic dish. Cover with a glass lid or foil and bake for 25 to 30 minutes, or until the cauliflower is just tender. (The other vegetables should still be crunchy.)

4. Garnish with the diced red pepper and parsley and serve hot or cold with a rice dish or green salad.

Matar Paneer

SERVES 4

1 tomato

16 ounces extra-firm tofu, cut into 1-inch cubes

2 tablespoons canola oil

¾ cup chopped yellow onions

2 cups frozen peas

1 cup chopped tomatoes

¾ cup unsweetened soy milk

3 teaspoons apple cider vinegar

½ cup finely chopped fresh cilantro

2 fresh green chile peppers, finely chopped

3 cloves garlic, crushed

2 teaspoons grated gingerroot

1 teaspoon ground coriander

1 teaspoon ground turmeric

¼ teaspoon chili powder

1½ teaspoons sea salt

1. Juice the tomato. Set aside ½ cup of the juice.

2. In a large frying pan, brown the tofu in the oil over high heat.

3. Add the onions and sauté for 2 to 3 minutes, or until the onions are soft.

4. Reduce the heat to medium-low, add the remaining ingredients, and simmer uncovered for an additional 5 minutes.

Sliced Tofu in Garlic Sauce

SERVES 2

Tofu
2 cups water
1 slice fresh ginger, peeled
16 ounces extra-firm tofu (block
    form)
3 scallions
½ teaspoon rice wine
1 clove garlic

Garlic Sauce
1 tablespoon Bragg's Liquid Aminos
1 tablespoon curry powder

1 tablespoon vegetable broth
1 tablespoon water
1 scallion, chopped
1 tablespoon minced garlic
⅛ teaspoon sea salt
1 tablespoon tamari sauce
1 teaspoon sesame oil
½ teaspoon honey
½ teaspoon chile oil or sesame oil

1. To prepare the tofu: In a medium saucepan, bring the water to a boil. Add the ginger, tofu block, scallions, wine, and garlic. Simmer for about 30 minutes.

2. Remove the tofu block from the cooking liquid. Set the liquid aside. Refrigerate the tofu to facilitate slicing. When cool, cut it into ribbon slices, then cut the slices into 2-inch squares.

3. To prepare the sauce: In a small saucepan, bring the aminos, curry powder, vegetable broth, and water to a boil. Remove from the heat. Add the remaining ingredients except for the final chile oil or sesame oil, mixing well. Set aside.

4. Bring the tofu cooking liquid to a boil. Place the tofu slices in the boiling liquid for about 5 to 7 seconds. Remove and drain. Pat dry with a paper towel.

5. Arrange the tofu on a platter. Pour the garlic sauce over. Sprinkle with chili oil or sesame oil to taste.

Good Shepherd's Pie
SERVES 2

1 large baking potato, peeled and
 diced
2 tablespoons sunflower seed oil
½ cup rice milk
1 tablespoon curry powder
¼ teaspoon celery salt
⅛ teaspoon ground black pepper
1 tablespoon olive oil
1 medium onion, chopped
1 scallion, chopped
1 clove garlic, chopped
½ pound vegetarian meat (textured
 vegetable protein, or TVP)

1 vegetable bouillon cube
3 ounces tomato paste
¼ teaspoon sage
1 tablespoon spelt flour
1 teaspoon parsley flakes
1 teaspoon thyme
1 teaspoon dried tarragon
¾ cup white wine (optional)
½ can adzuki beans
Pinch of paprika

1. Cook the potato in boiling salted water. Drain and mash, then add the sunflower oil and rice milk. Season with the curry powder, celery salt, and pepper.

2. Heat the olive oil and sauté the garlic, onion, and scallion until soft. Add the vegetarian meat and stir until brown and the flavors are married, about 5 minutes.

3. Crumble the bouillon cube and stir it into onion mixture. Stir in the tomato paste, sage, flour, parsley, thyme, and tarragon leaves. Add the wine and continue stirring for a few minutes. Cover and simmer on low for 10 additional minutes.

4. Preheat the oven to 350 degrees F. Lightly coat a souffle dish or loaf pan with oil.

5. Spread the mixture on the bottom of the dish. Follow with a layer of adzuki beans and then the mashed potatoes; sprinkle with paprika.

6. Bake for 30 minutes, then brown under the broiler for 1 minute. Serve.

Sesame and Spice Seitan

SERVES 2

2½ cups water
1 cup basmati rice
½ cup green peas
¼ tablespoon lemon or black
  peppercorns
4 teaspoons toasted sesame oil
1 pound seitan, cut into 1-inch cubes

4 cloves garlic, crushed
1 teaspoon celery seed
1 teaspoon dill
1 teaspoon mustard seed
Sea salt to taste
Orange wedges for garnish

1. Bring 2½ cups water in a large pot to a boil. Add the rice and simmer, covered, for 40 minutes or until the rice is done. Season with the green peas and peppercorns.

2. As the rice is cooking, heat the oil over high heat in a wok. Add the seitan and cook for 5 minutes. Add the garlic, celery seed, dill, mustard seed, and salt and cook for 5 minutes more.

3. Mix the rice and seasoned seitan together. Serve warm, decorated with orange wedges around the rim of the plate.

Cauliflower with Shiitake Mushrooms

SERVES 2

½ head cauliflower
¼ cup chopped and cooked shiitake
  mushrooms
¼ cup grated extra-firm tofu
½ cup egg substitute
½ teaspoon soy flour
½ teaspoon sea salt

½ cup soy or rice milk
1 tablespoon dry soy powder
2 tablespoons rice syrup
1 clove garlic
2 teaspoons grated lemon
Grated soy cheddar cheese for topping

1. Break off the cauliflower flowerets and cook the flowerets in slightly salted water until almost tender.

2. Oil a baking dish; arrange a bottom layer of cauliflower followed by a layer of mushrooms. Top with the grated tofu.

3. Preheat the oven to 325 degrees F. Blend the egg substitute, flour, salt, and soy milk (enriched with the soy powder), rice syrup, garlic, and lemon.

4. Pour the mixture over the mushroom layer in a baking dish. Sprinkle the top with cheese and bake until sauce thickens, approximately 25 minutes.

Eggplant Goulash

SERVES 2

1 medium eggplant, peeled and cubed
3 tablespoons tamari sauce
2 tablespoons olive oil
1 yellow onion, coarsely chopped
1/4 cup water
1 tablespoon paprika

1/2 green bell pepper, coarsely chopped
1 tablespoon red miso paste
1 teaspoon garlic powder
Yellow and orange bell pepper slices
    and carrot peels for garnish

1. Toss the eggplant in a bowl with the tamari and oil. Heat a sauté pan over medium heat and brown the eggplant.

2. Remove the eggplant and, in the same pan, sauté the onion.

3. Deglaze the pan with the water, then add the paprika, pepper, miso paste, and garlic powder. Simmer until the pepper is soft, then toss with the eggplant.

4. Serve over whole-wheat noodles or rice, garnishing with the yellow and orange pepper slices and carrot peels.

Stuffed Sweet-and-Sour Cabbage

SERVES 2

1 head cabbage
2 cups cooked brown rice
Sea salt to taste
Freshly ground black pepper to taste
1 teaspoon minced fresh garlic
1/8 teaspoon minced fresh ginger
1 teaspoon sesame oil
1/4 teaspoon soy sauce

1/4 cup peas
2 teaspoons honey
1 teaspoon tamari sauce
1 teaspoon dried mint
1/4 teaspoon dried oregano
1/4 cup grated firm tofu
Curly parsley for garnish

1. To remove the core from the cabbage, boil salted water and then cook the cabbage until tender. Drain the water and scoop out the center.

2. Season the rice with the salt, pepper, garlic, ginger, sesame oil, and soy sauce. Stuff the rice into the cabbage and add the peas. Place the cabbage in a deep baking dish.

3. To prepare the sweet-and-sour sauce: Mix together the honey, tamari, mint, and oregano.

4. Preheat the oven to 350 degrees F.

5. Cover the cabbage with the sweet-and-sour sauce and top with the grated tofu. Bake for 20 minutes. Garnish with the curly parsley.

Curry Potato Masala

SERVES 2

2 medium potatoes, cubed
1/4 cup fresh peas
2 large onions, diced
1/2 teaspoon turmeric
1 teaspoon sea salt
1/4 teaspoon cayenne
3 tablespoons grated fresh or dried
    unsweetened coconut
1/2 teaspoon powdered ginger

1 tablespoon toasted sesame oil
1/2 teaspoon mustard seeds
1 teaspoon cardamom
1 teaspoon anise
2 black peppercorns
1 teaspoon curry powder
Coriander and grated carrot for
    garnish

1. Cook the potatoes and peas in just enough water to cover, along with three-quarters of the diced onions, the turmeric, 1/2 teaspoon of the salt, and cayenne until half cooked, about 8 minutes.

2. Puree the coconut and ginger in a blender. Add to the potatoes and cook for 8 more minutes, until tender but not soft.

3. Heat the oil in a skillet and add the mustard seeds. Allow to sizzle for a few seconds until the popping stage, then add the remaining diced onions, cardamom, anise, and peppercorns and fry until golden. Stir into the potatoes.

4. Add the curry and remaining salt and garnish with the coriander and grated carrot.

Rice and Lentils (Dal)

SERVES 6

2 cups basmati rice
1 cup washed red or yellow lentils
1 cup button mushrooms
3 cloves garlic, thinly sliced
1 yellow onion, chopped
4 cups water

1 tablespoon soy sauce
3 tablespoons toasted sesame oil
1 teaspoon cumin seeds
2 teaspoons sea salt
Orange wedges for garnish

1. Combine the rice, lentils, mushrooms, garlic, and onion in a large bowl. Add enough water to cover. Soak for 1 hour, then drain and rinse.

2. Preheat the oven to 450 degrees F.

3. Place the rice mixture in a heavy ovenproof pan. Add the 4 cups water and soy sauce. Bring to a boil over medium heat. Cover, reduce heat, and simmer for 20 minutes.

4. Turn the oven *off* and place the tightly covered pan of cooked rice and lentils in the oven. Allow it to sit for 20 minutes to absorb the excess moisture.

5. In a small frying pan, warm the oil over medium heat. Add the cumin seeds and salt and sauté until brown and fragrant.

6. Serve the rice and lentils hot, topped with the cumin seasoning and garnished with the orange wedges around the rim of the plate.

A cup of ginger tea drunk 1 hour following this meal is an additional immune-booster.

Collards and Potatoes

SERVES 2

1 tablespoon olive oil
1 leek, chopped
½ small onion
1 clove elephant garlic or 3 regular
    cloves, chopped
2 cups chopped collard greens
1 cup chopped spinach
1 tablespoon finely chopped fresh
    parsley

1 bay leaf
⅛ teaspoon powdered thyme
2 russet potatoes, peeled and cubed
1 sweet potato, cubed
½ cup soy or rice milk powder with
    ¼ cup potato water
Paprika for garnish

1. In a sauté pan, heat the oil over medium heat. Sauté the leek, onion, and garlic until soft, 8 to 10 minutes.

2. Add the collard greens, spinach, and parsley. Cover and cook until tender, stirring frequently, 17 to 20 minutes.

3. In salted water with the bay leaf and thyme, boil the potatoes until they slide off a fork. Drain, reserving ¼ cup of the cooking water.

4. Place the potato cubes in a medium bowl and add the greens. Slowly add the reconstituted rice or soy milk until moderately thick.

5. Garnish with a sprinkle of paprika.

Mock Meatball Veggie Stew
SERVES 2

¼ teaspoon salt
⅛ teaspoon white pepper
Dash of Tabasco sauce
1 tablespoon Worcestershire sauce
1 teaspoon organic grated orange peel
½ teaspoon dried thyme
1 tablespoon curry powder
1 teaspoon tamari
1 stalk celery, chopped
1 scallion, chopped
2 tablespoons egg substitute
1 tablespoon Bragg's Liquid Aminos
4 ounces textured vegetable protein
　(TVP)

¼ cup spelt flour
1 tablespoon sunflower oil
1 cup sliced yellow squash
1 small turnip, boiled and cubed
1 medium red potato, boiled and
　shredded
1 cup peeled, cored, and chopped
　fresh tomato
1 leek, with top, sliced
4 cups vegetable bouillon
1 tablespoon chopped parsley

1. Combine the salt, pepper, Tabasco sauce, Worcestershire sauce, orange peel, thyme, curry, tamari, celery, scallion, egg substitute, aminos, and TVP. Shape into 1-inch balls and roll in the spelt flour.

2. Heat the oil in the skillet and brown the balls, using a fork and a spoon to turn them gently. Set aside. Save any drippings.

3. In a large saucepan, place the squash, turnip, potato, tomato, leek, and bouillon. Boil on medium heat for approximately 30 minutes.

4. Add the meatballs to the bouillon and reheat for 5 to 7 minutes. Sprinkle the parsley on top and serve with toasted homemade bread.

Exotic Rice

SERVES 2

1½ tablespoons sesame oil
1 medium onion (preferably Vidalia), chopped
1 small clove garlic, minced
½ inch cinnamon stick or ¼ teaspoon ground cinnamon
2 whole cloves
½ teaspoon sea salt

¼ teaspoon powdered ginger
1 cup jasmine or basmati rice, rinsed once and soaked for 5 minutes
1¾ cups boiling water
¼ teaspoon ground turmeric
¼ cup unsweetened coconut milk
¼ cup roasted cashews and pecans
1 tablespoon fennel seed

1. In a large saucepan, heat the sesame oil over low heat. Add the onion and garlic and cook until soft, about 10 minutes. Add the cinnamon, cloves, salt, and ginger.

2. Drain the rice and add it to the pan. Toss lightly to coat with the oil.

3. Add the boiling water to the rice mix. Bring to a full boil.

4. Add the turmeric, coconut milk, nuts, and fennel seed. Reduce the heat and simmer, covered, for 15 minutes.

5. Remove from the heat and leave covered for 5 to 10 more minutes before serving.

Red Beans with Rice

SERVES 2

½ medium yellow onion, chopped
2 cloves garlic, peeled and mashed
½ green bell pepper, chopped
1 tablespoon olive oil
1 cup cooked red kidney beans
2 cups water
1 tablespoon honey

¾ cup short-grain brown rice
1 tablespoon tamari sauce
Pinch of fresh ground pepper
Pinch of cumin
½ teaspoon sea salt
Colorful edible flowers or parsley for garnish

1. Sauté the onion, garlic, and bell pepper in the oil until golden. Place the sautéed ingredients in a saucepan, along with all of the remaining ingredients except for the flowers or parsley.

2. Simmer until the rice is al dente or to taste, about 35 minutes.

3. Garnish with the flowers or parsley and serve.

Galuska
SERVES 2

Soft Noodles
1 cup spelt flour
⅓ cup water
2 tablespoons egg substitute
½ teaspoon sea salt
½ teaspoon olive oil

Sauce
2 fresh tomatoes, cubed
½ green bell pepper, chopped
½ red bell pepper, chopped
½ onion, chopped

1. To prepare the noodles: Put the flour in a large bowl and make a well in the center. Add the water, egg substitute, salt, and oil to the well. Mix everything lightly until well blended.

2. Put a portion of the dough on a small, wet bread board. Flatten the dough. Using a wet knife, cut the dough into 1- × -3-inch pieces.

3. Push the dough pieces off the board into boiling salted water. They are done when they rise to the top. Skim the noodles out and pile them into a hot bowl or dish.

4. To prepare the sauce: Sauté the tomatoes, bell peppers, and onion for about 15 minutes. Serve over the noodles.

Caraway Soda Bread
MAKES 1 LOAF

1½ cups sifted rice flour
¼ cup sifted buckwheat flour
¼ cup sifted oat flour
⅓ cup honey plus additional to brush
    on bread
2 cups vanilla soy milk
1 teaspoon baking soda

½ teaspoon sea salt
1 tablespoon caraway seeds
½ teaspoon vanilla extract
Handful of raisins
Olive oil to grease bowl and pan (olive
    oil cooking spray preferred)

1. Preheat the oven to 350 degrees F.

2. In a bowl, mix all the ingredients except for the oil. Stir well to combine, and then turn the mixture into an oiled mixing bowl.

3. Lightly flour hands and blend the ingredients until a firm, ball-shaped dough forms. Place in an oiled metal baking pan. Dust a knife with flour and make an X on top of the loaf.

4. Bake for 45 to 60 minutes. Do not allow top to brown. About 5 minutes before the bread is done, use a pastry brush to coat the top with honey, if desired. Serve at room temperature.

Potato Pancakes

SERVES 2

3 new potatoes, peeled
½ cup rice milk
⅛ teaspoon sea salt

¼ cup egg substitute
¼ teaspoon cinnamon
2 tablespoons canola oil

1. Boil the potatoes until tender and then mash them.
2. Add the milk, salt, and egg substitute to the mashed potatoes and sprinkle in the cinnamon.
3. Shape into individual cakes. Heat the oil over medium-hot heat and sauté the cakes until golden brown.

Spelt Corn Bread

MAKES 1 LOAF

½ teaspoon sea salt
1 cup yellow cornmeal
1½ cups spelt flour
2 teaspoons rapid-rise yeast
½ cup fresh or frozen corn, slightly
    crushed

1 teaspoon honey
½ cup water
½ cup rice or soy milk
1½ teaspoons corn oil

1. Combine the salt, cornmeal, spelt flour, and yeast in a deep bowl. Add the corn.
2. Place the honey, water, milk, and oil in a pan and heat to 110 to 113 degrees F, or until it feels slightly warm to your wrist.
3. Mix the dry ingredients with the wet and shape into a ball. If the dough is too sticky, add more flour. Place the dough in a greased soufflé dish. Place in a warm spot away from drafts and allow to rise until doubled in bulk, approximately 1 to 1½ hours.
4. Preheat the oven to 350 degrees F.
5. After the dough has risen once, bake in the same dish for 30 minutes or until the loaf sounds hollow when tapped.

Pisto

SERVES 2

1 large yellow onion, chopped
2 green and red bell peppers, chopped
2 cloves garlic, chopped
¼ cup olive oil
½ large eggplant
1 zucchini, diced

2 large ripe tomatoes, peeled and
  chopped
Seasonings to taste: sea salt, paprika,
  chili powder, black pepper, garlic
  powder, onion powder, dried
  marjoram, dried oregano, cayenne

1. In a large saucepan, sauté the onion, bell peppers, and garlic in the oil until soft.

2. Add the eggplant, zucchini, tomatoes, and desired seasonings, and stir well. Cover and cook over medium heat for 30 to 40 minutes.

3. Remove from the heat. Let stand for a few minutes before serving.

Roasted Peppers with Vinaigrette

SERVES 2

2 large red and yellow bell peppers
½ tablespoon wine vinegar
2 teaspoons olive oil, plus additional
  to oil baking sheet

Sea salt to taste
Freshly ground black pepper to taste
1 artichoke heart, quartered
3 hearts of palm

1. Preheat the oven to 350 degrees F.

2. Bake the whole peppers on an oiled baking sheet for 25 to 30 minutes, turning every 10 minutes. Remove from oven.

3. To make the vinaigrette: In a small bowl, combine the vinegar, oil, salt, and pepper and set aside.

4. When the peppers are cool, peel them and cut them in half. Discard the seeds and cut the peppers into strips. Mix with the artichoke heart and hearts of palm. Pour the vinaigrette over the vegetables before serving.

Saffron Rice
SERVES 2

½ sweet red pepper, sliced thinly
½ sweet yellow pepper, sliced thinly
1 medium onion, chopped
2 cloves garlic, minced
2 tablespoons olive oil

2 cups basmati rice
3 cups boiling water
Pinch of saffron
1 teaspoon sea salt
½ cup cooked peas

1. In a saucepan, sauté the peppers, onion, and garlic in the oil until soft.

2. Add the rice and stir until grains are coated with oil. Add the water, saffron, and salt.

3. Cover and simmer for approximately 20 minutes until the rice is cooked and all the water is absorbed. Add the peas and fluff with a fork. Serve warm.

Seasoned Spaghetti with Garlic
SERVES 2

⅓ cup olive oil
5 cloves garlic, minced
¼ teaspoon crushed red pepper
¼ cup chopped parsley
¼ cup chopped arugula
¼ cup chopped basil leaves

2 tomatoes, chopped
3 black olives, pitted and chopped
1 tablespoon pine nuts
½ pound whole-wheat spaghetti,
    cooked according to package
    instructions

1. In a sauté pan, heat the oil over medium-high heat and add the garlic and red pepper, stirring constantly to keep from burning.

2. When the garlic starts to brown, stir in the parsley, arugula, basil, tomatoes, olives, and pine nuts. When the arugula is wilted, remove the mixture from the heat and toss with the cooked spaghetti.

Spicy Burritos

SERVES 2

1 fresh jalapeño, minced
4 cloves garlic, diced
1 tablespoon tamari sauce
1 teaspoon honey
1 pound firm tofu, cut into thin strips

4 medium-size flour tortillas
1 teaspoon olive oil
1 onion, thinly sliced
Salsa (optional)

1. In a bowl, combine the jalapeño, garlic, tamari, and honey. Add the tofu and marinate for 20 minutes.

2. Preheat the oven to 350 degrees F.

3. Stack the tortillas, wrap them in a slightly damp towel, and heat in the oven for 5 to 10 minutes.

4. In a small skillet, heat the oil over medium-high heat. Stir-fry the onion until translucent. Add the tofu with its marinade, stir well to combine, and cook for 5 minutes more.

5. Spoon some mixture onto each tortilla, roll, and serve with salsa, if desired.

Spanish Potato Omelet

SERVES 2

3 tablespoons canola oil
2 medium potatoes, peeled
Sea salt to taste
3 tablespoons chopped onion

½ cup egg substitute
Cayenne to taste
White pepper to taste

1. In a medium frying pan, heat 1 tablespoon of the oil over medium heat, add the potatoes and salt, and cook for 5 minutes.

2. Add the onion and continue cooking until the potatoes are soft but not brown. Remove the potatoes and onion from the oil and drain.

3. In a separate bowl, stir the egg substitute into the potatoes and onion and season to taste.

4. In another frying pan, heat the remaining 2 tablespoons of oil. Pour in the eggs and potato mixture and spread evenly in the pan.

5. Cook over medium heat for 2 to 3 minutes, shaking the pan occasionally. When the bottom of the omelet is firm, flip the omelet over and cook until golden brown.

Tempeh in Sherry Sauce

SERVES 2 to 3

3 tablespoons canola oil
1 pound tempeh or seitan, cut into
    chunks
1 medium yellow onion, diced
3 cloves garlic, chopped
2 teaspoons whole-wheat flour
1/4 cup vegetable broth

1 bay leaf
1 tablespoon chopped parsley
1/4 cup dry sherry
Sea salt to taste
Freshly ground black pepper to taste
Rice, cooked (optional)

1. In a large frying pan, heat the oil over medium heat. Sauté the tempeh for 2 to 3 minutes on both sides and remove from the pan.

2. Sauté the onion and garlic in the oil until the onion is translucent.

3. Stir in the flour, then add the vegetable broth and mix well.

4. Add the bay leaf, parsley, sherry, and salt and pepper to taste and simmer for 3 to 4 minutes. Add the tempeh, cover, and cook over low heat for 3 to 4 minutes.

5. Serve over rice, if desired.

Desserts

Fruit Salad
SERVES 2

1 orange
1 apple
1 banana
⅛ cup pecans or almonds, chopped
2 tablespoons date sugar

1 tablespoon freshly squeezed lemon
  juice
3 tablespoons shredded coconut
Fresh mint sprigs

1. Peel the orange, apple, and banana. Dice the fruit and mix together in a large, chilled bowl.
2. Add the nuts, sugar, lemon juice, and coconut and mix well.
3. Garnish with the mint leaves and serve.

Crispy Grapes
SERVES 2

½ cup date sugar
½ cup soy flour
⅛ teaspoon sea salt
¼ cup soy or rice milk
¼ cup vanilla extract

½ cup egg substitute
Canola oil for frying
½ pound fresh, ripe, hard grapes
½ teaspoon cinnamon

1. Blend the sugar in a blender on high speed for 2 minutes.
2. In a large bowl, mix the flour, ¼ cup sugar, salt, milk, and vanilla to form a smooth batter. Stir in the egg substitute.
3. Heat 3 inches of oil in a deep pan. Dip the grapes into the batter, making sure they are well coated. In small batches (so that the oil temperature remains hot), quickly plunge the grapes into the hot oil. Remove with a skimmer as soon as the fruit is browned and drain on paper towels.
4. Combine the remaining ¼ cup sugar with the cinnamon and sprinkle generously over the grapes. Serve warm.

Orange Glazed Apples

SERVES 2

2 large Red Delicious apples
¼ cup pure maple syrup
2 tablespoons grated orange zest

¼ cup orange juice
1½ teaspoons canola oil
1½ teaspoons ground cinnamon

1. Core and quarter the apples and set aside.

2. In a saucepan, combine the maple syrup, orange zest, orange juice, oil, and cinnamon. Simmer for 10 minutes.

3. Add the apples to the glaze, making sure to cover them well. Cook in a covered saucepan for 10 to 15 minutes. Serve immediately.

Flan

SERVES 2

¼ cup pure maple syrup
2 tablespoons water
1 teaspoon almond extract
1½ teaspoons vanilla extract

¾ cup rice or soy milk
¼ cup cornstarch
⅓ cup silken tofu
¼ cup pecan pieces, chopped

1. In a small nonstick saucepan, combine the maple syrup and water. Bring to a boil, then lower the heat to a simmer, making sure to swirl the mixture while it thickens and caramelizes.

2. Pour enough of the mixture into a flan mold to cover the bottom.

3. Preheat the oven to 350 degrees F.

4. Combine the almond and vanilla extracts, milk, cornstarch, tofu, and pecans and blend until smooth. Pour into the mold and cover with foil.

5. Place the mold in a pan. Fill the pan with water up to an inch below the top of the mold.

6. Bake for 40 to 50 minutes. Allow the flan to cool completely before removing it from the mold. Serve warm.

Sweet Rice on Papaya

SERVES 2

2¼ cups unsweetened coconut milk
⅓ cup honey
¼ teaspoon sea salt
1 cup basmati rice, rinsed

2 ripe, seeded papayas, cut in half
1 teaspoon fresh lemon juice
1 teaspoon sunflower seeds
Thick coconut cream (optional)
4 mint leaves for garnish

1. Bring the coconut milk and honey to a boil in a large saucepan, then add the salt and cook for 5 minutes. Add the rice, stir, and reduce the heat to simmer. Cover and check after 20 minutes. Remove from the heat when all the liquid has been absorbed.

2. Sprinkle each papaya half with lemon juice and sunflower seeds. Top with the rice mixture. Add a dollop of coconut cream, if desired, and garnish each half with one mint leaf.

Citrus Celebration

SERVES 2

3 tablespoons arrowroot powder
¼ cup freshly squeezed lemon juice
1½ cups freshly squeezed grapefruit
    juice
1 teaspoon lemon zest
2 teaspoons honey
1 pink or red grapefruit, peeled and
    sectioned

1 orange, peeled and sectioned
½ cup Nut Quick (available in health
    food stores)
¼ cup toasted coconut flakes
¼ cup pistachio nuts, chopped, for
    garnish

1. Whisk together the arrowroot powder, lemon and grapefruit juices, lemon zest, and honey in a saucepan. Bring to a boil, stirring constantly. Reduce the heat, simmer, and continue stirring for 5 minutes.

2. Gently fold in the grapefruit and orange sections. Simmer for 2 minutes more.

3. Fold in the Nut Quick and coconut and cook 5 minutes longer.

4. Pour into separate dessert cups or one large bowl.

5. Serve chilled, garnished with chopped pistachio nuts.

Flan de Calabaza

SERVES 2

Canola oil
3 tablespoons brown rice syrup
¼ cup honey
1 cup cooked pumpkin
¼ cup rice milk

Pinch of cinnamon
Pinch of salt
2 tablespoons arrowroot powder
3 teaspoons vanilla extract
1 teaspoon almond extract

1. Preheat the oven to 350 degrees F.
2. Oil a small baking dish and spread the brown rice syrup evenly on the bottom.
3. In a small bowl, combine all the other ingredients until smooth, then pour over the brown rice syrup.
4. Bake for 45 minutes. Refrigerate. Serve chilled.

Sangria Drink

SERVES 2

1 to 2 jalapeños, finely chopped
½ teaspoon finely chopped fresh dill
1 cup tomato juice
¼ cup lemon juice
½ cup orange juice
½ teaspoon paprika
½ teaspoon crushed coriander seed

½ teaspoon chili powder
⅛ teaspoon marjoram
⅛ teaspoon onion powder
⅛ teaspoon sea salt
⅛ teaspoon freshly ground black
   pepper
⅛ teaspoon crushed celery seed

Combine all of the ingredients in a blender and refrigerate for 3 to 4 hours before serving.

SPREADS AND DIPS

Date Spread
SERVES 2

1 cup cooked red kidney beans
½ cup ground cashews
3 tablespoons crystallized honey
2 teaspoons dates, finely chopped

¼ teaspoon sea salt
1 teaspoon dried mint
1 teaspoon almond extract
1 teaspoon vanilla extract

1. Rub beans through a food mill or a wire sieve to make a paste.
2. Add all of the other ingredients to the bean paste and stir to combine thoroughly. Refrigerate. Use on crackers or as a dip for vegetables.

Ginger Black Bean Paté
SERVES 2

1 cup cooked black beans
1 tablespoon tamari sauce
½ teaspoon chili paste
1 tablespoon spelt flour

2 tablespoons sesame oil
2 cloves garlic, minced
1 teaspoon minced ginger
¼ teaspoon sea salt

1. Mash the beans with a ricer or potato masher.
2. Add the tamari and chili paste and stir to combine well.
3. Stir in the flour and ½ tablespoon of the oil and mix well.
4. In a pan, heat the remaining 1½ tablespoons sesame oil and sauté the garlic, ginger, and salt. Cook, stirring constantly, for 2 minutes.
5. Add the garlic-ginger mixture to the beans, stirring to combine thoroughly.
6. Refrigerate but do not freeze.

Horseradish Sauce
SERVES 2

¼ cup freshly grated horseradish
1 teaspoon Bragg's apple cider vinegar
1 teaspoon rice wine vinegar
1 teaspoon dry white wine
⅛ teaspoon white powdered stevia,
   or ¾ teaspoon raw sugar

¼ teaspoon ground mustard
Pinch of sea salt
Pinch of garlic powder
¼ teaspoon curry powder
⅓ cup powdered soy milk mixed with
   2 tablespoons water

1. In a small bowl, mix the horseradish, vinegars, wine, stevia, mustard, salt, garlic, and curry powder.

2. Fold the reconstituted soy milk into the other ingredients. Chill for several hours.

Hot Peanut Sauce
SERVES 2

1 hot red chile pepper, seeded and
   diced, or ⅛ teaspoon cayenne
2 tablespoons lemon juice
4 whole scallions, diced

2 teaspoons honey
1 teaspoon sea salt
½ cup smooth peanut butter

1. In a blender or food processor, blend the chile pepper, lemon juice, scallions, honey, and salt to form a paste.

2. Blend together the paste and the peanut butter. Add hot water as needed to make a thick sauce. Serve warm with vegetables for dipping.

Tangy Carrot Dip
SERVES 2

½ carrot
¾ cup soft tofu
½ cup cubed or mashed steamed
   sweet potatoes

2 tablespoons apple cider vinegar
¼ teaspoon ground cinnamon

1. Juice the carrot. Set aside 2 tablespoons of the juice.

2. In a blender or food processor, combine the carrot juice with the remaining ingredients and blend for 2 minutes, or until smooth.

3. Serve cold with raw vegetables.

Anytime Salsa

SERVES 2

2 tablespoons diced white onion
1 teaspoon sea salt
½ teaspoon succanat
1 teaspoon finely chopped red bell pepper
Dash of cayenne
1 teaspoon finely chopped green bell pepper

1 tablespoon freshly squeezed lime juice
8 Roma tomatoes, diced
2 tablespoons finely chopped cilantro leaves

Mix all of the ingredients; serve chilled.

Lemon Egg-Substitute Sauce

SERVES 2

3 tablespoons egg substitute
1 teaspoon arrowroot powder or cornstarch
½ cup vegetable broth (vegetable bouillon plus water)

4 tablespoons fresh lemon juice, strained
½ teaspoon sea salt
½ teaspoon lemon zest

1. In a saucepan, whisk the egg substitute with the arrowroot and a small amount of vegetable broth, until the mixture is smooth and shiny.

2. Add the remaining broth, lemon juice, salt, and zest.

3. Cook over medium-low heat, whisking continuously until the sauce reaches desired thickness. Never permit the sauce to boil.

4. Serve over steamed vegetables, or potatoes.

Ginger or burdock drunk as a tea 1 hour prior to or 1 hour after a meal is an excellent addition for immune-boosting.

JUICES AND SHAKES

Honey Blue Moon
SERVES 2

1 pear
½ lemon (with ½ inch of zest left on)
2 tablespoons raw (unheated) honey
1 cup filtered water, or 1 cup soy or
    rice milk

1 cup ice
¼ cup blueberries

1. In a blender or food processor, combine all of the ingredients and blend until smooth.
2. Serve immediately.

Choco Shake
SERVES 2

2 pears
2 bananas, mashed
¼ cup raw unsalted walnuts
1 cup rice or soy milk

1½ tablespoons pure unsweetened
    cocoa or carob powder
1 teaspoon almond extract
1 cup ice

1. In a blender or food processor, combine all of the ingredients and blend for 2 minutes or until smooth.
2. Serve immediately.

Green Monster
SERVES 2

2 kiwis
1 pear
2 apples
1 bunch dandelion greens

4 stalks celery
1 inch gingerroot
½ cup blueberries

1. Juice the kiwis, pear, apples, dandelion greens, celery, and gingerroot.
2. In a blender or food processor, combine the juice with the blueberries and mix until smooth.
3. Serve immediately or refrigerate for a few hours.

Party Lemon
SERVES 3

2 peaches
1 pear
1 apple
2 tablespoons raw honey

½ lemon
1 cup ice
1 cup rice or soy milk

1. Juice the peaches, pear, and apple.
2. In a blender or food processor, combine the juice with the remaining ingredients and blend until smooth.
3. Serve immediately.

Purple Power
SERVES 2

3 cups watermelon (rind included)
3 stalks celery

1 cup Oregon red grapes

1. Juice the watermelon with its rind, celery, and grapes.
2. Drink immediately.

Papaya Almond Milk
SERVES 2

¼ cup fresh raw almonds
1½ cups filtered water

1 whole papaya

1. In a blender, combine the almonds with the water. Blend for 2 to 3 minutes, or until smooth.
2. Add the papaya; blend together.
3. Serve immediately or refrigerate for a few hours.

Thirst Quencher

SERVES 2

3 cups watermelon (rind included)   2 cups Oregon red grapes
¼ pineapple

1. Juice the watermelon with its rind, pineapple, and grapes.
2. Drink immediately, or serve chilled for a refreshing drink.

Tutti-Frutti

SERVES 2

½ cup blueberries   1 pear
1 cup strawberries   4 dried dates
1 apple   1 cup filtered water

1. In a blender or food processor, combine all of the ingredients and blend for 2 minutes, or until smooth.
2. Serve immediately.

Tropicalite

SERVES 3

½ pineapple   2 tangerines
1 kiwi   1½ cups ice
1 mango

1. Separately juice the pineapple, kiwi, mango, and tangerines.
2. In a blender or food processor, combine the juice with the ice and blend for 2 minutes, or until smooth.
3. Serve immediately.

Green Apple

SERVES 2

½ bunch Swiss chard   1 cucumber
1 cup sunflower or alfalfa sprouts   4 stalks celery
1 bunch watercress   1 inch gingerroot
3 to 4 leaves romaine lettuce   2 apples

1. Juice all of the ingredients together.
2. Drink immediately.

Crazy Beet
SERVES 2

4 stalks celery   1 cucumber
½ bunch kale   3 beets
½ bunch arugula   1 inch gingerroot
½ bunch parsley

1. Juice all of the ingredients together.
2. Serve immediately.

NOTE: You may want to add a little flaxseed oil to this. Put the juice and the oil in a blender or food processor and blend for 1 to 2 minutes. Drink immediately.

Nut Shake
SERVES 2

½ cup mixed cashews, almonds,   1 banana
    Brazil nuts, and hazelnuts   1 cup strawberries
1 cup filtered water   2 tablespoons raw honey, unheated
1 cup ice   ½ teaspoon vanilla extract

1. In a blender or food processor, combine all of the ingredients and blend for 2 minutes, or until smooth.
2. Serve immediately.

Very Berry Blue
SERVES 2

3 stalks celery   2 beets
½ head purple cabbage   1 inch gingerroot
1 bunch parsley   1 cup blueberries
1 red bell pepper

1. Juice all of the ingredients together except for the blueberries. Put the juice in a blender and add the blueberries. Blend for 2 minutes, or until smooth.
2. Serve immediately.

Banana Royal
SERVES 2

3 bananas
1 mango
1 pear

3 peaches
1 cup fresh or frozen strawberries
2 tablespoons cinnamon

1. Peel the bananas and freeze them. (Once frozen, they can be juiced.)
2. Put all of the fruit through the juicer.
3. Sprinkle with the cinnamon and serve immediately.

NOTE: This can also be enjoyed as a creamy dessert.

Avocado Surprise
SERVES 2 to 3

1 pear
¼ cup avocado
2 bananas
1 cup fresh or frozen blueberries

½ cup rice or soy milk
½ teaspoon almond extract
1 cup ice

1. Juice the pear.
2. In a blender or food processor, combine all of the remaining ingredients with the juice and blend together until smooth.
3. Serve immediately.

Papaya Blue
SERVES 2

2 slices papaya
2 apples
2 slices pineapple

½ cup blueberries
1 cup ice

1. Juice the papaya, apples, and pineapple.
2. In a blender or food processor, combine the juice with the remaining ingredients and blend until smooth.
3. Serve immediately.

Creamy Peach

SERVES 2

½ cup almonds
1 cup soy or rice milk
1 cup ice
1 banana

2 peaches
1 teaspoon almond extract
1 tablespoon unsweetened cocoa or
 carob powder

1. In a blender or food processor, combine all of the ingredients and blend for 2 minutes, or until smooth.

2. Serve immediately.

Sweet Dandelion

SERVES 2

2 apples
3 cups honeydew melon chunks
4 dried dates

½ bunch dandelion greens
½ bunch broccoli
1 inch ginger

1. Juice all of the ingredients.

2. Drink immediately.

Pineapple Date Shake

SERVES 2

½ pineapple
4 dried dates
3 tablespoons unsweetened shredded
 coconut

2 tablespoons raw unsalted pecans
½ cup soy or rice yogurt
½ teaspoon ground nutmeg
1 cup ice

1. Juice the pineapple.

2. In a blender or food processor, combine the juice with the remaining ingredients and blend for 2 minutes, or until smooth.

3. Serve immediately.

Happy Camper
SERVES 2

½ bunch watercress
1 medium bulb fennel
1 medium parsnip
3 stalks celery

1 cup alfalfa or sunflower sprouts
1 cucumber
½ bunch parsley
2 carrots

1. Juice all of the ingredients together.
2. Serve immediately.

Banana Split
SERVES 2

2 apples
2 bananas
½ cup walnuts
1 cup blueberries
1 cup ice

2 tablespoons unsweetened cocoa or
   carob powder
3 tablespoons unsweetened shredded
   coconut
1 teaspoon vanilla extract

1. Juice the apples.
2. In a blender or food processor, combine the juice with the remaining
ingredients. Blend for 2 minutes, or until smooth.
3. Serve immediately.

Wild World
SERVES 2

1 bunch dandelion greens
½ head cabbage
3 beets with tops
1 medium parsnip

½ bunch parsley
2 carrots
1 inch gingerroot
½ cup raspberries

1. Juice all of the ingredients together.
2. Drink immediately.

Some Like It Hot

SERVES 2

2 red peppers
1 head lettuce
½ cup radish sprouts
1 cup clover sprouts
4 stalks celery

4 leaves turnip greens
1 bunch spinach
2 radishes
2 apples
1 inch ginger

1. Juice all of the ingredients together.
2. Drink immediately.

Summertime

SERVES 3

1 papaya
2 peaches
2 apricots
4 pitted prunes
½ inch gingerroot

½ cup soy or rice yogurt
2 tablespoons unsweetened shredded
   coconut
2 cups ice

1. In a blender or food processor, combine all of the ingredients and blend for 2 minutes, or until smooth.
2. Serve immediately.

Strawberry Milk

SERVES 2

¼ cup fresh raw pecans
1 cup filtered water or soy or rice milk

2 cups strawberries
2 bananas

1. In a blender or food processor, combine all of the ingredients and blend for 2 to 3 minutes, or until smooth.
2. Serve immediately.

Macadamia Shake
SERVES 2

¼ cup raw unsalted macadamia nuts   1 cup blueberries
1 cup filtered water   4 figs
2 bananas   1 cup ice
1 pear   2 teaspoons lemon juice

1. In a blender or food processor, combine all of the ingredients and blend for 2 minutes, or until smooth.
2. Serve immediately.

Sweet 'n' Tangy
SERVES 2

3 carrots   ½ cup cranberries
2 apples   ½ cup raspberries
1 orange   1 teaspoon ground nutmeg
1 inch gingerroot

1. Juice the carrots, apples, orange, and gingerroot.
2. In a blender or food processor, combine the juice with the remaining ingredients.
3. Drink immediately.

Papayan Mango
SERVES 2

1 mango   2 cups ice
1 papaya   2 bananas
½ pineapple

1. Juice the mango, papaya, and pineapple.
2. In a blender or food processor, combine the juice with the bananas and ice and blend for 2 minutes, or until smooth.
3. Drink immediately.

Orange Passion
SERVES 2

1 inch gingerroot
2 oranges
2 large carrots
2 grapefruits

1 lemon
1 lime
2 tablespoons raw honey

1. Pass the gingerroot through a juicer. Then juice the other ingredients.
2. Drink immediately.

Raspberry Shake
SERVES 2

2 apples
2 bananas, mashed
3 tablespoons raw unsalted almonds
1 cup fresh or frozen raspberries

1 cup rice or soy milk
½ inch fresh lemon (with rind)
½ cup ice

1. Juice the apples.
2. In a blender or food processor, combine the juice with the remaining ingredients and blend for 2 minutes, or until smooth.
3. Serve immediately.

BUILDING THE IMMUNE SYSTEM:
THE ULTIMATE ANTI-AGING CHALLENGE

If there is one concept that is central to our entire understanding of health and disease, it is immune function. This is the unifying principle that ties together all of the elements needed for optimum health and longevity: detoxification, exercise, good diet, nutritional supplementation, stress management, hygiene, and emotional wellness. In many ways, health and immune fitness are one and the same thing. Due to the high media visibility of such illnesses as herpes and AIDS, the term *immune system* has become a commonplace of everyday speech. Everyone knows he or she's got one, that it can be compromised, and that such compromise can lead to illness or even death. But what are we really talking about when we speak of the immune system?

Actually, there is no single system or structure that corresponds to this term. Rather, the term represents the totality of all the stunningly complex and interrelated processes and structures that contribute to the maintenance of our health and vitality in the face of myriad hostile influences.

Elements of the immune system penetrate all of the tissues and organs of the body, vigilantly warding off every manner of threat. Tying them all together is a kind of cellular intelligence, in the form of exquisitely sophisticated electrical and chemical messaging systems. This brilliant communications system, which orchestrates all of our many defenses, amounts, in effect, to a sort of second brain, one that extends throughout the entire body.

It is interesting to note that centuries before Western medicine knew of an immune system, some concept of a protective force permeating the bodies of living organisms to help maintain well-being had already been appreciated by various cultures. For example, in traditional Chinese medicine there is the notion of "wey chi," a guardian energy that flows out of the pores of the skin from millions of subtle energy channels in the body, and extends beyond it to ward off harmful outside influences. What's more, the ancient Chinese understood that this energetic "shield" could be affected by our minds and that one could strengthen it via cultivation of a strong and peaceful spirit. Many modern Western doctors have only recently come to acknowledge this mind–immune system connection. Ortho-dox medicine has generally tended to dismiss the notion that there is a link between our thoughts and emotions and immunity. We now know, through the study of psychoneuroimmunology, not only that this connection exists, but that the mind can at times be the most potent of all the elements affecting immune competence.

Mission: Intelligent Destruction

The primary mission of the immune system is to identify and eliminate harmful cellular organisms and other materials foreign to the body. At the same time, it must leave unmolested our own normal cells and other elements integral to health. In other words, the immune system has to intelligently discriminate between those particles it reads as "nonself," which it is programmed to seek and destroy, and those it senses as "self," which are preserved.

The body's defenses against disease are not confined to any one, discrete anatomical system but are distributed among specialized tissues and cells throughout it. The first line of defense, although it's not usually considered part of the immune system, is actually the skin, in that it acts as an anatomical barrier that passively denies entrance to harmful outside influences. And the hydrochloric acid of the stomach, which neutralizes pathogens that enter through our mouths, could also legitimately be considered part of the immune system.

However, what is most often meant by the term *immune system* are those tissues, organs, cells, and molecules that are involved in the immune response, i.e., the complex chain of cellular and molecular actions that are mobilized against foreign invaders once they gain entrance to our bodies. The immune response is also involved in checking internally generated threats, such as cancer cells.

The immune response has two general aspects: nonspecific and specific immunity. The nonspecific immune response, also called the inflammatory response, is the body's initial reaction to any kind of injury, whether due to trauma, a foreign organism, a chemical toxin, or localized oxygen deprivation. It is this response that produces the swelling and fever that we may experience following an injury or infection. Sometimes the inflammatory response works a little too well, and then we have such disorders as allergies and autoimmune illnesses.

The specific immune response, which involves more specialized defenses against particular agents, itself has two branches. These are known as cell-mediated immunity and molecular immunity.

Cell-mediated immunity (or, more simply, cellular immunity) is conferred by special types of white blood cells that directly engulf and/or chemically destroy pathogens or abnormal body cells. Molecular immunity involves the action of antibodies that circulate in the blood. With the help of blood proteins, these antibodies bind offending cells and molecules to which they have been sensitized by prior exposure, thus aiding in their elimination.

It should be noted that although scientists divide living systems into subsystems, parts, and elements in order to understand them, in reality the divisions are somewhat artificial, because they all work closely together. So while we describe nonspecific versus specific immunity and cellular versus molecular immunity as if these were all independent processes, in reality they are intimately connected, coordinated, and often overlapping. For example, the inflammatory response involves elements and activities that are classified as belonging to both the cellular and molecular immune mechanisms. From a holistic point of view, we acknowledge that the whole is greater—and infinitely more subtle in its workings—than the sum of its parts.

Fighting the Good Fight: A Tour of Your Immune System

When we think of circulation in our bodies, we think of blood. But lymph is another circulating fluid that's just as important to our well-being. Indeed, the lymphatic system is the seat of the immune response that keeps us alive and well.

How Lymph Helps Life. Lymph is a generally colorless, watery fluid formed in tissue spaces throughout the body. The main function of this fluid, which is much like blood plasma in composition, is to carry away cellular waste products and debris that accumulate in the spaces between our cells. To accomplish this, the lymph flows through a vast network of channels, known as lymphatic vessels, that eventually empty into the bloodstream. Thus, the lymphatic system, which includes the lymphatic vessels and associated tissues and organs, can be thought of as the body's cellular sewage-disposal system.

But tissues and organs of the lymphatic system have another essential mission: They are central to the functioning of the immune response. In particular, they are critical to the growth, maturation, and activation of the body's white blood cells. Lymphatic (or lymphoid) tissues with immune activity include the thymus gland, the spleen, and the lymph nodes. The mucous membranes lining the respiratory and gastrointestinal tracts are also richly endowed with immune-related lymphatic tissue. For example, masses of lymphoid tissue encircle the upper end of the respiratory tract, where they form the tonsils and adenoids. The old way of thinking about tonsils and adenoids—that they are useless tissues that should be removed if infection is a problem—is being supplanted by an understanding that these lymphoid tissues, in fact, work *against* infection and should not, in the vast majority of cases, be removed.

The Thymus Gland. The thymus gland, located beneath the top of the breastbone, carries out a number of essential immune functions. Foremost among these is its production of T-lymphocytes, the all-important white blood cells that help direct the entire immune response. These cells are critical to the body's resistance to such invaders as yeast, fungi, parasites, and viruses. T-cells also help to monitor the body for developing cancer cells.

In addition to its T-cell function, the thymus gland secretes hormones that regulate immune activities. In a healthy individual, levels of these hormones increase in the face of any infection. However, their secretion tends to decline as we age. The levels of these hormones are also reduced in individuals with a depressed immune system. This includes people with recurring infections, those under chronic stress, and those with AIDS.

The thymus is at the core of much immune system controversy, in part because it involutes, or shrinks, as we age. Although the thymus becomes physically smaller, T-cells do continue to be produced and other thymus-related factors continue to function throughout life. However, certain stressors may accelerate the process of involution. In particular, the thymus gland is quite sensitive to the damage caused by free radicals. Therefore, an increase in free-radical activity in the body may speed up the shrinking of the thymus.

The Spleen. Think of the spleen as a kind of internal blood filter with important immune-system functions. Located on the upper left side of the abdominal cavity (under the lower ribs), the fist-size spleen is the largest area of lymphatic tissue in the body.

As an immune system organ, the spleen is a major site for the maturation and storage of lymphocytes, the primary cells involved in specific immunity. The spleen also produces monocytes, another type of immune cell, which destroy circulating pathogens as well as worn-out or abnormal red blood cells as they filter through. The spleen can also act as a reservoir for blood that may be needed during an emergency such as excessive bleeding.

Other Lymphatic Structures. Lymph nodes are small kidney-shaped structures found at intervals along the lymphatic vessels. There are over six hundred of them in our bodies, with particularly large concentrations found in the armpits, groin, and neck, and in the abdomen surrounding the intestines.

Like the much larger spleen, lymph nodes function like filters—in this case, filtering lymph fluid rather than blood. Like the spleen, they contain large numbers of lymphocytes and other immune cells that destroy microbes and abnormal cells as they pass through. Lymph nodes are similar to the spleen in one other way, too. They act as storage sites for immune cells ready to be mobilized elsewhere in the body as needed.

Finally, a large proportion of the body's lymphatic tissue is distributed in the form of small nodules within the membranes lining the respiratory and gastrointestinal tracts. These structures contain various immune cells that provide site-specific protection against the numerous pathogens that may enter our bodies as we breathe and eat. In the GI tract, these nodules are known as Peyer's patches. What they do is screen the contents of our digestive system for harmful invaders before they can be absorbed into the bloodstream. They also secrete messenger chemicals that communicate directly with the brain. Thus, we have a connection between our "gut feelings," our immunity, and our minds.

Bone Marrow. Present throughout the body, bone marrow is the "nursery" for all of our immune cells. Some emerge fully formed from the bone marrow. Others, such as certain lymphocytes and monocytes, migrate out of the bone marrow in an undifferentiated form to the lymphatic tissues, especially to the thymus gland, spleen, and lymph nodes, where they develop into their characteristic forms.

A Look at Leukocytes

All of the body's many types of immune cells are known collectively as leukocytes. This is simply the technical term, derived from the Greek, for what you know as white blood cells. In describing the actions of the immune system, it is most common to use the extended metaphor of war, with the leukocytes cast in the role of cellular soldiers in an immune army. This imagery is apt for characterizing the various functions of the leukocytes against "invading" particles: killing, destroying, poisoning, engulfing, and neutralizing.

However useful the war analogy may be, though, it is important to understand that this is only a metaphor. As holistic physician Dr. Ronald Hoffman cautions, "The invader/army image has become a limiting stereotype." In actuality, the immune system's job is much broader than merely fighting off "bad guys." Its wider mission is no less than to allow us to coexist with a complex and ever-shifting environment. This requires a precise and rapid ability to differentiate that which may cause harm from that which is beneficial or merely neutral. Hoffman views it as a way of processing information and achieving a balance, distinguishing between self and nonself, rather than simply as a kind of Star Wars defense system against external threats. Sickness, then, becomes not the enemy but a natural phase in the ebb and flow of optimal immunity.

Although there are a variety of types of leukocyte with different functions, in general these cells protect us from threats in one of three ways: They may engulf or "eat" invading particles, release chemicals that directly destroy them, or produce antibodies to neutralize the attackers. In addition to their immune functions, certain leukocytes also act as scavengers of damaged cells, which they engulf and "digest." This process is known as phagocytosis. White blood cells that act by "eating" microbes, damaged cells, and other particles are thus sometimes referred to as phagocytes.

To get to their targets, leukocytes maneuver through the body in an amoebalike fashion. Many are able to move independently and can penetrate body tissues. Thus, they are able to rapidly go where needed in response to an injury or threat and then return to the bloodstream. When not in action, some leukocytes stay in the circulating blood, some migrate to the lymph fluid, while others set up housekeeping in various lymphatic tissues and organs such as the spleen, lymph nodes, and Peyer's patches in the lining of the gut. When called into action in response to a threat to the body, some types of leukocytes respond immediately, some can take months to get into the battle, while yet others sit it out and then serve as the cleanup crew.

To some extent, the number and types of leukocytes seen in the blood at a particular time provide clues to a person's health status. Normally, there are some five thousand to ten thousand leukocytes per cubic millimeter of circulating blood. Many more are sequestered in body tissues to provide site-specific immunity or for later mobilization as needed to counter a threat. Elevated white blood cell counts, i.e., more than ten thousand per cubic millimeter, may signal the presence of an infection or disease process. On the other hand, a low blood leukocyte count (less than five thousand) may be a sign of an immunodeficient state or a severe or prolonged infection that has depleted white cell reserves.

All of the body's leukocytes fall into one of three categories: polymorphonuclear granulocytes, monocytes, and lymphocytes. Each of these has its own role to play in immune function:

Polymorphonuclear Granulocytes. The "polys," or polymorphonuclear granulocytes, are so named because these cells have multilobed nuclei and have prominent grainlike, or granular, structures. These granules contain various chemicals that may be released as part of the cell's immune functioning. (All the other white cells, i.e., monocytes and lymphocytes, lack the large granules found in the polys and are sometimes called agranulocytes.)

There are three main subtypes of polymorphonuclear granulocytes: these are neutrophils, eosinophils, and basophils.

Neutrophils. Accounting for some 55 to 70 percent of all leukocytes circulating in the bloodstream, the neutrophils are the body's workhorses against infection. Neutrophils attack their targets by "eating" them (phagocytosis). Once engulfed, materials incorporated into the neutrophils are digested by enzymes contained within specialized granules inside the cell called lysosomes.

Neutrophils are very mobile cells, capable of reaching every part of the body. When summoned to a particular tissue site, they are able to migrate out of the bloodstream to where they are needed by squeezing through the walls of the capillaries.

Neutrophils play a major role in the inflammatory response, and their population in the blood can increase rapidly in response to an acute injury or infection. In autoimmune conditions, though, neutrophils may begin attacking normal cells.

Eosinophils. These cells are normally a small minority of circulating leukocytes, comprising just 1 to 3 percent of the total. However, their numbers can increase markedly in asthma, hay fever, or other allergic reactions and also in response to certain parasitic infections.

Eosinophils are thought to act primarily through phagocytosis, digesting antigen-antibody complexes produced after an antibody "grabs hold" of an allergenic particle, or antigen. They also secrete an enzyme that breaks down histamine, thus helping to "cool down" allergic reactions (which are characterized by excessive histamine release).

Basophils. Basophils normally account for less than 1 percent of the white cells in the blood. Although they have no ability to "eat" foreign material, these cells are thought to play an important role in the nonspecific immune response due to their ability to release histamine and other chemicals. Basophils also secrete heparin, an anticoagulant, presumably as a natural modulator of the blood coagulation process.

Another type of cell important in the inflammatory response is the mast cell. They're similar to basophils, but mast cells do not circulate in the blood. Rather, they congregate around the blood vessels of the skin and in the bone marrow. These cells, which contain some twenty times more histamine than do basophils, are quite active in allergic reactions.

Monocytes. The largest cells in the bloodstream are monocytes. These cells—some 3 to 8 percent of all circulating leukocytes—perform a number of immune functions, but their main job is basically to "eat" offending cells and particles.

Young monocytes circulate in the bloodstream for about one day, after which they migrate into various tissues throughout the body. Once they have settled into a tissue, monocytes mature into long-lived cells called macrophages (literally "large eating cells").

Macrophages are found in large numbers in the liver, spleen, lymph nodes, air sacs in the lungs, and tonsils. They are also present in the brain, skin, bones, and other tissues.

Macrophages perform functions similar to those of the circulating monocytes; they swallow up and digest pathogenic organisms and cellular debris, as well as cancerous, damaged, or aging cells. In fact, along with the neutrophils, the macrophages—especially those that have taken up residence in the blood-filtering lymphatic tissues—are the body's major phagocytes. Think of them as tireless Pacmen, constantly seeking out and scavenging unwanted materials from the circulation.

Like neutrophils, monocytes and macrophages are major cellular players in the inflammatory, or nonspecific, immune response. This is the body's generalized "one size fits all" reaction to any sort of injury or infection, irrespective of cause. These leukocytes engulf and destroy invading organisms and damaged cells at the site of the insult and then help to clean up or scavenge the resulting debris. In addition, macrophages participate in both immediate and delayed allergic responses.

Monocytes and macrophages also play important roles in specific immunity, functioning as parts of both the cell-mediated and molecular immune responses. This involves close coordination with the all-important lymphocytes, which "talk" with the monocytes via a complex system of chemical messengers.

Indeed, chemicals released by monocytes and macrophages are central to the cells' participation in both the inflammatory and specific immune responses. For example, they secrete substances called monokines, which activate the specialized lymphocytes known as T-cells. These, in turn, are the major "orchestrators" of the many cellular and chemical players involved in specific immunity.

Monocytes and macrophages also release substances called chemotaxins, which are involved in mobilizing the inflammatory response. In effect, chemotaxins sound the alarm when an abnormal cell, injury, or infection is detected, thus attracting neutrophils and many more monocytes to the site.

Macrophages also release toxic chemicals such as hydrogen peroxide and other reactive oxygen molecules to directly destroy invading pathogens and tumor cells. Unfortunately, these very substances that help to protect us from harmful particles also generate free radicals. Since these free radicals may destroy or damage neighboring cells, they must be combated by antioxidants such as the enzymes superoxide dismutase, catalase, and glutathione peroxidase, which are also secreted by these busy cells.

Lymphocytes. The principal mediators of the immune system are lymphocytes, cells that are potentially capable of recognizing every antigen they come across. Lymphocytes are especially plentiful in the thymus, spleen, and lymph nodes, and they come in three types: B-cells, which make antibodies to invading antigens; T-cells, which oversee all aspects of immune functioning; and natural killer cells, which destroy cells that are cancerous or that contain a virus. As a group, the lymphocytes constitute 18 to 45 percent of white blood cells. This proportion may decrease as the number of neutrophils increases, when, for instance, the body fights off a bacterial infection.

B-lymphocytes. When a B-cell encounters an antigen, or foreign substance, in the blood or lymphatic system, it transforms into a lymphocytic plasma cell. This newly created cell manufactures immunoglobulin, commonly known as antibody, to counter that particular antigen. With complex antigens such as viruses, whole microbe cells, or large protein molecules, the B-cells must enlist the help of a particular type of T-lymphocyte, appropriately named the T-helper cell, to activate the antibody mechanism.

The B-cells produce antibodies as long as the antigen is present. Once the antigen molecules are destroyed or removed, another type of T-lymphocyte, the T-suppressor cell, shuts off the B-cell's antibody factory. At that point, the antibody level in the entire body should start to diminish.

The body, in its wisdom, takes some of the B-cells from this factory and converts them into B-memory cells, which then serve as the basis of our acquired immunity. If the same type of antigen enters the body again, the B-memory cells can rapidly crank up the antibody production factory.

T-lymphocytes. The all-important T-cells are named after the thymus gland, in which they mature. These cells control the body's immune response in three essential ways: They initiate, direct, and conclude the activity of the immune system.

The two main categories of T-lymphocytes are T-4 cells and T-8 cells. One subtype of T-4 cells—the T-helper cells—initiate the immune response of both T- and B-lymphocytes. The T-8 cells include two subtypes: T-cytotoxic cells kill any foreign or abnormal cells found in the body, while T-suppressor cells turn off the entire lymphocyte response once the threat is no longer present.

Natural killer cells. A third type of T-lymphocyte, called the natural killer cell, or null cell, kills certain target cells in the body, even when the cells in question do not have any relationship to a foreign invader. According to one major theory regarding natural-killer-cell functioning, these lymphocytes destroy tumor cells caused by the body's own cellular metabolism or by outside agents such as chemicals, radiation, and viruses.

Chemical Messengers

The immune system has access to nearly every cell in the body. Such a complex network requires an excellent communication system to coordinate the functions of various cells. The communications are carried out by special types of small-chain proteins, known as cytokines, which serve as chemical messengers throughout the immune system.

Some of these messengers are called lymphokines, and the most famous of these are the interleukins and interferons. One essential function of lymphokines is to stimulate or suppress T-cell activity. Lymphokines also prompt the production of antibodies and protect cells from infection by viruses and intracellular parasites.

Immunoglobulins and the Complement System. Immunoglobulins, or antibodies, are proteins that circulate in the blood until they are called into action. The B-cells produce an antibody to a particular antigen when it enters the body. The five groups of immunoglobulins are known as IgG, IgM, IgA, IgE, and IgD. Each has a different physical configuration and different immune functions to perform.

Once the immunoglobulin has been produced, it forms a "complex" with the antigen itself. This arrangement allows the antibody to neutralize the intruder. At that point the complex itself must be destroyed—another job for the immune system.

The antigen-antibody complex tends to work in tandem with another component of our cell-mediated immunity, called the complement system. This system includes more than twenty proteins, each with specific functions to perform in the immune response. The proteins circulate in the serum at all times and are activated according to a sequence called the complement cascade.

Once activated, the complement proteins execute certain tasks that help the elimination of the intruder, such as neutralizing a virus, binding to a phagocyte cell, or releasing certain chemicals, which are called chemotoxins and anaphylatoxins. Unfortunately, the complement system is also a major player in allergic and hypersensitivity reactions.

When a Virus Meets the Body

First, let's assume the virus invades the body through the mucous membranes of your nose. There it will be met by IgA, which attempts to deactivate the intruder from the outset. Next, macrophages are signaled into action in a six-step process to eliminate the invading virus. One of the macrophages' jobs is to produce interleukin-1, which activates T-cells and gamma-interferon. When you get a fever along with your cold, these two chemicals are the agents that cause the fever.

At this point, the T-cells begin to reproduce themselves. Meanwhile, the T-helper cells begin to make interleukin-2, which stimulates the growth and duplication of the new T-cells. They also stimulate B-cells by secreting interleukin-4. The B-cells participate in the immune response by producing antibodies. IgM comes first, followed several days later by IgG. These two antibodies each form a complex with their antigens, thereby entrapping the foreign particles and rendering them harmless.

However, the antibodies cannot actually kill the invading antigens. That's a job for the complement cascade, which IgG and IgM help to initiate. The complement cascade produces chemotoxins, which lure more phagocytes to the area. The cascade also produces anaphylatoxins, which prompt the release of histamine from the mast cells. Histamine causes inflammation.

The antibodies help to attach the antigens to phagocytes, which have the job of engulfing and digesting the antigens. Antibodies also draw more phagocytes to the area. In the final leg of the immune response, the T-cytotoxic cells are called into action to kill any cells infected by the virus. If virus particles are released in the process, they are destroyed via phagocytosis.

Once the immune system has cleared the body from the virus's presence, the T-helper cells direct the T-suppressor cells to deactivate all the participating immune cells. The only cells that remain are the T-memory cells. If the same antigen reappears in the future, these cells are ready to activate the immune system once again.

When the Immune System Breaks Down

One of the things that can go wrong with our immune system is that it can make the mistake of classifying benign components of its own body as "nonself," then go on to attack these tissues as if they were foreign invaders. The result is autoimmunity. Today, researchers are discovering that many degenerative diseases share an underlying pattern that qualifies them as autoimmune disorders. As Dr. Russell Jaffe, who has studied this field extensively, points out, at first glance these diseases seem to be unrelated. But on closer inspection they appear to have some common elements at the biochemical level.

Consider this example: In some patients who develop adult-onset diabetes, the illness may be related to an autoimmune process in which the immune system attacks the pancreas. Similarly, a condition called myasthenia gravis may stem from the immune system's attack on the muscle surface. In the past, few of us would have thought these two conditions were related. However, they may indeed share a common denominator: a poorly modulated immune system that causes the body to attack itself.

Other organs or systems may be attacked as well, leading to such disorders as lupus erythematosus, thyroiditis, thrombocytopenia (a blood platelet disorder), rheumatoid arthritis, multiple sclerosis, and the kidney disease glomerulonephritis. While most autoimmune illnesses are somewhat rare, millions of Americans suffer from common allergies that also stem from immune system overvigilance.

Jaffe explains that autoimmunity can attack the body on a variety of levels, depending on the disorder: It can attack intracellularly (inside the cell), outside the cell in a nearby receptor, the cell membrane, the plasma protein, or the circulating hormones. Jaffe stresses that looking at certain diseases from the autoimmune standpoint is a complete shift from the old school of thought, which classified a disease strictly by the organ it affects. The complex immune system extends throughout the body so that most immune syndromes have a far-reaching impact on body functioning. Lupus, for example, primarily affects the skin and the connective tissue, but it may eventually affect the internal organs as well.

What are the common elements of this destructive pattern? According to Jaffe, autoimmune disorders share three negative factors at the cellular level: The inside of the cells becomes too acidic, the electron-transport system does not function properly, and the nutrients that support the immune system are depleted. Indeed, this combination often exists with other moderate to severe immune disorders as well. These include chronic or recurring viral problems, recurring herpes outbreaks, cytomegalovirus, Epstein-Barr virus, and hepatitis.

How Is the Immune System Weakened? Jaffe identifies a number of basic factors that will predispose a person to immune problems. First, when the amount of antigens coming into the body exceeds the immune system's capacity to handle them, the result is immune system overload, and with this condition of weakened immunity, the body may eventually begin to attack itself. At the same time, it may not be able to control pathogens or disease agents from the outside. Another problem that may lead to compromised immunity down the road is maldigestion. When the digestive apparatus is sluggish or underactive, it does not assimilate nutrients or remove wastes efficiently. This takes a toll on the whole body, including our immune apparatus. Exposure to environmental toxins, such as heavy metals and pesticides, is obviously not going to be beneficial to immune wellness. And psychological stress is a big immunity buster. For many years it has been common folk wisdom that emotional stress can "make you sick." Now scientific studies are beginning to explain the biological basis of a mind-body relationship. The nervous and endocrine systems, both of which secrete chemicals when you are stressed, influence the immune system on a cellular level. That's because cells of one system have receptors for the chemicals produced by another.

The Free-Radical Scourge. A major factor in immunity reduction is free radicals, those troublesome electron-hungry molecules that researchers are coming to view as the nemesis of those who would like to stay youthful. Actually, concerning the immune system and free radicals, there are two sides to the story. On the one hand, a variety of immune system cells, including neutrophils, monocytes, and macrophages, can generate free radicals in the body. These immune cells depend on this mechanism in order to kill bacteria, and this is one example of the body's legitimate need for free radicals.

The flip side of this scenario, however, is the adverse effect free radicals can have on the immune response. When free radicals damage cell membranes, for example, the immune system cannot function properly. The reason: Its communication system depends on cell membranes, where the receptors for interleukins, hormones, and immunoglobulins are located. Also, two types of immunoglobulin help the phagocytes to "eat" foreign intruders by fixing them on the phagocyte's surface. A damaged cell membrane impairs this crucial immune response.

At this point a variety of serious disorders have been linked to free-radical pathology, including cancer, coronary artery disease, cataracts, arthritis, and neurological degeneration. What's more, as we've mentioned, the aging process itself seems to be connected to free-radical activity. Researcher Dr. Richard Passwater explains the connection as follows: Free radicals impair or destroy healthy cells. Eventually the cumulative loss of active cells can lead to a loss of the reserve function in various organs, or the amount of energy held in reserve for functioning beyond the body's daily needs.

In a nutshell, the loss of reserve function and the aging process are one and the same. Passwater, along with others, believes that the stability of living systems becomes progressively impaired not by the passage of time but rather through chemical reactions. If the rate of these deleterious reactions can be controlled, we can control aging.

Radical-Reduction Strategies. It is clear that we must continually strive to balance the events taking place in the molecules of our bodies. Fortunately, nature has given us a way to achieve this balance in the form of antioxidant enzymes and nutrients that remove free radicals before they can cause cellular damage.

The antioxidant enzymes include two forms of superoxide dismutase (SOD) as well as glutathione and catalase. Mineral cofactors are needed by these enzymes: SOD needs either manganese or a copper-zinc combination to do its work, and glutathione peroxidase requires selenium as its cofactor nutrient. Catalase depends on iron to carry out its antioxidant functions.

Likewise, antioxidant vitamins act as scavengers to remove various forms of free radicals from the body and prevent new ones from being formed. These potent nutrients include vitamin C, vitamin E, and beta-carotene, a precursor to vitamin A. In addition to trapping free radicals, all three of these antioxidants can "quench" the highly reactive singlet oxygen molecule. In essence, they absorb the molecule's altered energy state, thereby returning it to normal without harming the system. The bottom line in all of this is that intelligent consumption of antioxidant-rich foods and supplements, combined with stress-reducing lifestyle choices, is the best route to health maintenance.

The Misperceptions of Medicine

Unfortunately, the idea of taking control of our immune system's health by using antioxidants and other self-help strategies goes against the grain of what Western medicine has traditionally been about. The illness paradigm of conventional medicine has been one of "catching" a disease. A person goes around minding her own business and all of a sudden a disease comes along out of the blue in the form of germs that invade her body and so she catches that disease. It's a nice picture of a helpless victim who then must go to the doctor to get some miracle medicine to "knock out" the invading germ.

The problem is, it's not an accurate picture in most instances. In reality, our bodies are home to many bacteria and viruses and even cancer cells that are being held in check by our immune systems. It is only when the immune system gets weakened, through nutritional deficits, toxic input, or the biochemical effects of stress, that the pathogenic agents get the upper hand and their long-awaited chance to make us sick. The homeostasis, or state of balance in our bodies, finally gets upset, and suddenly it seems that we've "caught" something. In actuality, that something was there all along.

Once we do get sick, we in America are not patient patients. This society, with its get-the-job-done attitude, expects a fast solution to every problem, and that mentality extends into the medical model, where people expect to be provided with quick-and-easy solutions to their health problems. In some cases, the medical community can indeed supply that type of quick cure. Penicillin, for example, certainly does its job of killing some bacteria. But the success of such drugs as penicillin has unfortunately fueled the mentality that for every disease there is a magic curative bullet.

The burden then is on the physician to deliver better and faster magic bullets. At the same time we downplay the importance of each person's natural resistance to ailments and disease. If more focus were put on the immune system's health, we would learn to work with the body's wisdom and to support its natural ability to resist a bacterium, virus, or even cancer through its own defense system. "Take two aspirin and call me in the morning" might be replaced by "Eat two fruits and take a walk every morning"! We'd be a lot better off in the long term with this approach.

A Tale of Two Immune Systems

Consider two hypothetical individuals. They are the same age, live in the same polluted city, and work at the same type of stressful job. This is where the similarities end.

Person A comes down with multiple infections over the course of each year, including colds and the flu. He also has chemical sensitivities and allergies, and as he gets older, he starts to develop degenerative diseases, such as arthritis. Person A's doctor tells him that the different diseases and conditions he has are separate, unrelated, and unavoidable disorders, all of "unknown etiology."

Person B, though, hardly ever gets sick, and what's more, with the advancing years he's still energetic and disease-free.

What's the difference between the two of them? B is making an effort to feed his immune system and A isn't. Further, A is actually poisoning his immune system, through the foods he consumes and even his mode of interacting with the world.

Let's take a look at how each of these people lives. Person A, a man living the average American lifestyle, believes it's okay to do anything—in moderation. So in moderation he smokes; drinks alcohol; drinks coffee, colas, and other beverages laced with sugar or artificial sweeteners; eats the average American diet of denatured, refined foods; and eats hamburgers, chicken, and that favorite American vegetable, french fries. Once in a while he has an iceberg lettuce salad or a bit of fruit. He's about 10 percent over his ideal body weight but doesn't think much of it because most of the people he knows are, too.

Person A does exercise—in moderation. So on weekends, if it's sunny, he'll play a game of tennis. He'll take a walk—maybe once a season. Otherwise, he's sedentary, sitting at a desk or dining table, on a couch in front of a TV, or in his car.

When he's in his car going to work, sometimes people do things to make Person A mad. Other drivers will cut him off and Person A will yell and scream at them, sure that they have a personal vendetta against him and that he is honor-bound to retaliate. Sometimes at work Person A's boss will make him mad. Then he can't yell and scream, but he *can* hold his anger in and keep it there all day. He seems to be used to the chronic surge of anger-induced hormones, such as adrenaline, that are coursing through his bloodstream all day at work. At home, he hardly notices the anger, because he has the distractions of the TV, the telephone, the radio, the computer, and various interactions with his family, which, because of the pace of everyone's lives these days, always seem to be rushed.

Person B has a totally different approach to life. For instance, B follows the same route to work as A, so people cut him off, too, but B just figures that many of these people don't mean to cut him off, or if they do, so what? B listens to books on tape in his car, so he doesn't feel that his commute is wasted time. At work, when B's boss is unfair to him, he tries to talk to the boss calmly about the problem right away. If that is impossible, the situation is just not that big a deal to B as it is to A. Maybe that's because B knows he'll be doing something relaxing and meaningful at the end of the day, such as riding his bike through the park, where he'll be able to think things through and enjoy being out in nature. B tries to spend some time introspectively each day; he finds it helps him maintain his generally positive attitude. He also tries to spend some relaxed "downtime" with his family daily. He and his family discovered a long time ago that it's not necessary to shop as much as everyone thinks it is, and that if you shop less, life becomes less frantic.

There's a tremendous difference in the way A and B eat. B has done extensive reading about how antioxidants promote immune fitness, and he puts what he's learned to use every day in the kitchen. He eats many servings of organic vegetables—steamed, raw, or juiced—daily and many servings of organic fruit—raw or juiced—as well. The juice portion of this intake averages three to four glasses. B also eats whole grains, such as kamut, quinoa, and barley, because he knows that these all contain enzymes that are catalysts, acting like spark plugs to enhance metabolic activity. B's reading has helped him understand that since aging is characterized by generally slowed metabolism throughout the body, anything he can do to promote metabolic activity is going to help him stay young.

B understands the value of phytochemicals, the plant-based substances that help us fight disease, so his diet is rich in phytochemical-rich foods like blackberries, blueberries, raspberries, strawberries, watermelon, peaches, plums, sea vegetables, cabbage, Brussels sprouts, alfalfa sprouts, tomatoes, and soy foods. He consumes about 60 grams of fiber a day from a variety of sources. He eats about three to five servings of grains a day, two to three servings of legumes, a serving of nuts, and one of seeds. He also gets acidophilus from nondairy yogurt. B avoids dairy products and does not eat meat. He also avoids sugar; refined carbohydrates, such as white-flour-based baked goods; caffeine; and alcohol. His body, like his diet, is on the lean side.

Although he knows that food is the best source of nutrients, B also takes supplements. He periodically consults with his health-care practitioner about an immune-enhancing supplementation plan based on his individual needs. Here are some of the things he's taken on a daily basis at different times:

Alpha-lipoic acid—200 mg
Acetyl-L-carnitine—1000 mg
Coenzyme Q10—200–300 mg
Ginkgo biloba—100 mg
Calcium and magnesium from citrate—1400 mg
Vitamin C—3000–10,000 mg
Bioflavonoid complex—2000 mg
Garlic—3000 mg
Aloe vera—2–3 oz
Full-spectrum B-complex vitamin—50 mg
Selenium—200 micrograms
Zinc—at least 30 mg
MSM (methyl sulfonyl methane)—500 mg
Primrose oil—1500 mg
Trimethylglycine—500 mg
Glutathione, reduced—500 mg
Phosphatidyl choline—500 mg
Phosphatidyl serine—500 mg
NAC (N-acetylcysteine)—500–1000 mg
SAM (S-adenodylmethionine)—500 mg

This list of antioxidant supplements—although far from complete—is long, and in no way am I recommending that everyone should be taking all of these things every day. The point is that a person who is diligent about his or her immune system wellness might want to take some of these supplements after exploring with his or her health-care practitioner how they might help.

Let's look a little further into how B lives. He exercises aerobically forty-five minutes to an hour each day and he lifts weights as well. The many benefits of exercise, he knows, include its facilitating the circulation of lymphatic fluid. Also, he's made an effort to keep his home environment as clean as possible, getting rid of shag carpeting, sealing or shellacking any surfaces that were outgassing fumes, installing a water filter, using an air filter, and keeping street-soiled shoes from his floors (see "Your Personal Detoxification Program"). And it goes without saying that he would never smoke.

The outcome of B's lifestyle is that when his body is threatened by a virus, his immune system will be equipped with a full armamentarium of neutrophils, basophils, natural killer cells, and everything else necessary to neutralize it. He'll be able to stay healthy in many situations in which A will get sick, because he's nurtured his immune system all along. This is not to imply that this tale of two immune systems has to end sadly for A. No matter what stage of life he's in, it's not too late for him to start turning things around and fortifying his system. The first step in that process will have to be getting rid of the toxins that have accumulated in his body over the years. The next chapter, on detoxification, discusses how that can be done.

YOUR PERSONAL DETOXIFICATION PROGRAM

Getting healthy is like cleaning out your hall closet: You can't do a good job unless you get rid of the old stuff first. That's why I tell everyone who's really interested in making meaningful health changes, and not just dabbling in taking a few supplements, that they've got to start by detoxifying.

Unfortunately, many physicians who call themselves complementary, or holistic, haven't yet grasped this fact. So, too many of them are happy to quickly send their patients off with whatever is the popular natural remedy of the moment. This could be the phosphatidylserine or the ginkgo biloba for neurological function, the ozone for viruses, or the vitamin C drips for cancer—whatever is in and whatever is easy. This kind of "quick natural fix" mentality is not a far cry from the way some orthodox physicians prescribe antibiotics for everyone, whether they need them or not. What's missing is a truly holistic understanding of the patient's complete situation. That, and the knowledge that to really get healthy, a patient needs to start by devoting six months to two years to a complete detoxification program.

What's Involved in Detox?

Detoxification, or clearing the toxins from our bodies, is a complex process involving several bodily systems. The liver, one of our largest internal organs, counts among its functions the transformation of toxins, as well as metabolic by-products, into harmless substances. This underappreciated workhorse of the body is constantly filtering our blood and sending toxins to our other eliminatory organs. Prime among these are the large intestine, the conduit for solid wastes, and the kidneys, which eliminate such unwanted substances as urea, a protein metabolism by-product, excess mineral salts, and drugs that we may have in our bloodstream.

You may not have thought of your skin as an organ, but it's actually your largest one, and it plays a vital role, through perspiration, in the eliminatory process. Our lungs, too, help in the process, as we eliminate gaseous waste, such as carbon dioxide, with each exhalation. Finally, the lymphatic system is a big player in the body's detox process. This system has been compared to an internal ocean, because the lymphatic fluid, which constantly flows through the body, bathes our cells. In doing so it transports nutrients to our tissues, but it also removes toxins and metabolic waste and destroys harmful micro-invaders.

While these body systems are vital cleansing mechanisms, the detox process really goes beyond what our organs do physically to clean our insides. When a holistic health practitioner refers to detoxification, he or she is referring to nothing less than a multifaceted health program that takes into account the cleansing of the body, mind, emotions, and spirit. And any practitioner worth his or her salt (or herbal-mixture substitute!) will add that the detox process—while you can get it off to a running start with an intense few days of juice fasting—really has to be extended into a long-term program. To understand why, let's look at what we currently know about disease.

The Long Road to Ill Health

One of the most important paradigm shifts that have occurred in recent years is in our understanding of disease. We've gone from the idea that disease is, in general, something that you just "catch," or that mysteriously or uncontrollably befalls you, to an understanding that most adult disease in western culture is the result of gradual processes that are, to a large extent, modifiable. We now understand that continual exposure to low-level toxicity, e.g., through such means as pollutants in the air, water, and soil, or unwholesome foods, eventually causes our bodies to become overwhelmed. Then it's only a question of circumstance as to what will be the crisis—the emotional stress, the lack of exercise, the nutritional deficiency, the exposure to something toxic in the environment—that one day causes the system to no longer maintain homeostasis and to actively start to process disease. It is at this crisis stage that the body can no longer keep the viruses, bacteria, or cancer cells within it under surveillance and they become disease causing. It's as if there's a bunch of bad guys who have been hanging around the body all along, and the crisis stage is when the body finally says, "Okay, fellas, I guess you can go ahead and do your thing." That is when symptoms first appear.

What it boils down to is that, contrary to traditional medical dogma, by the time we actually see the result of a tumor or some other condition, it's actually the end stage of the disease process and not the beginning. The idea that we are either healthy because we have no disease symptoms or sick because we manifest a symptom, is passé. It may take ten, twenty, thirty, or even more years to collapse the system but surely any system that is not vigorously protected and fortified will collapse.

Unfortunately, much of what we do in our everyday routine is just the opposite of fortification; we're actually contributing to the disease process. Think of how we spend our days. We wake up after having slept all night next to the electromagnetic field of our alarm clock. We start the morning with caffeine and possibly a "meal" that's really just an overdose of fat and sugar. At work, we may be sitting too close to a computer, ingesting more caffeine, sugar, and fat, drinking chlorinated water, and eating denatured and highly refined excuses for food. Back at home, in an attempt to unwind, we may be adding alcohol to the toxic mix, as we sit back clicking our remote control after an exerciseless day. Other harmful things we routinely do without much thought include getting our teeth filled with mercury, exposing ourselves to unnecessary X rays, taking antibiotics excessively, and breathing in formaldehyde, benzene, and asbestos. Most Americans may assume that all these actions are a normal part of modern life, but our bodies have not caught up with our definition of normalcy, and these actions all exact a physical price.

Emotional assaults take their toll as well. If you get angry in traffic, for example, your adrenal glands will oversecrete the hormone adrenaline, because this is the way your body prepares to either do battle or run away. While this classic "fight or flight" response served a purpose in humankind's early days, when people needed to react physically to life-threatening situations in order to survive, in today's world this response usually does more harm than good. For most of the challenging situations encountered nowadays, a fight-or-flight response is physiological overkill. And it's the kind of overkill that can, with time, possibly kill *you*, because it raises your level of adrenaline, which in turn raises the level of cortisol, a stressor hormone that is not good for you.

Now, this is not to say that you should never get stressed. I'm not telling you to spend your life in a padded room listening to Muzak (unless that's your thing!). Stress is a part of life, and some people—those I call dynamic aggressives and dynamic assertives, for instance—actually thrive on stress because they know how to cope actively and positively with it and they genuinely enjoy molding challenge into opportunity. The problem comes when you are subjected to stressful situations that you feel you can do nothing about. If this is the case, your body is probably in chronic fight-or-flight mode, a condition that is going to totally deplete you after a few years. All of this is why true detoxification has to encompass your emotional state as well as physical factors.

Once we understand the gradual nature of the disease process, we can see that reversing the damage will be accomplished gradually, too. You're not going to detoxify the system from a lifetime accumulation of poisons overnight. Programs that promise immediate results using powders or other supplements, magnets, or any particular medical therapy are just not realistic. This is not to suggest that these remedies don't have benefits. They do. But detoxification is a slow process, one that may be difficult at times and for which there are no easy shortcuts available. A thorough approach, combined with patience and perseverance, are what it takes to detoxify successfully.

While there's no denying that—to adapt an old song lyric—cleaning up is hard to do, the payoff is that once you do detoxify, chances are that you're going to feel better than you have in a long time. People I have guided as they undertake this process report that after a period of detoxification—usually months long—they feel more energetic than they have in decades and that they need significantly less sleep than they did previously. Also, detoxification delivers real benefits to the way people look. Their skin becomes smoother and rosier, their eyes brighten, and their bodies become firmer. In short, they become younger-looking.

Most important, though, is that people's mental outlooks often change dramatically after they've undertaken a detoxification program. They feel more in control of their lives and more ready to meet the world than they ever have, at any age. So while their looks may become younger, their *outlooks* become better.

The other day, while running in Central Park, I crossed paths with a man who had recently completed one of my six-month detox programs. He came over to me and, grasping my shoulders and looking me in the eye, said, "Gary, I didn't believe that it would work, but I'm living proof that it does!" The man—a scientist, by the way—was sixty, but he told me that lately he had the energy of a teenager. He'd lost twenty-four pounds on the detox program, lowered his previously elevated PSA to a normal level, rid himself of his mood swings, and was so happy that, he reported, he bounced out of bed every morning. The interesting thing was that this man had done nothing more on the detox program than eliminate all the "bad stuff." I always recommend taking supplements in conjunction with detoxing, but he hadn't even done that. Still, he was obviously glowing with vitality.

It's not that I was surprised. Having completed more than thirty health study programs involving over five thousand individuals in the past five to six years, I'm familiar with the power of detoxification. When people take the time to approach their health in this rigorous way, the benefits are often dramatic, and likely to be lasting.

Testing . . . Testing . . .

Okay, so you've decided it's time to detoxify. The very first thing I recommend doing is getting a thorough evaluation of what is actually happening inside your body by taking some simple tests. The classic SMA-24 blood test supplies a lot of useful information. It will let you know, for example, whether you're too acid or too alkaline, and whether your uric acid, calcium, and cholesterol levels are in balance or not. In addition, an inexpensive blood test will identify any microorganisms that may be undermining your health. This is important because you could be doing all the right things, in terms of exercising, eating right, and taking supplements, and yet find yourself unable to maintain good health due to the parasites, bacteria, viruses, or fungi that call your body home.

You can also get allergy tests done to determine whether or not your fatigue, PMS, migraines, insomnia, or other problems are due to food sensitivities or chemicals or something else in the environment. And if your health practitioner suspects that you have candidiasis, or an overgrowth of the yeast *Candida albicans* that can cause fatigue and other symptoms, tests can be done to determine this.

Applied kinesiology is a field that offers tests that may prove useful. This discipline is based on the assumption that the body has its own innate intelligence and, therefore, knows exactly what it needs and what is harmful to it. According to practitioners, exposure to a particular food or some other substance will cause the body to become stronger or weaker. For example, sugar placed under the tongue may cause immediate weakness, while vitamin C may have a strengthening effect. Other substances will affect different individuals differently, and tests are done based on this principle.

Are valuable enzymes in your system being neutralized by such toxic substances as lead, cadmium, and mercury? Tests to determine the amount of heavy metals in your body can be valuable. You can also get tested to see if the silver amalgam fillings in your teeth are outgassing mercury. Some people for whom this is a problem report that after having these fillings properly removed—using holistic dental protocols—and replaced with a safer substance, their overall health improved.

You might want to take a glucose tolerance test (GTT) to measure blood levels of sugar that the body uses. Ideally, glucose is maintained at a relatively constant level by means of insulin and other hormones, but in an imbalanced system glucose levels can become too high or too low, resulting in lethargy, dizziness, and irritability. The GTT, a simple, inexpensive test, can help determine if your mood and energy fluctuations are connected to blood sugar problems.

Another test to consider is the impedance test, which measures how much body fat you have. Did you know that you can be overfat even if you are not overweight according to the charts? On the other hand, the charts can brand you as overweight when in reality your body composition is ideal. That's because lean muscle tissue weighs more than fat. With an impedance test it takes just two seconds to determine the percentage of body fat, lean muscle tissue, and water in your body. Healthy men should be between 10 and 21 percent fat; women should be around 12 and 23 percent fat. Most people, however, are 5 to 10 percentage points above these targets. Ideally, you want more lean muscle and less fat, not only for aesthetic reasons or because you'll be aerobically more fit, but because many toxins—from pesticide and herbicide residues to heavy metals such as lead and cadmium—get trapped and stored in fat. The fatter you are, in other words, the more toxic you're likely to be.

Getting tested will give you an objective baseline assessment of where you are healthwise and let your health-care practitioner know what you must do to get rid of substances that can lessen the quality of life and ultimately cause disease. It's your start of the path to wellness.

Helping Ourselves to Health

Once your doctor or other health-care professional has guided you through the testing and evaluation process, you can get started with a personal detoxification program tailored to your individual needs. I want to stress here that if you are going to do any sort of rigorous detoxing, this is not the time to go it alone. Let a holistically oriented doctor guide you and keep him or her filled in on how you're doing. I say this because the significant dietary changes you make on a detox program, while helpful to people in general, may be harmful to certain individuals, such as those with a particular medical condition, those taking certain medications, or pregnant women. So be sure to keep your doctor in your detox loop.

Of course, when it comes down to actually making the changes needed to detoxify, you have to do that for yourself. The exciting thing about this, according to certified nutritionist Linda Berry, is that there *are* so many effective changes you can make. Berry, the author of a book on detoxification, *Internal Cleansing: Rid Your Body of Toxins Return to Vibrant Good Health,* stresses the centrality of the digestive system as the key to our well-being. "If we think about our digestive system," she says, "the colon is like the septic tank. If your sewerage gets blocked up in your house, what happens? You get a raving mess inside your home. We need to keep the septic system moving so that the food that's processed, starting in our mouths . . . gets fully metabolized and then properly eliminated through the colon." Berry offers several hints on how to help our detoxification processes work optimally.

Have healthy thoughts. It sounds like a corny platitude, but sometimes true things do, and the fact remains that having a healthy, happy attitude toward life is the most important thing you can do for yourself. As we've mentioned, stress adversely affects hormones, which results in a less than optimal bodily balance. Conversely, happy thoughts keep our hormone levels in optimal balance. "One of the easiest and simplest ways to begin to cleanse," Berry advises, "is to smile more, lifting the corners of your mouth and making sure your eyes crinkle when you smile. That's what's necessary, researchers say, to get those 'joy juices' flowing. Then we're in a state where our body can be vibrantly healthy and optimally functioning so that we can absorb, digest, and eliminate."

Breathe fully. Think about when life's stresses are building up. Say you're worried about what's required of you at work, whether you're going to pass that test, how you're going to feed your family, or how you're going to get all your urgent errands done. At times like these, you're probably taking shallow breaths high in your chest. This may contribute to an acidic system that's receptive to disease. To keep your system in a healthy, alkaline state, learn to breathe deeply and slowly into your abdomen. If you don't know how to breathe properly, enroll in a yoga class, where techniques for deep breathing and total relaxation can be learned. The results—acid/base balance, better digestion and elimination, and increased ability to relax—will be immediately rewarding.

There are a variety of approaches taught by holistic practitioners to optimize breathing. One involves a series of three breaths. First, inhale deeply through your nose. Then, using your abdominal muscles, push the air out through your mouth. Take a second breath the same way, sucking the air in through the nose and blowing out forcefully through the mouth. On the third breath, inhale and then hold the air a few seconds without creating stress. This exercise is said to be great for stimulating lymphatic flow, but you should not do it to the point of dizziness.

Brush up on skin brushing. Another way to stimulate lymphatic flow is dry brush skin massage. Use a dry vegetable bristle brush, one that's stiff enough to stimulate your skin but not one that's going to scratch. Then, before a shower, brush your skin in the direction of your heart. Brush up your legs and arms, up your back, and across your abdomen. (Avoid, though, the delicate skin of your neck and face.) Use this technique gently but regularly and you'll be aiding lymphatic circulation and helping to remove trapped toxins.

A different route to lymphatic system boosting involves rebounding on a rebounder, which is a minitrampoline. An effective lymphatic system is one that's kept moving, but, unfortunately, most Americans have sluggish lymphatic action due to inactive lifestyle. Therapists recommend using a trampoline as an enjoyable way to counter lymphatic stagnation. Those who are unable to jump up and down can benefit just by sitting on the rebounder and bouncing.

Do *sweat the small stuff.* If you haven't already, add exercise to your life and keep it there. Exercise is a great way not only to get your lymphatic system moving and get yourself aerobically fit, but to get yourself to sweat and thereby eliminate heavy metals and other toxins. If your doctor gives you the okay, make cardiovascular exercise part of your routine. Try jogging, running, jumping rope, dancing, swimming, rowing, race walking, or rebounding, if you like. The key is to do what you like, so that you'll keep doing it.

Taking a weekly sauna, if you've got medical clearance to do so, is another great way to induce sweating and speed detoxification. Be sure that you're adequately hydrated while indulging in a sauna. To protect the circulation to your head and prevent faintness, wrap a cold towel around your head. An even easier way to induce sweating is to soak in a hot tub. Pouring one to three cups of Epsom salts into the bathwater will aid you further by supplying magnesium to your cells and facilitating cell cleansing. Adding equal parts of baking soda to the water will produce a more alkalizing effect. Soaking in a hot bath like this for fifteen or twenty minutes is an excellent way to relax at the end of a tension-filled day. By the way, another benefit of a hot bath or a sauna is that you're raising your body core temperature, which helps kill pathogens. Again, though, be sure you get your doctor's go-ahead before you do this, particularly if you have heart disease, hypertension, diabetes, or another chronic condition, and do not use these body-temperature-raising techniques if you're pregnant.

Become a drinker. Of water, that is. A great majority of toxins are water-soluble and can be expelled via the kidneys through the urine, so be sure to drink plenty of pure water. And since drinking a lot of water is good for the skin and other eliminatory organs themselves, you'll get a double benefit.

Always keep in mind that thirst is not generally a sufficient indicator of how much water people need, especially as they age. If you are detoxifying, it is recommended that you drink half your body's weight in ounces, so for a 140-pound person that would be seventy ounces, or almost nine glasses. If you are exercising regularly and sweating, add more water each day.

One more thing about water: If you're fighting toxins, make sure your water, which should be part of the solution, isn't adding to the problem. The water you drink, cook with, and bathe in should be as free as possible of fluoride, chlorine, metals, bacteria, and viruses. Have your water tested and, if necessary, install a home purification system. These are not that expensive and are well worth their cost in health benefits and peace of mind. After all, your body is two-thirds water, so if you clean up your water, you're cleaning up *you*!

Eat fiber-rich foods. In addition to water, fiber is another essential element of any cleansing diet. Nowadays, Americans are increasingly aware of the importance of fiber. Sadly, though, they're not acting on their knowledge, and many are still getting only a small percentage of what is needed. For optimal health, make fresh, live foods the mainstay of your diet and try to get between forty and sixty grams of fiber daily. In addition to eating several servings of fruits and vegetables, you'll want to start the day with cooked, whole-grain cereals. Ideally, you should rotate grains, choosing from amaranth, barley, buckwheat, bulgur, millet, oatmeal, quinoa, rice, rye, and triticale. You can get additional fiber by adding rice bran, oat bran, barley bran, flaxseeds, or psyllium to your diet.

Fiber helps us stay healthy by decreasing the time it takes fecal matter to leave the body. With the standard American diet, undigested food can remain in the body for up to four days, and the results can be toxic. When fecal matter stays stuck in the intestinal tract, food rots and becomes toxic to the system. Then dangerous microbes begin to work on it, and this undermines good health. Over time, carcinogenic substances are produced. As colon cancer is one of the major causes of death in this country, we want to be sure we are getting all the fiber we need to help our colons eliminate in a timely and thorough fashion.

Eating more fiber has several other advantages, too. It helps to make the feces softer, lessening pressure on the colon walls and resulting in easier bowel movements. For people with blood sugar instabilities, fiber may help to normalize blood sugar levels. In addition, fiber has been shown to lower cholesterol levels. Studies also suggest that a small percentage of arthritic conditions may be related to pathogenic microorganisms in the bowel. For some people, then, clearing the bowel of toxic chemicals can have the added benefit of lessening joint pain.

Important to effective detoxification is the ability to listen to your body and go to the bathroom when necessary. It's easy to get absorbed in your daily activities and ignore the urge for as long as possible. But that's not good for your colon—or for your overall health. Over time, this habit may make the ability to eliminate more difficult. Always respect your body's needs and go to the bathroom when it tells you to.

Sometimes, holistic health practitioners recommend drinking an intestinal cleansing beverage before bedtime to really get things moving. Recipes differ, but an example is: ½ teaspoon of powdered psyllium husks, 1 tablespoon of ground flax or chia seeds, and ½ tablespoon of liquid bentonite clay, which is a substance that traps and binds toxins. These are mixed into a base of 8 ounces of organic apple juice or water; the beverage is then consumed immediately, because it will gel quickly. It's very important to consume extra fluids with high-fiber beverages like this. Getting enough water into your system can mean the difference between alleviating constipation and creating intestinal compaction, so remember to drink. Garlic capsules (500 to 2000 mg), vitamin C (500 to 2000 mg), caprylic acid, and natural acidophilus are also good every other night instead of the fiber.

NOTE: Whenever you're going to depart dramatically like this from your usual eating and drinking habits, seek medical advice first. This is particularly vital if you're pregnant or elderly, are taking medication, or have a hypertensive or heart condition.

Jettison the Junk

As you're getting rid of the old poisons in your system, it makes no sense to take in new ones. So now is the time to start saying "No, thank you" to caffeine and alcohol, not to mention cigarettes. Beyond these obvious no-no's, though, are many others that we in America have come to think of as acceptable food sources, but which, in reality, are undermining our health.

A first simple rule to remember as you clean up your dietary act is this: Shun sugar. Americans, on average, eat the equivalent of more than half a cup of this refined carbohydrate a day, which adds up to a whopping 149 pounds of sugar a year. What's so bad about this? Well, consider that every time you eat as little as two teaspoons of sugar, you can upset the calcium/phosphorus ratio in your body. You can start to tip the body's pH toward the acid, rather than the alkaline, which is not desirable because the body seems to do better in a slightly alkaline state. We can't digest as well in an acidic state, and our immune systems become compromised.

Besides sugar, there are other refined carbohydrates you should stay away from, such as white flour. Actually, you should stay away from all of them, not that this is easy, since refined foods are so pervasive in our culture. Refinement of foods is an example of modern society's not knowing when to leave well enough alone. We take perfectly good grains and mechanically strip them of their outer shell, the bran, which contains most of the fiber. We also often take away the core of the grain, the germ, which provides important B vitamins. We bleach, puff, flake, dry, fry, and otherwise process foods until they are nutrient-poor shadows of their original selves. We do all this in the name of convenience and shelf life. But what could be more convenient than staying healthy by eating pure foods? And what's shelf life compared to *your* life?

As you begin choosing fresh produce and whole grains over processed foods, take it one step further and start buying organic produce and grains rather than nonorganic choices. In this way you'll be forgoing pesticides and artificial fertilizers. In addition, you're going to want to cut down on or, ideally, eliminate, meat and dairy products. This will enable you to cut out a lot of fat, and you'll be avoiding the toxic drugs, pesticides, and other chemicals that farm animals in our country are routinely exposed to. If you feel you must eat animal foods, however, choose organic meat, eggs, or dairy products. These will be antibiotic-, artificial-hormone-, and pesticide-free, and the animals will generally have been more humanely treated than nonorganically raised factory-farm animals.

Other foods to avoid: the pickled and the salted. You won't need these unhealthy flavor boosts when you're concentrating on fresh whole foods seasoned with delicious herbs. Other flavor boosters that you should have nothing to do with are MSG and aspartame, which are called excitotoxins because they overstimulate brain cells. Also avoid artificial colorings and preservatives, irradiated produce and herbs, produce treated with wax, and overcooked foods. And if it's canned, can it! Canned food tends to be over-salted, sugared, and nutritionally and enzymatically weak.

Finally, there's a big, fat category of substances to stay away from, and that's saturated fat. There should be no mystery about which fat is saturated—it's the kind that's solid at room temperature. Think of lard. Other examples are the marbling in meat, the fat in butter and chocolate, and the whitish shortening that comes in cans and that's supposed to be good to bake with. It's not, but that doesn't stop most commercial producers of baked goods from using such products. You should know that many so-called unsaturated fats, the ones labeled "hydrogenated," have for all intents and purposes become saturated through the hydrogenation process. What they actually become is something called trans fatty acids, which you may have heard referred to as trans fats and as something to stay away from like the plague. This is a good idea, since trans fatty acids have been shown to elevate cholesterol and increase the incidence of heart disease.

The bottom line on saturated fat is that you're going to have to steer clear of most animal products and commercially baked offerings. But if you like delicious goodies, don't despair, because vegetarian cookbooks can guide you in creating your own, using liquid oils instead of shortening as well as egg substitutes, chocolatelike carob, and sweeteners that are more wholesome than white sugar.

One more note on fats: Restaurants often reuse frying fats over and over again to the point of rancidity. This kind of fat is particularly unhealthful.

Out with indoor irritants. You may think that the only toxins in your home are those found in your kitchen cabinets, but guess what, those very cabinets themselves may be harboring toxins! That's because the pressed wood that cabinetry and other modern furniture are frequently made of often contains formaldehyde, a substance also found in treated fabrics, such as no-iron sheets and curtains.

If you're making a clean sweep of toxins at home, you might want to start doing so literally, with your floor. Do you have wall-to-wall carpeting? Many environmentally oriented health practitioners recommend having bare floors, perhaps with a few area rugs, rather than wall-to-wall carpeting because of the massive microorganism and pollutant loads carpeting carries. One study revealed up to ten million microorganisms in a square foot of carpeting. Another problem is the toxic chemicals that outgas from new carpets as well as from their rubber or latex padding and from glue. If you do opt for wall-to-wall, look for carpeting that hasn't been chemically treated and has natural fiber padding.

A step you can take whether you have carpets or bare floors is to use a vacuum cleaner with a HEPA filter. Regular vacuums suck up dirt and then exhaust the air back into your home; with that exhausted air come very small particle pollutants, including lead. HEPA filters trap most of these particles. It's also important to have the people who enter your home remove their shoes at the door. I've made this a practice for years, and while a few of my visitors claim to find it "silly," they're the ones who are ridiculous, when you think about it. Consider what our shoes pick up on the street: lead, motor oil, and other poisons from car exhaust; soot and soil; and animal and even human wastes. Do you really want these substances tracked all over your house? You can reduce your family's exposure to lead just by employing the shoe-removal strategy.

In another area of home detoxification, look for sources of electromagnetic fields that you can eliminate. For example, unplug your bedside digital alarm clock and replace it with a mechanical one. Finally, when we do home cleanup chores, we tend to think in terms of things that people walk on, eat off, or sleep in. At least as important are the things people touch. Remember to disinfect—using alcohol or another antibacterial—such things as doorknobs, telephone handsets, TV and radio knobs and remote controls, stove knobs, faucets, and refrigerator handles. If you've got kids, give them the project of listing all such heavy-touch items in your home. This can be a real eye-opener for everyone and lead to implementation of another simple toxin-reduction technique—having everyone in the home wash their hands more frequently.

Toss the Toxic Talkers, Too

It's all well and good to jettison the toxic foods and chemicals from your life, but don't forget to jettison the toxic people, too. You know who they are—the folks who can never seem to communicate without projecting negativity, anger, or bitterness. I realize that sometimes these people are related to you, are your boss, or live next door, so you can't cut them off completely. But that doesn't mean that you are obligated to play a part in the negative scenarios that make up their world. When you have to interact with such people, make it a point to keep the interactions short and sweet. Cut off your conversations with them, whether these are in person or on the phone, as soon as you can. Other people's toxic emotions can drag you down just as surely as a toxic diet can, and there's no reason that you have to let that happen.

One other thing: Some people who aren't particularly negative will suddenly get that way when they see that you're starting to make health-giving or self-empowering changes. They feel threatened, afraid, perhaps, that you're going to leave them behind or that they'll look bad in comparison with you.

What I recommend is that you level with them. Tell them that you don't appreciate their negativity, because you've made up your mind to improve your life. Then encourage them to join you in making changes if they want, but reassure them that you won't judge them if they don't.

Then live up to your word and see what happens. I have friends who eat all different ways, ranging from strict vegans to fast-food devotees. What I don't have are friends who are chronically negative.

Deal with Your Allergies

Certain foods, for certain people, have adverse effects and should be eliminated from the diet or eaten less frequently. To discover which foods these are for you, you may, as we discussed earlier, have a doctor conduct tests for this purpose. On your own, you can keep a diary of what you eat for two weeks and write down any symptoms you experience—headaches, bloating, or gas pains, for example. Sometimes effects are immediate, but at other times they may appear hours, or even days, later. This can complicate matters, but over time patterns should become apparent that tell you what foods are upsetting your system. Commonly, these culprits include wheat, dairy products, soy, and citrus fruits.

For getting allergens out of your system and for general detoxification, holistic therapist Dr. Philip Hodes recommends a transitional cleansing diet that works up to a fast and then gradually reverses to solid foods. On this diet, which you should only follow with medical clearance, you begin by eating steamed and raw foods for several days. Then you drink only soups and raw juices for two days. Watermelon juice is an excellent cleanser but should be taken alone, Hodes notes. He recommends that for one week you take in just raw juices, protein drinks, and pure water. During the process, it's important to get lots of rest. One colonic irrigation or an enema by an experienced practitioner is also good to have at this time.

Then follow the program in reverse. Go from having raw juices and water to watermelon and soups and then to steamed and raw foods. But don't, Hodes warns, go back to eating the junk foods that made you toxic in the first place.

Once you start eating food again, Hodes recommends going on a four- to five-day rotational diet in order to avoid overloading the immune system and developing allergic addictions to any foods. In other words, if you eat wheat on Sunday, don't eat it again until Thursday.

So What *Should* You Eat?

There are so many foods to avoid if you're health conscious that sometimes it may seem difficult to know what *to* eat. It's not. What you should concentrate on are fruits, vegetables, legumes, nuts, seeds, and whole grains in as fresh and natural a state as possible. That means you'll be eating, for example, fresh vegetables rather than canned ones, fresh fruits rather than sugared canned ones, whole-grain breads rather than white, and brown rice rather than white. Also, these foods should be organically grown, if possible, so you'll be eating foods grown without man-made chemicals and grown, generally, using soil-preserving methods rather than soil-depleting ones.

That said, let me steer you to some dietary detoxification aids. To start with something you may never have tried, be sure to eat sea vegetables. Their names include kombu, wakame, hijiki, nori, agar, kuzu, algin, alaria, sea palm, and dulce, and you should try to include them in your diet about four times a week. These nutritional gold mines are rich in protein, calcium, potassium, and a number of important trace minerals lacking in our soil today. Sea vegetables may take some getting used to, but many vegetarian cookbooks can guide you in their use in tasty soups and salads.

Cruciferous vegetables, such as broccoli, cauliflower, and brussels sprouts, are known to fight cancer. Add flavor to these vegetables with garlic, onions, leeks, and other members of the onion family to cleanse the system and promote good health.

Include plenty of healthful fruits, raw or dried, for digestive wellness. Watermelon helps the kidneys; papayas and, in particular, blueberries, aid digestion; prunes combat constipation; and apples are an overall tonic. But don't buy the shiny apples that got that way through waxing! Fungicides added to the paraffin or shellac will not do you any good. Look for organic fruit, and remember to eat fruit alone for the best effect.

Eat salads often, combining a rainbow of ingredients—celery, radish, red, yellow, and green pepper, dandelion, and tomato, for example. (Did you know that the lycopene in tomatoes—the phytochemical that gives them their red color—provides your skin cells with protection from sun damage?) Season your salads with a delicious homemade dressing of healthful cold-pressed olive or flaxseed oil and lemon juice or apple cider vinegar.

Go for the green. Having just mentioned a rainbow of vegetable choices, let's zero in on one color from that rainbow, green. Green foods are great because they're rich in chlorophyll, the ultimate blood purifier. This easily absorbed substance is known to cure various infections in the respiratory tract, and it can nullify the effects of pollutants. In addition, it can turn an acidic pH more alkaline. (By the way, you can place a pH test strip in a urine sample each morning to see if it reads in the ideal range of somewhere near 6.8. Deviations upward from that number mean that foods eaten the previous day were alkaline, and downward deviations indicate that they were acidic. Acidic foods can be especially irritating and can contribute to numerous diseases. Cutting down on these foods, and eating lots of fruits and vegetables instead, will support health.)

For good sources of chlorophyll, I recommend barley grass, wheat grass, and earthrise spirulina. Both of these are superrich in vitamins, minerals, amino acids, and trace elements, and they're high in the antioxidant enzyme superoxide dismutase. You can blend these grasses into your freshly made juices, which brings me to the next important detoxification strategy you should know about.

Rejuvenate with Juice

I'm always railing against processing, but there's one kind of processing that you can do yourself and that I highly recommend, and that's juicing. In fact, I feel that every household should have an electric juice extractor and use it daily, because raw juices enable you to flood your body with an easily usable mix of nutrients. Try juicing any combination of organic produce, adding in small amounts of dark green vegetables for cleansing. You can also add a small amount of wheat grass for its powerful cleansing properties.

Juice fasts for the fast track. Many people like to go on a juice fast as the first, fast-track step of their detox program. We've already discussed juice fasts as a way of minimizing allergies, but I wholeheartedly recommend them also as the best way to jump-start your detox. In fact, when I lead detox groups, we usually do start out with several juice-only days because I've found that, all other things being equal, people who use juice fasting at the beginning of the detox process do better several months down the line than people who don't. I do have to inject the caveat here, though, that your health-care practitioner should be providing guidance, particularly if you are pregnant, elderly, have high blood pressure, or are taking medications. Although the high levels of phytonutrients in juices are generally health-enhancing, there may be some circumstances in which they're contraindicated (for example, if you are on medication for high blood pressure).

Once you've got your doctor's go-ahead, invest in a good juicing-oriented vegetarian cookbook for inspiration. Two of mine are *The Joy of Juicing* and *The International Vegetarian Cookbook,* or you can find other good choices at your bookstore. Then begin the several days' adventure of creating the most delicious, healthful juices you can come up with.

As a general guideline for a juice fast, think in terms of drinking about eight ten-ounce glasses of juice a day. Three days is a good length of time for a juice fast, provided that you do not have a blood sugar problem or other medical condition that would contraindicate this. You don't have to stick slavishly to any particular recipes, but the backbone of your juices should be such watery sources as apple, celery, cucumber, or cabbage. To these you'll be adding smaller amounts of the more concentrated dark-green vegetables, e.g., parsley and spinach. Dilute carrot juice with water (4 to 1, water to juice), to temper the sweetness. Remember that you can use sprouts in your creations as well. And consume your juices slowly, savoring them like the gourmet meals they are. You won't be cheating yourself out of taste enjoyment this way, and you'll be kinder to your kidneys and bladder.

When you come off a juice fast, do so gradually. Reintroducing solids all at once is too much of a shock to your system.

Don't Overlook Supplements

In the best of all possible worlds, food would be our only source of vitamins and other nutrients. Unfortunately, today's food falls short when you're seeking sufficient amounts of nutrients for optimal health. So we need to get extra protection from antioxidant supplements, such as vitamin E. Other antioxidants we may need include vitamin A, alpha lipoic acid, beta carotene, the B vitamins, choline and inositol (which together make up lecithin), vitamin C, bioflavonoids, quercetin, rutin, and pygnogenol. In addition, vitamin C drips are something you may want to explore as a way of maximizing your immunity, not to mention keeping your skin looking good. C helps skin partly by supporting the health of the collagen underneath.

Also important are minerals and enzymes, which Nina Anderson, the author of *Over Fifty, Looking Thirty!*, stresses as two key anti-aging factors. She recommends taking the crystalloid forms of each, for maximum benefit to your cells. Enzymes, in case you were unsure, are catalysts; that is, they make possible the chemical reactions that make our bodies run. You can have all the vitamins and minerals you need, but without adequate enzymes to help things happen, your body isn't going to function optimally. Glutathione peroxidase, superoxide dismutase, and catalase are three important enzymes that offer antioxidant benefits.

Antioxidant minerals to be particularly conscious of are selenium and zinc. The former will help protect you against cancer as well as detoxify your system of environmental pollutants. The latter is essential to the immune system and helps normalize insulin activity and vitamin A usage, among other functions.

Additionally, be sure to include the essential fatty acids, omega 3 and omega 6, in your diet.

Some supplements to consider taking on a daily basis include:

Vitamin E—200–400 IU
Vitamin C—500–5,000 mg
Pygnogenol—200 mg
Quercetin—500–2000 mg
NAC (n-acetyl cysteine)—1000 mg
Glutathione—200 mg

But avoid the temptation to start buying up whole medicine cabinetsful of supplements and taking them indiscriminately. Consult your doctor or nutritionist about what's right for you.

Chelation

While following a healthy lifestyle is always important, we sometimes need additional intervention to more fully detoxify. One valuable modality is chelation. This technique is used to remove excess metals, as well as excess calcium, from the blood, and in the process to improve the circulatory system. Traditionally, people have been led to believe that there is no real way of helping the heart. You simply have to take your medications and accept your condition or undergo risky bypass operations that offer no hope of lasting change. But chelation therapy, used to treat patients with circulatory problems, often produces great and lasting success. Many heart patients who were not expected to live are fully alive today and leading normal, healthy, and productive lives. One such patient, for example, reports that after several bypass operations his cardiologist had given up on him. But he didn't give up on himself and turned to chelation therapy. The result: a dramatic improvement in his health, to the point where he does not take any heart medication and is able to work, and play, with vigor.

How does this therapy work? In Greek, *chele* means to claw or to bind, and that's the root of the word *chelation*. What's involved is a molecule that is able to grab on to, deactivate, and eliminate toxic metals from the body. The process involves the intravenous infusion of the synthetic amino acid ethylenediaminetetraacetic acid (EDTA) into the body, usually over a period of three to four hours. The EDTA moves through the blood vessels and removes excesses of calcium, as well as iron, copper, lead, and various other metals that are implicated in disease. But the EDTA is not metabolized at all. Its "miracle molecules" simply come in, grab minerals, and go out through the urine.

The therapeutic effects of this detoxifying process don't happen suddenly; you have to go through a series of treatments and you have to clean up your lifestyle in general. But the benefits are definite, and various. Chelation reduces the risks of stroke, Alzheimer's disease, diabetes, and intermittent claudication as it strengthens the heart and blood vessels. It removes excess calcium from arteries and soft tissues, a real boon because, while we want this mineral in our bones, it causes problems in these other places. Many doctors I know around the country are using this therapy with great success, particularly when they combine it with a comprehensive program of health-habit changes. It's a great therapy because it goes beyond treating symptoms to treating the underlying causes of illness. You should know that in addition to the IV method of chelation, there are some oral chelating agents you can take. Among these is cracked chlorella, chlorella being an alga that helps to bind heavy metals.

While chelation is approved for the removal of heavy metals, it is not usually used in conventional medicine except in cases where lead levels in the body are very, very high. The problem with this thinking is that since toxic substances like lead are quite dangerous and have no biological function, they don't belong in the body at all and should be removed at any level. Unfortunately, heavy metals do not reveal their tremendous burden on the body until a great deal of harm has already been done. Only when damage is in its acute phase will symptoms like headaches and dizziness appear. But why wait until this happens? The approximately eight hundred chelation therapists in the United States are convinced that this therapy is the pound of prevention that's worth a hundred pounds of cure. You can get a list of them from the American College of the Advancement of Medicine at (800) 532–3688.

Herbs for Cleansing

Unlike chelation, herbal therapy is really beginning to be accepted by the American mainstream. Many pharmaceutical companies are adding herbals to their line of products, and neighborhood drugstores and even supermarkets are fairly bursting with these new offerings. The latest news, an issue being debated in newspapers and medical journals, is that a lot of mainstream physicians are now selling herbal remedies to their patients. Unhappy with the way managed-care organizations are curbing their incomes, and realizing that their patients often prefer herbal remedies to prescription pharmaceuticals for things like lowering cholesterol and hormone replacement, these doctors are running sideline, over-the-counter businesses right in their offices.

While those of us in the alternative movement may have mixed feelings about these developments—ranging from "It's about time!" to "They're only doing it to cash in on a trend"—the generally increased availability of herbals is, all in all, a welcome thing. Herbs are wonderful aids to any detoxification program, and the more people who can reap their benefits, the better.

While many herbs can now be easily purchased over the counter, for the best results you should work with a knowledgeable doctor or an herbalist. This is someone who can steer you to herbs based on your individual cleansing needs, prescribe correct dosages, and warn you of possible contraindications. But whatever you choose to do, the following are some herbal strategies you should know about.

Give your liver a lift. As we've mentioned, the liver is vital to detoxification, and bitter greens and herbs have traditionally been used to keep this organ in tip-top shape. You can make a tea with a gentle bitter flavor that will stimulate bile flow and thus cleanse the liver. What you do is: Combine, in a pot, 2 teaspoons of dandelion root, 2 teaspoons of organic grape root, 1 teaspoon of gingerroot, 1 teaspoon of licorice root, and 3 cups of water. Cover the pot, bring the mixture to a boil, and then lower the heat and simmer for 15 minutes, or even longer if you want a strong but still tasty liver tonic. Strain the mixture; you can then drink three cups of this tea spaced throughout the day. Fifteen to thirty minutes before each meal is ideal, and you can do this for two to three weeks at a time.

Herbs that can protect liver cells from chemical toxicity and even foster rejuvenation of a damaged liver are called antihepatoxics. One of the best antihepatoxics is milk thistle, a nontoxic herb with a centuries-long history of helping to reverse liver damage. You can grind up milk thistle seeds, steeping about half a teaspoon in hot water to make a tea that you drink twice a day. Also helpful to the liver are the Chinese herbs bupleurum,

Siberian ginseng, schizandra, and licorice—the latter only if high blood pressure is not a problem. And some people like to stimulate the liver with a breakfast drink of grapefruit juice to which is added some lemon juice, 1 tablespoon of olive oil, and a clove of garlic, crushed.

Liver-cleansing salad greens include chicory, escarole, dandelion, water-cress, endive, arugula, radicchio, and broccoli rabe.

For bowel health. A wide variety of herbs are available to improve bowel function, including senna and cascara sagrada. But be careful to avoid overuse, as these are as physically addictive as any laxative. Long-term use—meaning, generally, use over a year or two—may result in your inability to have a bowel movement on your own. Safer herbs to consider are dandelion root and yellow dock.

For kidney health. There are several herbs to choose from if you want to keep your kidneys functioning well. Some, such as dandelion leaf, promote diuresis. Others, like corn silk, soothe inflammation of the urinary tract and stimulate secretion. The antimicrobial herb bearberry, also known as uva-ursi, may also help relieve pain from bladder stones and gravel, and help where bedwetting is a problem.

To make a gentle kidney-cleansing tea, and to alleviate water-retention problems, try the following: Pour 1 cup of boiling water over 1 teaspoon of dried dandelion leaf and 1 teaspoon of marshmallow root. Cover and let it steep until it reaches room temperature. Then strain, add natural sweetening if you want, and drink. You can do this several times throughout the day, always waiting for the tea to cool down if you want the best diuretic effect. The great thing about this tea is that, unlike synthetic diuretics, it doesn't disturb your natural mineral balance. In fact, it's rich in minerals, especially potassium.

Other natural diuretics, by the way, are asparagus and watermelon. And if you're concerned about not stressing your kidneys, stay away from alcohol and caffeine.

For the lymphatic system. Red clover is recommended by herbalists for lymph system optimization. The ever-popular echinacea is also good for this purpose. Finally, ginkgo biloba, known for its ability to protect cerebral function, is a liver protector as well.

For the lungs. Try elecampane tea to quiet a cough or overcome respiratory ailments. This is a good herb for ex-smokers. A little less strong, vapors from mullein flowers will help clear nasal congestion.

For the skin. Concentrate on diaphoretics such as nettles, cleavers, and burdock for skin health.

Antiviral herbs. Herbs that combat viruses include garlic, echinacea, and St. John's wort, an herb you've probably heard about lately in relation to its antidepressant effect. (St. John's wort should be used as an antiviral only on a temporary basis. Garlic, on the other hand, should be taken every day, and more than once a day if you like.)

Antifatigue herbs. Cleaning up is hard work, and when you're in the detox process, particularly at the beginning, you can feel tired. Tonic herbs can provide the adrenal support to counter fatigue. Try astragalus—10 to 12 drops one to three times a day, as you need it. Alternatively, you can make the ground form of this herb into a tea, using ⅓ teaspoon per cup, or you can add the astragalus that comes in strip form to soups. Gotu kola is another good energizing herb, and licorice is also recommended as a tonic, although licorice is not for those with high blood pressure.

Other Therapies

Beyond supplements, herbs, and chelation, there are numerous ways to enhance the detoxification process that you should be familiar with.

Ozone. Ozone therapy is something you may want to use in conjunction with your detox process if there are particular health conditions you are concerned about. This modality is based on the fact that when ordinary oxygen is mixed with ozone, an allotrope, or different form, of the element, a substance results that has unique healing properties that are only beginning to be appreciated in this country. Used more extensively in Europe and Cuba, ozone therapy combats a whole variety of health problems ranging from the bacterial to the viral, and even including cancer and AIDS. It's also used protectively, to ward off viral invaders and to check the free radicals that cause degeneration and disease. In Europe, autohemotherapy is a commonly used method of administering ozone; what this involves is drawing some blood out of the body, mixing a dose of the oxygen-ozone mixture into that blood, and then returning it via the same intravenous cathether into the patient. In this country, rectal insufflation is the method most commonly used, with the ozone mixture entering the bloodstream via the walls of the large intestine. This is obviously a medically supervised therapy, but since it's nontoxic, with many people reporting good results, it's worth looking into.

Colonic therapy. Colonic therapy can be helpful at the beginning of a detoxification regimen because it gets the debris in the intestines moving. This procedure is done to cleanse, heal, rebuild, and in time restore the large intestine, or the colon, to its natural size, normal shape, and correct function.

The first step of this therapy involves cleansing, a thorough washing of the large intestine. The colon is irrigated with gently infused water that is made to flow in and out at steady intervals. Through this method water is allowed to travel the entire length of the colon, all the way around to the cecum area. A good colon therapist will use from 10 to 15 gallons of water, but only 1 or 2 pints at a time. The walls of the colon are washed and old encrustation and fecal material are loosened, dislodged, and swept away. This toxic-waste material has very often been attached to the bowel walls for a long time. It is laden with millions of bacteria, which set up the perfect environment for disease. As all this body pollution is eliminated, a whole variety of conditions—from skin disorders to breathing difficulties, depression, chronic fatigue, severe constipation, and arthritis—may be significantly reduced. This is especially so when colon therapy is augmented with dietary changes and other treatment modalities.

After the basic washing procedure, a colon therapist goes on to the next treatment phase, which involves healing. Materials are infused into the bowel to soothe inflamed areas and strengthen weak sections on the colon wall. Flax-ET, white oak bark, and slippery elm bark are all substances used for this purpose. Also, herbal teas may be taken orally to help repair the bowel. And people receiving colon therapy are often told to double their habitual intake of water as part of a long-term lifestyle change.

To help rid the bowel of toxins, some therapists recommend charcoal, a substance that has the ability to absorb many times its weight in toxins and one that's available in any drugstore. And if intestinal parasites are a problem, natural remedies may be able to help. For worms, the sage-family herb wormwood can be taken in controlled doses several times daily; it contains volatile oils that combat these parasites. Short one-to-three-day tropical-fruit fasts, using watermelon, pineapple, and papaya, are a way of countering amoebas, or you can use supplements based on these, such as papain, the digestive enzyme from papaya. You take a tablet of this enzyme three times a day, always between meals. For yeast overgrowth, caprylic acid, an extract of a fatty acid from coconut, is recommended. You can also use undecyclinic acid, or, if you need to, turn to the pharmaceutical Mystatin.

After colon therapy, after you've dealt with yeast overgrowth, or after a round of antibiotics, you may need to replenish the colonic flora. To do this, live acidophilus is often recommended. Particularly good for restoring the inner ecosystem is the yogurtlike drink called kefir. While this is a dairy product, it's a predigested one, so it's easy to assimilate. In addition to being rich in the good-to-your-insides kind of bacteria, kefir contains calcium, magnesium, protein, and a full range of B vitamins.

Yet more therapies to look into. Are you a person who likes the idea of exercise but thinks something like step aerobics or rope jumping a little too fast and frantic? You might want to try the Chinese discipline of T'ai Chi, a type of exercise that's slow, relaxing, and meditative.

Speaking of meditation, you can call it either a therapy or a way of life, but everyone ought to try meditation and then decide for themselves. Other therapies to familiarize yourself with include visualization and affirmations; these are ways of mentally focusing on what you want and where you want to be that have helped a lot of people. With visualization, you mentally "see" a desired outcome; and affirmations involve verbalizing what you ideally want to be experiencing. You say, for instance, "My mind and body are relaxed," the idea being that the positive statements you make will actually trigger natural endorphins to flow into the body and effect this result.

You may have noticed that relaxation is a prime aim of many complementary therapies. This might lead some people to think that these therapies aren't to be taken seriously; after all, what difference does relaxation really make? The answer is: It makes a great deal of difference to your health. That's because when you relax, your blood vessels get larger. Now you've got the same volume of blood, but it's in a more spacious system, so the pressure is off. The blood can get through more easily, so oxygen and other nutrition can be delivered more deeply into your organs and glands, helping them to work more effectively. These results—lowered blood pressure and increased organ effectiveness—are some pretty significant benefits.

Fortunately, the list of what you can do to help yourself relax these days seems to go on and on. Lie in a flotation tank; soothe yourself in a sauna; look into homeopathy, acupuncture, magnets, reiki, chiropractic, or aromatherapy; explore biofeedback, Swedish massage, music therapy, or polarity therapy; receive rolfing; venture into color therapy, Bach flower remedies, or dipoles to help the brain's bioelectric field function better. See a vision therapist, someone who can help you to reorganize the way you perceive space and think. Read up on different therapies, try a few for yourself, and remember that you don't have to rely on the trendy; something as classic as walking on the beach can be beneficial. A combination of techniques, as opposed to just one, will be more likely to foster relaxation, help the detox process, and promote better all-around functioning.

SELECTED BIBLIOGRAPHY

AUTHOR'S NOTE: Due to space considerations, this bibliography was shortened from over 4,000 entries to a general sampling of peer-reviewed scientific papers, books, and articles.

Abbey, et al., "Dietary Supplementation with Orange and Carrot Juice in Cigarette Smokers Lowers Oxidation Products in Copper-Oxidized Low-Density Lipoproteins," *Journal of the American Dietary Association*, 95, 1995, p. 671–675.

Abe, Y., et al., "Effect of Green Tea Rich in Gamma-aminobutyric Acid on Blood Pressure of Dahl Salt-Sensitive Rats," *American Journal of Hypertension*, 8 (1), January 1995, p. 74–79.

Agnoli, A., et al., "CBF and Cognitive Evaluation of Alzheimer Type Patients Before and After MAO-B Treatment: A Pilot Study," *European Neuropsychopharmacol*, 2 (1), March 1992, p. 31–35.

Albanes, D., et al., "Effects of Alpha-Tocopherol and Beta-Carotene Supplements on Cancer Incidence in the Alpha-Tocopherol Beta-Carotene Cancer Prevention Study," *American Journal of Clinical Nutrition*, 62 (Suppl), 1995, p. 1427S–1430S.

Alberts, D.S., et al., "Positive Randomized, Double Blinded, Placebo Controlled Study of Topical Difluoromethyl Ornithine (DFMO) in the Chemoprevention of Skin Cancer," *Proceedings of the Annual Meeting of the American Society of Clinical Oncology*, 15, 1996, p. A342.

Ali, M., et al., "A Potent Thromboxane Formation Inhibitor in Green Tea Leaves," *Prostaglandins Leukot Essent Fatty Acids*, 40 (4), August 1990, p. 281–283.

Allard, M., [Treatment of the Disorders of Aging with Ginkgo Biloba Extract. From Pharmacology to Clinical Medicine], *Presse Med*, 15 (31), September 25, 1986, p. 1540–1545.

Allman, M. A., et al., "Supplementation with Flaxseed Oil Versus Sunflowerseed Oil in Healthy Young Men Consuming a Low Fat Diet: Effects on Platelet Composition and Function," *European Journal of Clinical Nutrition*, 49 (3), March 1995, p. 169–178.

Amagase, H., et al., "Dietary Rosemary Suppresses 7,12-dimethylbenz(a)anthracene Binding to Rat Mammary Cell DNA," *Journal of Nutrition Carnosol*, 126 (5), May 1996, p. 1475–1480.

Ambrosio, G., et al., "Reduction in Experimental Infarct Size by Recombinant Human Superoxide Dismutase: Insights into the Pathophysiology of Reperfusion Injury," *Circulation*, 74 (6), December 1986, p. 1424–1433.

Anderson, R. A., "Chromium, Glucose Tolerance, and Diabetes," *Biological Trace Element Research*, 32, January–March 1992, p. 19–24.

Angeles, A. P., et al., "Chondrocyte Growth Inhibition Induced by Homogentisic Acid and its Partial Prevention with Ascorbic Acid," *Journal of Rheumatology*, 16 (4), April 1989, p. 512–517.

Araki, R., et al., "Chemoprevention of Mammary Preneoplasia. In Vitro Effects of a Green Tea Polyphenol," *Annals of the New York Academy of Science*, 768, September 30, 1995, p. 215–222.

Austin, S., "Recent Progress in Treatment and Secondary Prevention of Breast Cancer with Supplements," *Alternative Medicine Review*, 2 (1), 1997, p. 4–11.

Avorn, J., et al., "Reduction of Bacteriuria and Pyruia after Ingestion of Cranberry Juice," *JAMA*, 271 (10), March 9, 1994, p. 751–754.

Baba, K., et al., [Antitumor Activity of Hot Water Extract Dandelion,Taraxacum Officinale—Correlation Between Antitumor Activity and Timing of Administration], *Yakugaku Zasshi*, 101 (6), 1981, p. 538–543.

Banderet, L. E. and Lieberman, H. R., "Treatment with Tyrosine, a Neurotransmitter Precursor, Reduces Environmental Stress in Humans," *Brain Research Bulletin*, 22 (4), April 1989, p. 759–762.

Barak, Y., et al., "Inositol Treatment of Alzheimer's Disease: A Double Blind, Cross-over Placebo Controlled Trial," *Progress in Neuropsychopharmacology and Biological Psychiatry*, 20 (4), May 1996, p. 729–735.

Behl, C., et al., "Vitamin E Protects Nerve Cells from Amyloid Beta Protein Toxicity," *Biochem Biophys Res Commun*, 186 (2), July 31, 1992, p. 944–950.

Belaiche, P. and Lievoux, O., "Clinical Studies on the Palliative Treatment of Prostatic Adenoma with Extract of Urtica Root," *Phytotherapy Research*, 5, 1991, p. 267–269.

Belford-Courtney, R., "Comparison of Chinese and Western Uses of Angelica Sinensis," *Australian Journal of Med Herbalism*, 5 (4), 1993, p. 87–91.

Bellizz, M. C., et al., "Vitamin E and Coronary Heart Disease: The European Paradox," *European Journal of Clinical Nutrition*, 48 (11), November 1994, p. 822–831.

Bengtsson, B. A., et al., "Treatment of Adults with Growth Hormone (GH) Deficiency with Recombinant Human GH," *Journal of Clinical Endocrinology and Metabolism*, 76 (2), February 1993, p. 309–317.

Bertuglia, S., et al., "Effect of Vaccinium Myrtillus Anthocyanosides on Ischemia Reperfusion Injury in Hamster Cheek Pouch Microcirculation," *Pharmacol Research*, 31 (3–4), March–April 1995, p. 183–187.

Bhargava, U. C. and Westfall, B. A., "Antitumor Activity of Julans Nigra (Black Walnut) Extractives," *Journal of Pharm Science*, 57 (10), 1968, p. 1674–1677.

Birdsall, T. C., "The Biological Effects and Clinical Uses of the Pineal Hormone Melatonin," *Alternative Medicine Review*, 1 (2), 1996, p. 94–102.

Birkenhager-Gillesse, E. G., et al., "Dehydroepiandrosterone Sulfate (DHEAS) in the Oldest Old, Aged 85 and Over," *New York Academy of Science*, 1994, p. 543–552.

———. "Births and Deaths: United States, 1996," *Monthly Vital Statistics* 46 (1).

Blackwell, G. J., et al., "Inhibition of Human Platelet Aggregation by Vitamin K," *Thromb Research*, 37 (1), January 1, 1985, p. 103–114.

Bodnar, A. G., et al., "Extension of Life-Span by Introduction of Telomerase into Normal Human Cells," *Science*, January 16, 1998.

Boucher, F., et al., "Oral Selenium Supplementation in Rats Reduces Cardiac Toxicity of Adriamycin During Ischemia and Reperfusion," *Nutrition*, 11 (5 Suppl), September–October 1995, p. 708–711.

Braeckman, J., "The Extract of Seronoa Repens in the Treatment of Benign Prostatic Hyperplasia: A Multicenter Open Study," *Current Therapeutic Research*, 55 (7), July 1994, p. 776–785.

Breithaupt-Grogler, K., et al., "Protective Effect of Chronic Garlic Intake on Elastic Properties of Aorta in the Elderly," *Circulation*, 96 (8), October 21, 1997, p. 2649–2655.

Brinckerhoff, C. E., et al., "Effect of Retinoids on Rheumatoid Arthritis, a Proliferative and Invasive Non-malignant Disease," *Ciba Found Sympathy*, 113, 1985, p. 191–211.

Brinker, F., "Larrea Tridentata (D. C.) Colville (Chaparral or Creosote Bush)," *British Journal of Phytotherapy*, 3 (1), 1993–1994, p. 10–30.

Brittenden, J., et al., "L-arginine Stimulates Host Defenses in Patients with Breast Cancer," *Surgery*, 115 (2), February 1994, p. 205–212.

Brzeski, M., et al., "Evening Primrose Oil in patients with Rheumatoid Arthritis and Side-effects of Non-steroidal Anti-inflammatory Drugs," *British Journal of Rheumatology*, 30 (5), October 1991, p. 370–372.

Bul'on, V. V., et al., "The Use of L-DOPA for Treating Myocardial Infarct Patients," *Eksp Klin Farmakol*, 56 (2), March–April 1993, p. 28–30.

Cai, F., et al., [Preliminary Report of Efficacy of Diabetic Polyneuropathy Treated with Large Dose Inositol], *Hua Hsi I Ko Ta Hsueh Hsueh Pao*, 21 (2), June 1990, p. 201–203.

Cai, Q., et al., "Antioxidative Properties of Histidine and its Effects on Myocardial Injury During Ischemia/Reperfusion in Isolated Rat Heart," *Journal Cardiovascular Pharmacology*, 25 (1), January 1995, p. 147–155.

Caprioli, A., et al., "Acetyl-L-Carnitine: Chronic Treatment Improves Spatial Acquisition in a New Environment in Aged Rats," *J Gerontol A Biol Sci Med Sci*, 50 (4), July 1995, p. B232–B236.

Carbin, B. E., et al., "Treatment of Benign Prostatic Hyperplasia with Phytos-terols," *British Journal of Urology*, 66, 1990, p. 639–641.

Casamenti, F., et al., "Phosphatidylserine Reverses the Age-dependent De-crease in Cortical Acetylcholine Release: A Microdialysis Study," *European Journal of Pharmacology*, 194 (1), February 26, 1991, p. 11–16.

Cassady, J. M., et al., "Use of a Mammalian Cell Culture Benzo(a)pyrene Me-tabolism Assay for the Detection of Potential Anticarcinogens from Natural Products: Inhibition of Metabolism by Biochanin A, an Isoflavone from Tri-folium pratense L," *Cancer Research*, 48, November 15, 1988, p. 6257–6261.

Chabanov, M. K., et al., [Effect of an Intravenously Administered Phosphati-dylserine Emulsion on Blood Coagulation and Blood System Indices], *Far-makol Toksikol*, 42 (3), May–June 1979, p. 257–261.

Chang, H. M. and But, P. P., *Pharmacology and Applications of Chinese Materia Medica*, Vol 1. Hong Kong: World Scientific, 1986.

Chen, M. D., et al., "Effects of Zinc Supplementation on the Plasma Glucose Level and Insulin Activity in Genetically Obese (ob/ob) Mice," *Biol Trace Element Research*, 61 (3), March 1998, p. 303–311.

Chevallard, M., et al., "Effectiveness and Tolerability of Ketoprofen Lysine, Once a Day, in Patients with Rheumatic Disorders," *Drugs Exp Clinical Re-search*, 13 (5), 1987, p. 293–296.

Chew, B. P., et al., "Effects of Lutein from Marigold Extract on Immunity and Growth of Mammary Tumors in Mice," *Anticancer Research*, 16 (6B), November–December 1996, p. 3689–3694.

Chopra, S., et al., "Propolis Protects Against Doxorubicin-induced Myocardio-pathy in Rats," *Exp Mol Pathol*, 62 (3), June 1995, p. 190–198.

Chuang, S. E., et al., "Curcumin (CCM) Decreases the Level of Proliferation Cellular Nuclear Antigen (PCNA), and Retards the Process of Diethylnitro-samine (DEN)-induced Mouse Hepatocarcinogenesis," *Proceedings of the An-nual Meeting of the American Association of Cancer Researchers*, 38, 1997, p. A2479.

Chui, J. and Chen, K. J., [American Ginseng Compound Liquor on Retard-aging Process], *Chung Hsi I Chih*, 11 (8), August 1991, p. 457–460.

Chwang, L. C., et al., "Iron Supplementation and Physical Growth of Rural Indonesian Children," *American Journal of Clinical Nutrition*, 47 (3), March 1988, p. 496–501.

Cinar, M. G., et al., "Effects of Vitamin E on Vascular Responses of Thoracic Aorta in Rat Experimental Arthritis," *Gen Pharmacol*, 31 (1), July 1998, p. 149–153.

Clark, W. F., et al., "Flaxseed: A Potential Treatment for Lupus Nephritis," *Kidney Int*, 48 (2), August 1995, p. 475–480.

Clarkson, P., et al., "Oral L-arginine Improves Endothelium-dependent Dilation in Hypercholesterolemic Young Adults," *Journal of Clinical Investigation*, 97 (8), April 15, 1996, p. 1989–1894.

Clemmensen, O. J., et al., "Psoriatic Arthritis Treated with Oral Zinc Sulphate," *British Journal of Dermatology*, 103 (4), October 1980, p. 411–415.

Clinton, S. K., et al., "Cis-trans Isomers of Lycopene in the Human Prostate: A Role in Cancer Prevention?" *FASEB Journal*, 9 (3), 1995, p. A442.

Cohen-Salmon, C., et al., "Effects of Ginkgo Biloba Extract (EGb 761) on Learning and Possible Actions on Aging," *J Physiol Paris*, 91 (6), December 1997, p. 291–300.

Cong, K., et al., "Calcium Supplementation During Pregnancy for Reducing Pregnancy Induced Hypertension," *Chinese Medical Journal*, 108 (1), January 1995, p. 57–59.

Conlay, L. A., et al., "Tyrosine Increases Blood Pressure in Hypotensive Rats," *Science*, 212 (4494), May 1, 1981, p. 559–560.

Cordatos, E., "Taraxacum Officinale," *Aust Journal of Medical Herbalism*, 3 (4), 1991, p. 64–73.

Cotzias, G. C., et al., "Prolongation of the Life-span in Mice Adapted to Large Amounts of L-Dopa," *Proceedings of the National Academy of Science*, 71, June 1971, p. 2466–2469.

Das, S., "Vitamin E in the Genesis and Prevention of Cancer: A Review," *Acta Oncol*, 33 (6), 1994, p. 615–619.

Davis, R. H. and Maro, N. P., "Aloe Vera and Gibberellin. Anti-inflammatory Activity in Diabetes," *Journal of the American Podiatry Medical Association*, 79 (1), January 1989, p. 24–26.

Dean, W. and Morgenthaler, J., *Smart Drugs & Nutrients*. Menlo Park, CA: Health Freedom Publications, 1990.

Dean, W., Morgenthaler, J. and Fowkes, S. W., *Smart Drugs II: The Next Generation*. Petaluma, CA: Smart Publications, 1993.

Deijen, J. B., et al., Vitamin B-6 Supplementation in Elderly Men: Effects on Mood, Memory, Performance and Mental Effort," *Psychopharmacology*, 109 (4), 1992, p. 489–496.

Delafuente, J. C., et al, "Immunologic Modulation by Vitamin C in the Elderly," *International Journal of Immunopharmacology*, 8 (2), 1986, p. 205–211.

Deschner, E. E., et al., "Quercetin and Rutin as Inhibitors of Azoxymethanol-induced Colonic Neoplasia," *Carcinogenesis*, 12 (7), July 1991, p. 1193–1196.

Deucher, G. P., "Antioxidant Therapy in the Aging Process," *EXS*, 62, 1992, p. 428–437.

De La Cruz, J. P., et al., "Effect of Evening Primrose Oil on Platelet Aggregation in Rabbits Fed an Atherogenic Diet," *Thromb Research*, 87 (1), July 1, 1997, p. 141–149.

di Padova, C., "S-adenosylmethionine in the Treatment of Osteoarthritis. Review of the Clinical Studies," *American Journal of Medicine*, 83 (5A), November 20, 1987, p. 60–65.

Ding, D. Z., et al., [Effects of Red Ginseng on the Congestive Heart Failure and its Mechanism], *Chung Kuo Chung Hsi I Chieh Ho Tsa Chih*, 15 (6), June 1995, p. 325–327.

Donzelle, G., et al., "Curing Trial of Complicated Oncologic Pain by D-phenylalanine," *Anesth Analg,* 38 (11–12), 1981, p. 655–658.

Douillet, C., et al., "A Selenium Supplement Associated or not with Vitamin E Delays Early Renal Lesions in Experimental Diabetes in Rats," *Proceedings of the Soc Exp Biol Med*, 211 (4), April 1996, p. 323–331.

Edmonds, S. E., et al., "Putative Analgesic Activity of Repeated Oral Doses of Vitamin E in the Treatment of Rheumatoid Arthritis. Results of a Prospective Placebo Controlled Double Blind Trial," *Annals Rheum Disease*, 56, 1997, p. 649–655.

el-Saadany, S. S., et al., "Biochemical Dynamics and Hypocholesterolemic Action of Hibiscus Sabdariffa (Karkade)," *Nahrung*, 35 (6), 1991, p. 567–576.

Elliott, J. F., et al., "Immunization with the Larger Isoform of Mouse Glutamic Acid Decarboxylase (GAD67) Prevents Autoimmune Diabetes in NOD Mice," *Diabetes*, 43 (12), December 1994, p. 1494–1499.

Engler, M. M., "Comparative Study of Diets Enriched with Evening Primrose, Black Currant, Borage or Fungal Oils on Blood Pressure and Pressor Responses in Spontaneously Hypertensive Rats," *Prostaglandins Leukot Essent Fatty Acids*, 49 (4), October 1993, p. 809–814.

Ernst, E. and Pittler, M. H., "Yohimbine for Erectile Dysfunction: A Systematic Review and Meta-analysis of Randomized Clinical Trials," *Journal of Urology*, 159 (2), February 1998, p. 433–436.

Feldman, D., et al., "Vitamin D and Prostate Cancer," *Adv Exp Med Biol*, 375, 1995, p. 53–63.

Fitzpatrick, D. F., et al., "Endothelium-dependent Vasorelaxing Activity of Wine and Other Grape Products," *American Journal of Physiology*, 265 (2 Pt 2), August 1993, p. H774–H778.

Flagg, E. W., et al., "Dietary Glutathione Intake and the Risk of Oral and Pharyngeal Cancer," *American Journal of Epidemiology*, 139 (5), March 1, 1994, p. 453–465.

Flindt-Hansen, H., et al., "The Effect of Short-term Application of PABA on Photocarcinogenesis," *Acta Derm Venereol*, 70 (1), 1990, p. 72–75.

Folkers, K., et al., "Therapy with Coenzyme Q_{10} of Patients in Heart Failure Who Are Eligible or Ineligible for a Transplant," *Biochem Biophys Res Commun*, 182 (1), January 15, 1992, p. 247–253.

Fortes, C., et al., "The Effect of Zinc and Vitamin A Supplementation on Immune Response in an Older Population," *Journal of the American Geriatric Society*, 46 (1), January 1998, p. 19–26.

Fortes, C., et al., "Zinc Supplementation and Plasma Lipid Peroxides in an Elderly Population," *European Journal of Clinical Nutrition*, 51 (2), February 1997, p. 97–101.

Fossel, M., *Reversing Human Aging*. New York: Ballantine, 1996.

Fossel, M., "Telomerase and the Aging Cell: Implications for Human Health," *JAMA*, 279 (21), June 3, 1998, p. 1732–1735.

Fregly, M. J. and Fater, D. C., "Prevention of DOCA-induced Hypertension in Rats by Chronic Treatment with Tryptophan," *Clin Exp Pharmacol Physiol*, 13 (11–12), November–December 1986, p. 767–776.

Fregly, M. J., et al., "Effect of Chronic Dietary Treatment with L-tryptophan on the Development of Renal Hypertension in Rats," *Pharmacology*, 36 (2), 1988, p. 91–100.

Fuhrman, B., et al., "Licorice Extract and Its Major Polyphenol Glabridin Protect Low-density Lipoprotein Against Lipid Peroxidation: In Vitro and Ex Vivo Studies in Humans and in Atherosclerotic Apolipoprotein E-deficient Mice," *American Journal of Clinical Nutrition*, 66 (2), August 1997, p. 267–275.

Gaby, A. R., "The Role of Coenzyme Q_{10} in Clinical Medicine: Part 1," *Alternative Medicine Review*, 1, 1996, p. 11–17.

Galati, E. M., et al., "Biological Effects of Hesperidin, a Citrus flavonoid. (Note III): Antihypertensive and Diuretic Activity in Rat," *Farmaco*, 51 (3), March 1996, p. 219–221.

Galli, G. and Fratelli, M., "Activation of Apoptosis by Serum Deprivation in a Teratocarcinoma Cell Line: Inhibition by L-acetylcarnitine," *Exp Cell Res*, 204 (1), January 1993, p. 54–60.

Garland, C. F., et al., "Can Colon Cancer Incidence and Death Rates Be Reduced with Calcium and Vitamin D?" *American Journal of Clinical Nutrition*, 54 (1 Suppl), July 1991, p. 193S–201S.

Gatti, C., et al., "Effect of Chronic Treatment with Phosphatidyl Serine on Phospholipase A1 and A2 Activities in Different Brain Areas of 4 Month and 24 Month Old Rats," *Farmaco*, 40 (7), July 1985, p. 493–500.

Gerard, G., [Anticancer Therapy and Bromelain] *Agressologie*, 13 (4), 1972, p. 261–274.

Gerber, G. S., et al., "Saw Palmetto (Serenoa repens) in Men with Lower Urinary Tract Symptoms: Effects on Urodynamic Parameters and Voiding Symptoms," *Urology*, 51 (6), June 1998, p. 1003–1007.

Gerster, H., "Antioxidant Vitamins in Cataract Prevention," *Z Ernahrungswiss*, 28 (1), March 1989, p. 56–75.

Gerster, H., "The Potential Role of Lycopene for Human Health," *Journal of the American College of Nutrition*, 16 (2), April 1997, p. 109–126.

Geusens, P., et al., "Long-term Effect of Omega-3 Fatty Acid Supplementation in Active Rheumatoid Arthritis. A 12-month, Double-blind, Controlled Study," *Arthritis Rheum*, 37 (6), June 1994, p. 824–829.

Gilliland, S. E., et al., "Assimilation of Cholesterol by Lactobacillus Acidophilus," *Appl Environ Microbiol,.* 49 (2), February 1985, p. 377–381.

Gnhannam, N., et al., "The Antidiabetic Activity of Aloes," *Hormone Research,* 24, 1986, p. 288–294.

Golczewski, J. A., "Effect of 2-mercaptoethylamine on Proliferation and Lifespan of WI-38 Cells," *Exp Gerontol,* 19 (1), 1984, p. 7–11.

Goldin, B. and Gorbach, S. L., "Alterations in Fecal Microflora Enzymes Related to Diet, Age, Lactobacillus Supplements, and Dimethylhydrazine," *Cancer,* 40 (5 Suppl), November 1977, p. 421–426.

Goldstein, N., et al., "Bromelain as a Skin Cancer Preventive in Hairless Mice," *Hawaii Medical Journal,* 54 (3), 1975, p. 91–94.

Grad, B. R., et al., "The Effect of Concord Grape Extracts on the Survival of Mice Bearing Ehrlich Ascites Tumors," *Proceedings of the American Association of Cancer Researchers,* 17, 1976, p. 165.

Hale, L. P. and Haynes, B. F., "Bromelain Treatment of Human T Cells Removes CD44, CD45RA, E2/MIC2, CD6, CD7, CD8, and Leu 8/LAM1 Surface Molecules and Markedly Enhances CD2-mediated T-Cell Activation," *Journal of Immunology,* 149 (12), December 15, 1992, p. 3809–3016.

Halks-Miller, M., et al., "Vitamin E-enriched Lipoproteins Increase Longevity of Neurons in Vitro," *Brain Research,* 254 (3), October 1981, p. 439–447.

Hayflick, L., *How and Why We Age,*: Ballantine, New York: 1994, p. 137–149.

Head, K. A., "Ascorbic Acid in the Prevention and Treatment of Cancer," *Alternative Medicine Review,* 3 (3), June 1998, p. 174–186.

Heiny, B. M., et al., "Mistletoe Extract Standardized for the Galactoside-specific Lectin (ML-1) Induces Beta-endorphin Release and Immunopotentiation in Breast Cancer Patients," *Anticancer Research,* 14 (3B), May–June 1994, p. 1339–1342.

Hemila, H., "Vitamin C and Common Cold Incidence: A Review of Studies with Subjects under Heavy Physical Stress," *International Journal of Sports Medicine,* 17 (5), July 1996, p. 379–383.

Heptinstall, S., et al., "Inhibition of Platelet Behaviour Folia by Feverfew: A Mechanism of Action Involving Sulphydryl Groups," *Haematol Int Mag Klin Morphol Blutforsch,* 15 (4), 1988, p. 447–479.

Heseker, [Antioxidative Vitamins and Cataracts in the Elderly], *Z Ernahrungswiss,* 34 (3), September 1995, p. 167–176.

Hida, W., et al., "N-acetylcysteine Inhibits Loss of Diaphragm Function in Streptozotocin-treated Rats," *American Journal of Respiratory Critical Care Medicine,* 153 (6 Pt 1), June 1996, p. 1875–1879.

Hishikawa, K., et al., "L-arginine as an Antihypertensive Agent," *Journal of Cardiovascular Pharmacol,* 20 (Suppl 12), 1992, p. S196-S197.

Hoedt-Schmidt, S., et al., "Histomorphological Studies on the Effect of Recombinant Human Superoxide Dismutase in Biochemically Induced Osteoar-thritis," *Pharmacology*, 47 (4), October 1993, p. 252–260.

Hsueh-Chang, C. and Ming, H., "Pumpkin Seed (Cucurbita Moschata) in the Treatment of Acute Schistosomiasis," *Chinese Medical Journal*, 80, February 1960, p. 115–120.

Huang, M. T., et al., "Inhibitory Effects of Curcumin on in Vitro Lipoxygenase and Cyclooxygenase Activities in Mouse Epidermis," *Cancer Research*, 51 (3), February 1, 1991, p. 813–819.

Ickes, G. R., et al., "Antitumor Activity and Preliminary Phytochemical Exami-nation of Tagetes Minuta (Compositae)," *Journal of Pharm Science*, 62 (6), p. 1009–1011.

Iishi, H., et al., "Protection by Oral Phenylalanine Against Gastric Carcinogene-sis Induced by N-methyl-N'-nitro-N-nitrosoguanidine in Wistar Rats," *Brit-ish Journal of Cancer*, 62 (2), August 1990, p. 173–176.

Ip, C., et al., "The Efficacy of Conjugated Linoleic Acid in Mammary Cancer Prevention Is Independent of the Level or Type of Fat in the Diet," *Carcino-genesis*, 17 (5), May 1996, p. 1045–1050,

Jackson, C. V., et al., "Vitamin E and Alzheimer's Disease in Subjects with Down's Syndrome," *Journal of Mental Deficit Research*, 32 (Pt 6), December 1988, p. 479–484.

Janssen, K., et al., "Effects of the Flavonoids Quercetin and Apigenin on He-mostasis in Healthy Volunteers: Results from an in Vitro and a Dietary Sup-plement Study," *American Journal of Clinical Nutrition*, 67 (2), February 1998, p. 255–262.

Janssen, Y. J., et al., "A Low Starting Dose of Genotropin in Growth Hormone-Deficient Adults," *Journal of Clinical Endocrinol Metab*, 82 (1), January 1997, p. 129–135.

Jantti, J., et al., "Evening Primrose Oil in Rheumatoid Arthritis: Changes in Serum Lipids and Fatty Acids," *Annals of Rheumatic Disease*, 48 (2), February 1989, p. 124–127.

Jellinger, K., et al., "Levodopa in the Treatment of (pre) Senile Dementia," *Mech Ageing Dev*, 14 (1–2), September–October 1980, p. 253–264.

Jingum, K., et al., "Protective Effect of L-cysteine Upon Leukopenic Syndrome due to Radiotherapy," *Nippon Gan Chiryo Gakkai Shi*, 16 (4), 1981, p. 681–693.

Jorgensen, J. O., et al., "Growth Hormone Versus Placebo Treatment for One Year in a Growth Hormone Deficient Adults: Increase in Exercise Capacity and Normalization of Body Composition," *Clinical Endocrinology*, 45 (6), De-cember 1996, p. 681–688.

Julius, M., et al., "Glutathione and Morbidity in a Community-based Sample of Elderly," *Journal of Clinical Epidemiology*, 47 (9), September 1994, p. 1021–1026.

Kahler, W., et al., "Results of Adjuvant Antioxdant Supplementation," *Z Gesamte Inn Med*, 48 (5), May 1993, p. 223–232.

Kahn, M. J. and Morrison, D. G., "Chemoprevention for Colorectal Carcinoma," *Hematol Oncol Clin North Am*, 11 (4), August 1997, p. 779–794.

Kamei, T., et al., "Experimental Study of the Therapeutic Effects of Folate, Vitamin A, and Vitamin B12 on Squamous Metaplasia of the Bronchial Epithelium," *Cancer*, 71 (8), April 15, 1993, p. 2477–2483.

Katsuki, T., [Experimental Studies on the Combination Use of Vitamin B_2-Butyrate and Coenzyme Q_{10} ($CoQ_{(10)}$) To Protect Against Adriamycin-induced Cardiac Mitochondrial Disorders," *Kurume Igakkai Zasshi*, 44 (12), 1981, p. 869–883.

Kawashima, K., et al., "Antihypertensive Action of Melatonin in the Spontaneously Hypertensive Rat," *Clinical Exp Hypertens*, 9 (7), 1987, p. 1121–1131.

Kelly, G. S., "Clinical Applications of N-acetylcysteine," *Alternative Medicine Review*, 3 (2), April 1998, p. 114–127.

Kelly, G. S., "Folates: Supplemental Forms and Therapeutic Applications," *Alternative Medicine Review*, 3 (3), 1998, p. 208–220.

Khansari, D. N. and Gustad, T., "Effects of Long-Term, Low-Dose Growth Hormone Therapy on Immune Function and Life Expectancy in Mice," *Aging Dev*, 57 (1), January 1991, p. 87–100.

Khaw, K. T. and Woodhouse, P., "Interrelation of Vitamin C, Infection, Haemostatic Factors, and Cardiovascular Disease," *British Medical Journal*, 310 (6994), June 17, 1995, p. 1559–1563.

Khwaja, T. A., et al., "Recent Studies on the Anticancer Activities of Mistletoe and its Alkaloids," *Oncology*, 43 (Suppl. 1), 1986, p. 42–50.

Kieler, J. and Biczowa, B., "The Effects of Structural Analogues of the Effect of Structural Analogues of Alpha-Lipoic Acid on the Growth and Metabolism of L-Firboblasts and Ehrlic Cells," *Arch Immunol Ther Exp*, 15 (1), 1967, p. 106–111.

Kilbourn, R. G., et al., "NG-methyl-L-arginine, an Inhibitor of Nitric Oxide Synthase, Reverses Interleukin-2-Induced Hypotension," *Crit Care Med*, 23 (6), June 1995, p. 1018–1024.

Kiremidjian-Schumacher, L., et al., "Supplementation with Selenium Augments the Functions of Natural Killer and Lymphokine-activated Killer Cells," *Biological Trace Element Research*, 52 (3), June 1996, p. 227–239.

Knekt, P., et al., "Dietary Antioxidants and the Risk of Lung Cancer," *American Journal of Epidemiology*, 134 (5), September 1, 1991, p. 471–479.

Knuckey, N. W., et al., "N-acetylcysteine Enhances Hippocampal Neuronal Survival after Transient Forebrain Ischemia in Rats," *Stroke*, 26 (2), February 1995, p. 305–311.

Koifman, B., et al., "Improvement of Cardiac Performance by Intravenous Infusion of L-arginine in Patients with Moderate Congestive Heart Failure," *Journal of the American College of Cardiology*, 26 (5), November 1, 1995, p. 1251–1256.

Komada, H., et al., "Effect of Dietary Molybdenum on Esophageal Carcinogenesis in Rats Induced by N-methyl-N-benzylnitrosamine," *Cancer Research*, 50 (8), April 15, 1990, p. 2418–2222.

Konig, B., "A Long-term (two years) Clinical Trial with S-adenosylmethionine for the Treatment of Osteoarthritis," *American Journal of Medicine*, 83 (5A), November 20, 1987, p. 89–94.

Kotegawa, M., et al., "Protective Effects of Riboflavin and Its Derivatives Against Ischemic Reperfused Damage of Rat Heart," *Biochem Mol Biol Int*, 34 (4), October 1994, p. 685–691.

Koutsikos, D., et al., "Biotin for Diabetic Peripheral Neuropathy," *Biomed Pharmacotherapy*, 44 (10), 1990, p. 511–514.

Kremer, J. M., "Clinical Studies of Omega-3 Fatty Acid Supplementation in Patients Who Have Rheumatoid Arthritis," *Rheum Dis Clin North Am*, 17 (2), May 1991, p. 391–402.

Krzeski, T., et al., "Combined Extracts of Urtica diocia and Pygeum Africanum in the Treatment of Benign Prostatic Hyperplasia: Double-Blind Comparison of Two Doses," *Clinical Therapeutics*, 15 (6), 1993, p. 1011–1020.

Kubo, I., et al., "Cytotoxic Anthraquinones from Rheum Palmatum," *Phytochemistry*, 31, 1992, p. 1063–1065.

Lagrua, G., et al., "A Study of the Effects of Procyanidol Oligomers on Capillary Resistance in Hypertension and in Certain Nephropathies," *Sem Hop*, 57, 1981, p. 1399–1401.

Le Bars, P. L., et al., "A Placebo-controlled, Double-blind, Randomized Trial of an Extract of Ginkgo Biloba for Dementia. North American EGb Study Group," *JAMA*, 278 (16), October 22–29, 1997, p. 1327–1332.

Lee, I. M., et al., "Exercise Intensity and Longevity in Men. The Harvard Alumni Health Study," *JAMA*, 273, 1995, p. 1179–1184.

Lepran, I. and Szekeres, L., "Effect of Dietary Sunflower Seed Oil on the Severity of Reperfusion-induced Arrthymias in Anesthetized Rats," *Journal of Cardiovascular Pharmacology*, 19 (1), January 1992, p. 40–44.

Leszek, P., et al., "A Randomized Crossover Trial of Levodopa in Congestive Heart Failure," *Journal of Cardiac Failure*, 2 (3), September 1996, p. 163–176.

Lieberman, S., "A Review of the Effectiveness of Cimicifuga Racemosa (black cohosh) for the Symptoms of Menopause," *Journal of Women's Health*, 7 (5), June 1998, p. 525–529.

Lietti, A., et al., "Studies on Vaccinium Myrtillus Anthocyanosides. I. Vasoprotective and Antiinflammatory Activity," *Arzneimittelforschung*, 26, 1976, p. 829–832.

Linde, K., et al., "St John's Wort for Depression—an Overview and Meta-analysis of Randomised Clinical Trials," *British Medical Journal,* 313 (7052), August 3, 1996, p. 253–258.

Linos, A., et al., "The Effect of Olive Oil and Fish Consumption on Rheumatoid Arthritis—A Case Control Study," *Scandinavian Journal of Rheumatology,* 20 (6), 1991, p. 419–426.

Lipworth, L., et al., "Olive Oil and Human Cancer: An Assessment of the Evidence," *Prev Med,* 26 (2), March–April 1997, p. 181–190.

Lithander, A., "Intracellular Fluid of Waybread (Plantago major) as a Prophylactic for Mammary Cancer in Mice," *Tumour Biology,* 13 (3), 1992, p. 138–141.

Liu, C. X., et al., "Recent Advances on Ginseng Research in China," *Journal of Ethnopharmacology,* 36 (1), February 1992, p. 27–38.

Luettig, B., et al., "Macrophage Activation by the Polysaccharide Arabinogalactan Isolated from Plant Cell Cultures of Echinacea Purpurea.," *Journal of National Cancer Institute,* 81 (9), May 3, 1989, p. 669–675.

Luo, J., et al., "Masoprocol (nordihydroguaiaretic acid): A New Antihyperglycemic Agent Isolated from the Creosote Bush (Larrea tridentata)," *European Journal of Pharmacology,* 346 (1), April 3, 1998, p. 77–79.

Lopez, I., et al., [Treatment of Mucositis with Vitamin E During Administration of Neutropenic Antineoplastic Agents], *Ann Med Interne,* 145 (6), 1994, p. 405–408.

Ma, L., [Experimental Study on the Immunomodulatory Effects of Rhubarb], *Chung Hsi I Chieh Ho Tsa Chih,* 11 (7), July 1991, p. 418–419.

Maggioni, M., et al., "Effects of Phosphatidylserine Therapy in Geriatric Patients with Depressive Disorders," *Acta Psychiatr Scand,* 81 (3), March 1990, p. 265–270.

Maitra, et al., "Alpha-Lipoc Acid Prevents Buthionine Sulfoximine-Induced Cataract Formation in Newborn Rats," *Free Radical Biol Med,* 18 (4), April 1995, p. 823–829.

Mantero-Atienza, E., et al., "Vitamin B6 and Immune Function in HIV Infection," *International Conference on AIDS,* 6 (2), June 20–23, 1990, p. 432.

Marshal, M. E., et al., "Treatment of Metastatic Renal Cell Carcinoma with Coumarin (1,2-Benzopyrone) and Cimetide: A Pilot Study," *Journal of Clinical Oncology,* 5 (6), June 1987, p. 862–866.

Marshall, S., "Zinc Gluconate and the Common Cold. Review of Randomized Controlled Trials," *Canadian Family Physician,* 44, May 1998, p. 1037–1042.

Massie, H. R., et al., "Effect of Vitamin A on Longevity," *Exp Gerontol,* 28 (6), November–December 1993, p. 601–610.

Mateve, M., et al., [Clinical Trial of a Plantago Major Preparation in the Treatment of Chronic Bronchitis], *Vutr Boles,* 21 (2), 1982, p. 133–137.

Maucher, A., et al., "Evaluation of the Antitumour Activity of Coumarin in

Prostate Cancer Models," *Journal of Cancer Research and Clinical Oncology*, 119, 1993, p. 150–154.

Maurer, K., et al., "Clinical Efficacy of Ginkgo Biloba Special Extract EGb 761 in Dementia of the Alzheimer Type," *Journal of Psychiatric Res*, 31 (6), November–December 1997, p. 645–655.

McCarty, M. F., "Longevity Effect of Chromium Picolinate—'Rejuvenation' of Hypothalamic Function?" *Medical Hypotheses*, 43 (4), October 1994, p. 253–265.

Meck, W. H., et al., "Pre- and Postnatal Choline Supplementation Produces Long-term Facilitation of Spatial Memory," *Developmental Psychobiology*, 21 (4), May 1988, p. 339–353.

Metori, K, et al., "The Preventive Effect of Ginseng with Du-zhong Leaf on Protein Metabolism in Aging," *Biol Pharm Bull*, 20 (3), March 1997, p. 237–242.

Millar, J. H. D., et al., "Double Blind Trial of Linolate Supplementation of the Diet in Multiple Sclerosis," *British Medical Journal*, I, 1973, p. 765–768.

Mimori, Y., et al., "Thiamine Therapy in Alzheimer's Disease," *Metab Brain Disease*, 11 (1), March 1966, p. 89–94.

Mishima, Y., et al., "A Multiclinic Double-blind Trial of Pyridinolcarbamate and Inositol Niacinate in Ischemic Ulcer Due to Chronic Arterial Occlusion," *Angiology*, 28 (2), February 1977, p. 84–94.

Miyakawa, M. and Yoshida, O. "Protective Effects of DL-Tryptophan on Benzidine-induced Hepatic Tumor in Mice," *Gan*, 71 (2), 1980, p. 265–268.

Mochizuki, M., et al., "Inhibitory Effect of Tumor Metastasis in Mice by Saponins, Ginsenoside-Rb2, 20(R)- and 20(S)-ginsenoside-Rg3, of Red Ginseng," *Biol Pharm Bull*, 18 (9), September 1995, p. 1197–1202.

Morley, J. E., et al., "Nutrition in the Elderly," *Annals of Internal Medicine*, 109 (11), December 1, 1988, p. 890–904.

Mortola, J. F. and Yen, S. S., "The Effects of Oral Dehydroepiandrosterone on Endocrine-Metabolic Parameters in Postmenopausal Women," *Journal of Clinical Endocrinology Metabolism*, 71 (3), September 1990, p. 696–704.

Mouret, J., et al., "L-tyrosine Cures, Immediate and Long Term, Dopamine-dependent Depressions. Clinical and Polygraphic Studies," *C R Acad Sci III*, 306 (3), 1988, p. 93–98.

Mowrey, D. B., *The Scientific Validation of Herbal Medicine*. New Canaan, CT: Keats Publishing, 1986.

Murakami, T. and Uchikawa, T., "Effect of Glycrrhizine on Hyperkalemia Due to Hyporeninemic Hypoaldosteronism in Diabetes Mellitus," *Life Sciences*, 53 (5), 1993, p. 63–68.

Murakoshi, M., et al., "Inhibitory Effects of Alpha-carotene on Proliferation of the Human Neuroblastoma Cell Line GOTO," *Journal of the National Cancer Institute*, 81 (21), November 1, 1989, p. 1649–1652.

Nagasawa, H., et al., "Effects of Motherwort (Leonurus sibiricus L) on Preneo-plastic and Neoplastic Mammary Gland Growth in Multiparous GR/A Mice," *Anticancer Research*, 10 (4), July–August 1990, p. 1019–1023.

Nakadaira, H., et al., "Distribution of Selenium and Molybdenum and Cancer Mortality in Niigata, Japan," *Arch Environ Health*, 50 (5), October–September 1995, p. 374–380.

Narisawa, T., et al., "Inhibitory Effects of Natural Carotenoids, Alpha-carotene, Beta-carotene, Lycopene and Lutein, on Colonic Aberrant Crypt Foci For-mation in Rats," *Cancer Letters*, 107 (1), October 1, 1996, p. 137–142.

Nattakom, T. V., et al., "Use of Vitamin E and Glutamine in the Successful Treatment of Severe Veno-Occlusive Disease Following Bone Marrow Trans-plantation," *Nutrition Clinical Practice*, 10 (1), Feb 1995, p. 16–18.

The New England Centenarian Study Website, Harvard Medical School, 1998, *http://www.med.harvard.edu/programs/necs/background.htm*

Newnham, R. E., "Essentially of Boron for Healthy Bones and Joints," *Environ-mental Health Perspectives*, 102 (Suppl 7), November 1994, p. 83–35.

Nishino, H., et al., "Berberine Sulfate Inhibits Tumor-Promoting Activity of Teleocidin in Two-Stage Carcinogenesis on Mouse Skin," *Oncology*, 43, 1986, p. 131–134.

Nishiyama, N., et al., "An Herbal Prescription, S-113m, Consisting of Biota, Ginseng and Schizandra, Improves Learning Performance in Senescence Accelerated Mouse," *Biol Pharm Bull*, 19 (3), March 1996, p. 388–393.

Norbiato, G., et al., "Effects of Potassium Supplementation on Insulin Binding and Insulin Action in Human Obesity: Protein-Modified Fast and Refeed-ing," *European Journal of Clinical Investigations*, 1984, p. 414–419.

Nuraliev, I. and Avezov, G. A., "The Efficacy of Quercetin in Alloxan Diabetes," *Eksp Klin Farmakol*, 55 (1), January–February 1992, p. 42–44.

Okamoto, H., et al., "Effect of CoQ_{10} on Structural Alterations in the Renal Membrane of Stroke-prone Spontaneously Hypertensive Rats," *Biochem Med Metab Biol*, 45 (2), April 1991, p. 216–226.

Oldroyd, K. G. and Dawes, P. T., "Clinically Significant Vitamin C Deficiency in Rheumatoid Arthritis," *British Journal of Rheumatology*, 24 (4), November 1985, p. 362–363.

Ooms, M. E., et al., "Prevention of Bone Loss by Vitamin D Supplementation in Elderly Women: A Randomized Double-blind Trial," *Journal of Clinical Endocrinol Metab*, 80 (4), April 1995, p. 1052–1058.

Oshima, G., et al., "Anticoagulant Effect of Inositol Hexasulfate as Measurable by Clotting Times of Fibrinogen and Recalcified Plasma," *Thromb Research*, 58 (3), May 1, 1990, p. 243–250.

Oshima, Y., et al., "Isolation and Hypoglycemic Activity of Quinquefolans A, B, and C, Glycans of Panax Quinquefolium Roots," *Journal of Natural Products*, 50 (2), March–April 1987, p. 198–190.

Ostman-Smith, I., et al., "Dilated Cardiomyopathy due to Type II X-linked 3-methylglutaconic Aciduria: Successful Treatment with Pantothenic Acid," *British Heart Journal*, 72 (4), October 1994, p. 349–353.

O'Sullivan, M. G., et al., "Modulation of Colon Cell Proliferation in Monkeys by Isoflavone-rich Soy Protein- and Grape Phenol-based Diets," *Proceedings of the Annual Meeting of the American Association of Cancer Researchers*, 38, 1997, p. A738.

Ozturk, Y., "Testing the Antidepressant Effects of Hypericum Species on Animal Models," *Pharmacopsychiatry*, 30 (Suppl 2), September 1997, p. 125–128.

Palan, P. R., et al., "Beta-carotene Levels in Exfoliated Cervicovaginal Epithelial Cells in Cervical Intraepithelial Neoplasia and Cervical Cancer," *American Journal of Obstetrics and Gynecology*, 167 (6), December 1992, p. 1899–1903.

Pangrekar, J., et al., "Effects of Riboflavin Deficiency and Riboflavin Administration on Carcinogen-DNA Binding," *Food Chem Toxicol*, 31 (10), October 1993, p. 745–750.

Panigrahi, M., et al., "Alpha-Lipoic Acid Protects Against Reperfusion Injury Following Cerebral Ischemia in Rats," *Brain Research*, 717 (1–2), April 22, 1996, p. 184–188.

Panteleimonova, T. N. and Zapadniuk, V. I., [Effect of Trimethylglycine on Lipid Metabolism in Experimental Atherosclerosis in Rabbits], *Farmakol Toksikol*, 46 (4), July–August 1983, p. 83–85.

Panzer, A. and Viljoen, M., "The Validity of Melatonin as an Oncostatic Agent," *Journal of Pineal Research*, 22 (4), May 1997, p. 184–202.

Paradies, G., et al., "The Effect of Aging and Acetyl-L-carnitine on the Activity of the Phosphate Carrier and on the Phospholipid Composition in Rat Heart Mitochondria," *Biochim Biophys Acta*, 1103 (2), January 31, 1992, p. 324–326.

Pence, B. C., et al., "Protective Effects of Calcium from Nonfat Milk Against Colon Carcinogenesis in Rats," *Nutrition and Cancer*, 25 (1), 1996, p. 35–45.

Peng, S. Y., et al., "Decreased Mortality of Norman Murine Sarcoma in Mice Treated with the Immunomodulator, Acemannan," *Mol Biother*, 3 (2), June 1991, p. 79–87.

Penland, J. G., "Dietary Boron, Brain Function, and Cognitive Performance," *Environmental Health Perspectives*, 102 (Suppl 7), November 1994, p. 65–72.

Penn, N. D., et al., "The Effect of Dietary Supplementation with Vitamins A, C and E on Cell-mediated Immune Function in Elderly Long-stay Patients: A Randomized Controlled Trial," *Age Aging*, 20 (3), May 1991, p. 169–174.

Perdigon, G., et al., "Systemic Augmentation of the Immune Response in Mice by Feeding Fermented Milks with Lactobacillus Casei and Lactobacillus Acidophilus," *Immunology*, 63 (1), January 1988, p. 17–23.

Petkov, V., "Plants with Hypotensive, Antiatheromatous and Coronary Dilating Action," *A.J. Chinese Medicine*, 7, 1979, p. 197, 236.

The Physician's Guide to Life Extension Drugs. Hollywood, FL: Life Extension Foundation.

Pietri, S., et al., "Cardioprotective and Anti-oxidant Effects of the Terpenoid Constituents of Ginkgo Biloba Extract (EGb 761)," *Journal of Mol Cell Cardiology*, 29 (2), February 1997, p. 733–742.

Plaitakis, A., et al., "Pilot Trial of Branched-chain Aminoacids in Amyotrophic Lateral Sclerosis," *Lancet*, 1 (8593), May 7, 1988, p. 1015–1058.

Poeggeler, B., et al., "Melatonin, Hydroxyl Radical-Mediated Oxidative Damage, and Ageing: A Hypothesis," *Journal of Pineal Research*, 14, 1993, p. 151–168.

Polasek, J., "Acetylsalicylic Acid and Vitamin E in Prevention of Arterial Thrombosis," *Can J Cardiol*, 13 (5), May 1997, p. 533–535.

Poltronieri, R., et al., "Protective Effect of Selenium in Cardiac Ischemia and Reperfusion," *Cardioscience*, 3 (3), September 1992, p. 155–160.

Prasad, K., "Dietary Flax Seed in Prevention of Hypercholesterolemic Atherosclerosis," *Atherosclerosis*, 32 (1), July 11, 1997, p. 69–76.

Prasad, K. N., et al., "Vitamin K3 (Menadione) Inhibits the Growth of Mammalian Tumor Cells in Culture," *Life Science*, 29 (13), 1981, p. 1387–1392.

Rapoport, B., et al., "Inhibitory Effect of Dietary Iodine on the Thyroid Adenylate Cyclase Response to Thyrotropin in the Hypophysectomized Rat," *Journal of Clinical Investigations*, 56 (2), August 1975, p. 516–519.

Rao, C. V., et al., "Chemoprevention of Azoxymethane-induced Colon Cancer by Ascorbylpalmitate, Carbenoxolone, Dimethylfumarate and p-methoxyphenol in Male F344 Rats," *Anticancer Research*, 15 (4), July–August 1995, p. 1199–1204.

Raszejowa, W. and Szpunarowna, K., "Consituents of the Bark of Viburnum Opulus and Some Pharmacodynamic Properties Thereof," *Acta Polon Pharm*, 16, 1959, p. 131–139.

Rayner, T. E., et al., "Purified Omega-3 Fatty Acids Retard the Development of Proteinuria in Salt-loaded Hypertensive Rats," *Journal of Hypertension*, 13 (7), July 1995, p. 771–780.

Reddy, B. S. and Rivenson, A., "Inhibitory Effect of Bifidobacterium Longum on Colon, Mammary, and Liver Carcinogenesis Induced by 2-amino-3-methylimidazo[4,5-f]quinoline, a Food Mutagen," *Cancer Research*, 53 (17), September 1, 1993, p. 3914–3918.

Rector, T. S., et al., "Randomized, Double-blind, Placebo-controlled Study of Supplemental Oral L-arginine in Patients with Heart Failure," *Circulation*, 93 (12), June 15, 1996, p. 2135–2141.

Regland, B., et al., "Vitamin B_{12}–induced Reduction of Platelet Monoamine Oxidase Activity in Patients with Dementia and Pernicious Anemia," *European Archives of Psychiatry and Clinical Neuroscience*, 240 (4–5), 1991, p. 288–291.

Reider, A., et al., "Delay of Diethylnitrosamine-Induced Hepatoma in Rats by Carrot Feeding," *Oncology*, 40, 1983, p. 120–123.

Reilly, D. K., et al., "On-off Effects in Parkinson's Disease: A Controlled Investigation of Ascorbic Acid Therapy," *Advances in Neurology*, 37, 1983, p. 51–60.

Reiter, R. J. "Oxygen Radical Detoxification Processes During Aging: The Functional Importance of Melatonin," *Aging*, 7 (5), October 1995, p. 340–351.

Reiter, R. J., "The Pineal Gland and Melatonin in Relation to Ageing: A Summary of the Theories and of the Data," *Exp Gerontol*, 30 (3–4), May 1995, p. 199–212.

Reiter, R. J., et al., "A Review of the Evidence Supporting Melatonin's Role as an Antioxidant," *Journal of Pineal Research*, 18 (1), January 1995.

Ricci, A., et al., "Oral Choline Alfoscerate Counteracts Age-dependent Loss of Mossy Fibres in the Rat Hippocampus," *Mech Aging Dev*, 66 (1), 1992, p. 81–91.

Rimm, E. B., et al., "Folate and Vitamin B6 from Diet and Supplements in Relation to Risk of Coronary Heart Disease among Women," *JAMA*, 279, 1998, p. 359–364.

Rong, Y., et al., "Pycnogenol Protects Vascular Endothelial Cells from t-butyl Hydroperoxide Induced Oxidant Injury," *Biotechnol Ther*, 5 (3–4), 1994–1995, p. 117–126.

Rose, D. P. and Connolly, J. M., "Effects of Dietary Omega-3 fatty Acids on Human Breast Cancer Growth and Metastases in Nude Mice," *Journal of the National Cancer Institute*, 85 (21), November 3, 1993, p. 1743–1747.

Rosenkranz, E. R., et al., "Safety of Prolonged Aortic Clamping with Blood Cardioplegia. III. Aspartate Enrichment of Glutamate-blood Cardioplegia in Energy-depleted Hearts after Ischemic and Reperfusion Injury," *Journal of Thoracic Cardiovascular Surgery*, 91 (3), March 1986, p. 428–435.

Rozencweig, M., et al., "N-(Phosphonacetyl)-L-Aspartate (PALA): Current Status, Recent Results," *Cancer Research*, 74, 1980, p. 72–77.

Rozewicka, L., et al., "Protective Effect of Selenium and Vitamin E Against Changes Induced in Heart Vessels of Rabbits Fed Chronically on a High-fat Diet," *Kitasato Arch Exp Med*, 64 (4), December 1991, p. 183–192.

Ruggy, G. H. and Smith, C. S., "A Pharmacological Study of the Active Principal of Passiflora Incarnata," *Journal of the American Pharmaceutical Association*, 29, 1947, p. 245–249.

Sabate, J., et al., "Effects of Walnuts on Serum Lipid Levels and Blood Pressure in Normal Men," *New England Journal of Medicine*, 328, 1993, p. 603–607.

Sabir, M. and Bhide, N., "Study of Some Pharmacologic Actions of Berberine," *Indian Journal of Phys Pharm*, 15, 1971, p. 111–132.

Sage, J. I. and Mark, M., "Nighttime Levodopa Infusions to Treat Motor Fluctuations in Advanced Parkinson's Disease: Preliminary Observations," *Annals of Neurology*, 30 (4), October 1991, p. 616–617.

Sakane, T., et al., "Effects of Methyl-B$_{12}$ on the in Vitro Immune Functions of Human T Lymphocytes," *Journal of Clinical Immunology*, 2 (2), April 1982, p. 101–109.

Salikhova, R. A. and Poroshenko, G. G., [Antimutagenic Properties of Angelica Archangelica L], *Vestn Ross Akad Med Nauk*, (1), 1995, p. 58–61.

Sanchiz, F., et al., "Prevention of Radioinduced Cystitis by Orgotein: A Randomized Study," *Anticancer Research*, 16 (4A), July–August 1996, p. 2025–2058.

Sandyk, R., "Possible Role of Pineal Melatonin in the Mechanisms of Aging," *International Journal of Neuroscience*, 52 (1–2), May 1990, p. 85–92.

Sasaki, H., et al., "Vitamin B$_{12}$ Improves Cognitive Disturbance in Rodents Fed a Choline-deficient Diet," *Pharmacol Biochem Behav*, 43 (2), October 1992, p. 635–639.

Scambia, G., et al., "Inhibitory Effect of Quercetin (Q) on Primary Ovarian and Endometrial Cancer and Synergistic Activity with Cis -Diamminedichloroplatinum(II) (CDDP)," *Proceedings of the Annual Meeting of the American Society of Clinical Oncology*, 11, 1992, p. A760.

Scheller, S., et al., "Antitumoral Property of Ethanolic Extract of Propolis in Mice-bearing Ehrlich Carcinoma, as Compared to Bleomycin," *Z Naturforsch*, 44 (11–12), November–December 1981, p. 1063–1065.

Schmidt, U., et al., "Wirksamkeit des Extrak-tes LI 132 (600 mg/Tag) bei achitowchiger Therapie," *Munch. med. Wschr*, 136 (Suppl 1), 1994, p. S13–S19.

Schonheit, K., et al., "Effect of Alpha-Lipoic Acid and Dehydrolipoic Acid on Ischemia/Reperfusion Injury of the Heart and Heart Mitochondria," *Biochem Biophys Acta*, 1271 (2–3), June 9, 1995, p. 335–342.

Sen, C. K., et al., "A Positively Charged Alpha-lipoic Acid Analogue with Increased Cellular Uptake and More Potent Immunomodulatory Activity," *Biochem Biophys Res Commun*, 247 (2), June 18, 1998, p. 223–228.

Serraino, M. and Thompson, L. U., "Flaxseed Supplementation and Early Markers of Colon Carcinogenesis," *Cancer Letters*, 63 (2), April 15, 1992, p. 159–165.

Shamsuddin, A. M., "Inositol Phosphates Have Novel Anticancer Function," *Journal of Nutrition*, 125 (3 Suppl), March 1995, p. 725S–732S.

Sheela, C. G. and Augusti, K. T., "Antidiabetic Effects of S-allyl Cysteine Sulphoxide Isolated from Garlic Allium Sativum Linn," *Indian Journal of Experimental Biology*, 30 (6), June 1992, p. 523–526.

Shigenaga, M. K., et al., "Oxidative Damage and Mitochondrial Decay in Aging," *Proceedings of the National Academy of Science*, 91 (23), November 8, 1994, p. 10771–10778.

Shimizu, N., et al., "Experimental Study of Antitumor Effect of Methyl-B12,"*Oncology*, 44 (3), 1987, p. 169–173.

Shimon, I., et al., "Improved Left Ventricular Function after Thiamine Supplementation in Patients with Congestive Heart Failure Receiving Long-term Furosemide Therapy," *American Journal of Medicine*, 98 (5), May 1995, p. 485–490.

Shneider, A. B., [Anti-ischemic Heart Protection Using Thiamine and Nicotinamide], *Patol Fiziol Eksp Ter*, (1), January–February 1991, p. 9–10.

Shochat, T., et al., "Melatonin—the Key to the Gate of Sleep," *Ann Med*, 30 (1), February 1998, p. 109–114.

Skubitz, K. M. and Anderson, P. M., "Oral Glutamine to Prevent Chemotherapy Induced Stomatitis: A Pilot Study," *Journal of Laboratory Clinical Medicine*, 127 (2), February 1996, p. 223–228.

Slonim, A. E., et al., "Modification of Chemically Induced Diabetes in Rats by Vitamin E: Supplementation Minimizes and Depletion Enhances Development of Diabetes," *Journal of Clinical Investigation*, 71 (5), May 1983, p. 1282–1288.

Smart, C. R., et al., "An Interesting Observation on Nordihydroguaiaretic Acid (NSC-4291; NDGA) and a Patient with Malignant Melanoma—A Prelimary Report," *Cancer Chemotherpay Reports*, 53 (2), April 1969, p. 147–151.

Smidt, L. J., et al., "Influence of Thiamin Supplementation on the Health and General Well-being of an Elderly Irish Population with Marginal Thiamin Deficiency," *Journal of Gerontology*, 46 (1), January 1991, p. M16–22.

Sobala, G. M., et al., "Ascorbic Acid in the Human Stomach," *Gastroenterology*, 97 (2), August 1989, p. 357–363.

Soni, K. B. and Kuttan, R., "Effect of Oral Curcumin Administration on Serum Peroxides and Cholesterol Levels in Human Volunteers," *Indian Journal of Physiol Pharmacol*, 36 (4), October 1992, p. 273–275.

Spagnoli, A., et al., "Long-term Acetyl-L-carnitine Treatment in Alzheimer's Disease," *Neurology*, 41 (11), November 1991, p. 1726–1732.

Stampfer, M. J., et al., "Effects of Beta-carotene Supplementation on Total and Prostate Cancer Incidence among Randomized Participants with Low Baseline Plasma Levels: the Physicians' Health Study," *Proceedings of the Annual Meeting of the American Society of Clinical Oncology*, 16, 1997, p. A1467.

Steinberg, F. M. and Chait, A., "Antioxidant Vitamin Supplementation and Lipid Peroxidation in Smokers," *American Journal of Clinical Nutrition*, 68 (2), August 1998, p. 319–327.

Steinmuller, C., et al., "Polysaccharides Isolated from Plant Cell Cultures of Echinacea Purpurea Enhance the Resistance of Immunosuppressed Mice Against Systemic Infections with Candida Albicans and Listeria Monocytogenes," *International Journal of Immunopharmacol*, 15 (5), July 1993, p. 605–614.

Stewart, S., et al., "Managing Patients with Acute Myocardial Ischemia and Reperfusion Injury with N-acetylcysteine," *Dimens Crit Care Nurs*, 16 (3), May–June 1997, p. 122–131.

Stojko, A., et al., "Biological Properties and Clinical Application of Propolis. VIII. Experimental Observation on the Influence of Ethanol Extract of Propolis (EEP) on the Regeneration of Bone Tissue," *Arzneimittelforschung*, 28 (1), 1978, p. 35–37.

Stoll, S., et al., "The Potent Free Radical Scavenger Alpha-lipoic Acid Improves Memory in Aged Mice: Putative Relationship to NMDA Receptor Deficits," *Pharmacol Biochem Behav*, 46 (4), December 1993, p. 799–805.

Sugiura, H., et al., [Effects of Exercise in the Growing Stage in Mice and of Astragalus Membranaceus on Immune Functions], *Nippon Eiseigaku Zasshi*, 47 (6), February 1993, p. 1021–1031.

Suzuki, F., et al., "Inhibitory Effect of Glycyrrhizin (GR), an Active Component of Licorice Roots, on an Experimental Pulmonary Metastasis in Mice Inoculated with B16 Melanoma," *Proceedings of the Annual Meeting of the American Association of Cancer Researchers*, 38, 1997, p. A802.

Suzuki, Y., et al., "A Case of Diabetic Amyotrophy Associated with 3243 Mitochondrial tRNA(leu; UUR) Mutation and Successful Therapy with Coenzyme Q10," *Endocr Journal*, 42 (2), April 1995, p. 141–145.

Svedjeholm, R., et al., "Glutamate and High-dose Glucose-insulin-potassium (GIK) in the Treatment of Severe Cardiac Failure after Cardiac Operations," *Ann Thorac Surg*, 59 (2 Suppl), February 1995, p. S23–S30.

Svendsen, L., et al., "Testing Garlic for Possible Anti-ageing Effects on Long-term Growth Characteristics, Morphology and Macromolecular Synthesis of Human Fibroblasts in Culture," *Journal of Ethnopharmacology*, 43 (2), July 8, 1994, p. 125–133.

Takeo, S., et al., "Beneficial Effects of Yohimbine on Posthypoxic Recovery of Cardiac Function and Myocardial Metabolism in Isolated Perfused Rabbit Hearts," *Journal Pharmacol Exp Ther*, 258 (1), July 1, 1991, p. 94–102.

Tanaka, T., et al., "Chemoprevention of 4-nitroquinoline 1-oxide-induced Oral Carcinogenesis by Dietary Curcumin and Hesperidin: Comparison with the Protective Effect of Beta-carotene," *Cancer Research*, 54 (17), September 1, 1994, p. 4653–4659.

Taussig, S. J. and Nieper, H. A., "Bromelain: Its Use in Prevention and Treatment of Cardiovascular Disease—Present Status," *Journal of the International Academy of Preventive Medicine*, VI, 1979, p. 139–150.

Taylor, P. R., et al., "Prevention of Esophageal Cancer: The Nutrition Intervention Trials in Linxian, China: Linxian Nutrition Intervention Trials Study Group," *Cancer Research*, 54 (7 Suppl), April 1, 1994, p. 2029s–2031s.

Tixier, J. M., et al., "Evidence by in Vivo and in Vitro Studies that Binding of Pycnogenols to Elastin Affects Its Rate of Degradation by Elastases," *Biochem Pharmacol*, 33 (24), December 15, 1984, p. 3933–3939.

Torun, M., et al., "Evaluation of Serum Beta-carotene Levels in Patients with

Cardiovascular Diseases," *Journal of Clinical Pharm Therapy*, 19 (1), February 1994, p. 61–63.

Tramontano, D., et al., "Iodine Inhibits the Proliferation of Rat Thyroid Cells in Culture," *Endocrinology*, 125 (2), August 1989, p. 984–992.

Tseng, T. H., et al., "Inhibitory Effect of Hibiscus Protocatechuic Acid on Tumor Promotion in Mouse Skin," *Cancer Letters*, 126 (2), April 24, 1998, p. 199–207.

Tsujiuchi, T., et al., "Prevention by Methionine of Enhancement of Hepatocarcinogenesis by Coadministration of a Choline-deficient L-amino Acid-defined Diet and Ethionine in Rats," *Japanese Journal of Cancer Research*, 86 (12), December 1995, p. 1136–1142.

Uccella, R., et al., [Action of Evening Primrose Oil on Cardiovascular Risk Factors in Insulin-dependent Diabetics], *Clin Ter*, 129 (5), June 15, 1989, p. 381–388.

Ulus, I. H., et al., "Restoration of Blood Pressure by Choline Treatment in Rats Made Hypotensive by Haemorrhage," *British Journal of Pharmacology*, 116 (2), September 1995, p. 1911–1917.

Urban, T., et al., "Neutrophil Function and Glutathione-Peroxidase (GSH-px) Activity in Healthy Individuals after Treatment with N-acetyl-L-cysteine," *Biomed Pharmacother*, 51, 1997, p. 388–390.

van den Berg, M., et al., "Combined Vitamin B6 Plus Folic Acid Therapy in Young Patients with Arteriosclerosis and Hyperhomocysteinemia," *Journal of Vascular Surgery*, 20 (6), December 1994, p. 933–940.

Voskresenskii, O. N., et al., [Effect of Ascorbic Acid and Rutin on the Development of Experimental Peroxide Atherosclerosis], *Farmakol Toksikol*, 42 (4), July–August 1979, p. 378–382.

Visioli, F. and Galli, C., "The Effect of Minor Constituents of Olive Oil on Cardiovascular Disease: New Findings," *Nutrition Review*, 56 (5 Pt 1), May 1998, p. 142–147.

Watson, R. R., et al., "Effect of Beta-Carotene on Lymphocyte Subpopulations in Elderly Humans: Evidence for a Dose-response Relationship," *American Journal of Clinical Nutrition*, 53 (1), January 1981, p. 90–94.

Weber, P., "Management of Osteoporosis: Is There a Role for Vitamin K?" *International Journal of Vitamin and Nutrition Research*, 67 (5), 1997, p. 350–356.

Weber, P., et al., "Vitamin E and Human Health: Rationale for Determining Recommended Intake Levels," *Nutrition*, 13 (5), May 1997, p. 450–460.

Wei-min, H., et al., "Beneficial Effects of Berberine on Hemodynamics During Acute Ischemic Left Ventricular Failure in Dogs," *Chinese Medical Journal*, 105 (12), 1992, p. 1014–1019.

Whelton, P. K., et al., "Effects of Oral Potassium on Blood Pressure. Meta-analysis of Randomized Controlled Clinical Trials," *JAMA*, 277 (20), May 28, 1997, p. 1624–1632.

Wiethop, B. V. and Cryer, C. V., "Alanine and Terbutaline in Treatment of Hypoglycemia in IDDM," *Diabetes Care*, 16 (8), August 1993, p. 1131–1136.

Wilcken, D. E., et al., "Folic Acid Lowers Elevated Plasma Homocysteine in Chronic Renal Insufficiency: Possible Implications for Prevention of Vascular Disease," *Metabolism*, 37 (7), July 1988, p. 697–701.

Williamson, L. M., et al., "Effect of Feverfew on Phagocytosis and Killing of Candida by Neutrophils," *Inflammation*, 12 (1), February 1988, p. 11–16.

Wood, S. M., "Effects of Beta-Carotene and Selenium Supplementation in Aged Humans," *Dissertation Abstracts International*, 55 (4), 1994, p. 1387.

Xiaoguang, C., et al., "Cancer Chemopreventive and Therapeutic Activities of Red Ginseng," *Journal of Ethnopharmacology*, 60 (1), February 1998, p. 71–78.

Yan, L., et al., "Effect of Dietary Supplementation of Selenium on Pulmonary Metastasis of Melanoma Cells in Mice," *Proceedings of the Annual Meeting of the American Association of Cancer Researchers*, 38, 1997, p. A730.

Yatzidis, H. Y., et al., "Biotin in the Management of Uremic Neurologic Disorders," *Nephron*, 36 (3), 1984, p. 183–186.

Yen, S. S., et al., "Replacement of DHEA in Aging Men and Women. Potential Remedial Effects," *Annals of the New York Academy Science*, 774, December 29, 1995, p. 128–142.

Yen, T. T. and Knoll, J., "Extension of Lifespan in Mice Treated with Dinh Lang (Policias fruticosum L.) and (-)deprenyl," *Acta Physiol Hung*, 79 (2), 1992, 119–124.

You, W. C., et al., "Allium Vegetables and Reduced Risk of Stomach Cancer," *Journal of the National Cancer Institute*, 81 (2), January 18, 1989, p. 162–164.

Yuan, W. L., et al., "Effect of Astragalus Membranaceus on Electric Activities of Cultured Rat Beating Heart Cells Infected with Coxsackie B-2 Virus," *Chinese Medical Journal*, 103 (3), March 1990, p. 177–182.

Yue, D. K., et al., "Abnormalities of Ascorbic Acid Metabolism and Diabetic Control: Differences Between Diabetic Patients and Diabetic Rats," *Diabetes Research Clinical Practice*, 9 (3), July 1990, p. 239–244.

Zaman, Z., et al., "Plasma Concentrations of Vitamins A and E and Carotenoids in Alzheimer's Disease," *Age Aging*, 21 (2), March 1992, p. 91–94.

Zhan, Y., et al., [Protective Effects of Ginsenoside on Myocardiac Ischemic and Reperfusion Injuries], *Chung Hua I Hsueh Tsa Chih*, 74 (10), October 1994, p. 626–628.

Zhao, X. Z., [Antisenility Effect of Ginseng-rhizome Saponin], *Chung Hsi I Chieh Ho Tsa Chih*, 10 (10), October 1990, p. 586–589.

Zhao, X. Z., [Effects of Astragalus Membranaceus and Tripterygium Hypoglancum on Natural Killer Cell Activity of Peripheral Blood Mononuclear in Systemic Lupus Erythematosus], *Chung Kuo Chung Hsi I Chieh Ho Tsa Chih*, 12 (11), November 1992, p. 669–671.

Zhou, Y. P. and Zhang, J. Q., "Oral Baicalin and Liquid Extract of Licorice

Reduce Sorbitol Levels in Red Blood Cell of Diabetic Rats," *Chinese Medical Journal*, 102 (3), March 1989, p. 203–206.

Zhuang, X. X., [Protectuve Effect of Angelica Injection on Arrhythmia During Myocardial Ischemia Reperfusion in Rat], *Chung Hsi I Chieh Ho Tsa Chih*, 11 (6), June 1991, p. 360–361, 326.

Zou, Q. Z., et al., "Effect of Motherwort on Blood Hyperviscosity," *American Journal of Chinese Medicine*, 17 (1–2), 1989, 65–70.

SUBJECT INDEX

Acetylcholine, 130
Acetyl-L-carnitine, 154–56, 274, 385
Acid balance, 541, 543, 551
Acidophilus, 156, 158, 274, 558
Action, taking, 372–73
Acupuncture, 29, 308
Adaptive supportive energy, 363–64
Adaptogenic herbs, 231
Adenoids, 521–22
Adipose tissue, 258
Adrenal gland, 342
Adrenaline, 268, 539
Aduki beans/Adzuki beans, 327
Aerobics, 253, 254, 275, 286, 290–99. *See also* Exercise
Age spots, 118
Aging, 3–13, 357
  and appearance, 359
  of body, 125–34
  early evidence of, 23–27
  fight against, 379
  is changing, 3–13
  oxidative stress as cause of, 262, 263
  plan to stop, 14–31
  rate of, 127
  symptoms associated with, 119
  theories of, 117–24
Aging process, 5, 120, 131
  damage theories of, 117–20, 123
  diseases in, 4, 126
  free radicals in, 30
  mental changes, 126
  physical changes, 126, 133–34
  programmed theories of, 117, 120–24
  retarding/reversing, 5, 7, 11, 15, 21–23, 123, 342, 357
  study on reversing, 10–11
Agribusiness, 311–12
AIDS, 9, 522. *See also* HIV
  herbs in treatment of, 221, 226, 239
  nutrients in treatment of, 195, 205, 212, 219
Air pollutants/pollution, 133, 258, 266, 267
Alanine, 241
ALC (acetyl-L-carnitine), 154–56, 385
Alcohol, 9, 119, 262, 263
Aldosterone, 131
Allergies/allergic reactions, 525, 528, 530, 549–50

Allergy tests, 541
Allopathic medicine, 31, 260, 382
Aloe vera, 9, 220–21, 273, 388
Alpha-carotene, 156–57
Alpha-lipoic acid, 157, 274, 389, 552
Alpha-tocopherol, 214, 215–16
Alternative healing modalities, 29–31, 379, 380
  scientific evidence for, 382
Alternative health practitioners, 27–29
Aluminum, 260
Alzheimer's disease, 4, 118, 120, 122, 130
  and chelation therapy, 554
  heavy metals in, 260
  nutrients in treatment of, 154, 155, 166, 168, 182, 192, 198, 201, 209–10
  smart drugs in treatment of, 144, 146, 150, 153
Amantadine, 174
Amaranth, 319
American College for Advancement in Medicine, 554
American creosote bush, 221
American Dietetic Association (ADA), 137, 138
American Medical Association, 31, 381
Amino acids, 321, 322, 333
  essential, 245–47
  in grains, 320
  therapeutic, 241–45
Aminoguanidine, 144
Anaerobics, 286, 298
Anaphylatoxins, 529
Anderson, Nina, 553
Androgens, 131
Angelica, 221
Anger, 269, 366, 367, 368
Antacid tablets, 260
Anti-aging program, 12, 14–31, 251–57
Anti-aging protocol, 4–13, 23, 35, 259, 263
  success and failure in, 7–8, 10, 11–12
Antibiotics, 258, 260–61, 380
  fed to cattle, 312
Antibody production, 527, 528–29
Antioxidants, 9, 118, 119–20, 157, 262, 274
  enzymes, 526–27, 531–32
  supplements, 9, 273, 552–53
Antiviral herbs, 557

RECIPE INDEX